Advanced Practice Nursing
Changing Roles and Clinical Applications

DATE DUE

APR - 1 1996	
JUN 1 4 1996	
OCT 2 9 1996	
NOV 2 2 1996	
JAN 2 9 1997	
NOV 1 3 1997	
MAY 2 6 1998	
AUG 1 7 1998	
DEC 1 5 1998	
APR - 1 1999	
Prince Rupert	
due Mar 25/01	
NOV 27 2001	
OCT 1 6 2002	

BRODART   Cat. No. 23-221

Advanced Practice Nursing

Changing Roles and Clinical Applications

Joanne V. Hickey, PhD, ANP, CNRN
Assistant Professor
School of Nursing
Director, Acute Care Nurse Practitioner Program
Attending Nurse, Neuroscience Nursing
Duke University Medical Center
Durham, NC

Ruth M. Ouimette, MSN, RN, ANP
Assistant Clinical Professor
School of Nursing
Senior Fellow, Center for Aging And Human Development
Duke University Medical Center
Durham, NC

Sandra L. Venegoni, PhD, RN
Clinical Assistant Professor
Virginia Commonwealth University
School of Nursing
Richmond, VA
  and
Chesterfield County Health Center Commission
Director of Health Services
Lucy Corr Nursing Home
Chesterfield, VA

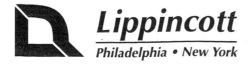

Lippincott
Philadelphia • New York

Sponsoring Editor: Margaret Belcher
Coordinating Editorial Assistant: Emily Cotlier
Project Editor: Erika Kors
Design Coordinator: Melissa Olson
Production Manager: Helen Ewan
Production Coordinator: Patricia McCloskey
Indexer: Victoria Boyle

Library of Congress Cataloging in Publication Data

Advanced practice nursing: changing roles and clinical applications/
[edited by] Joanne V. Hickey, Ruth M. Ouimette, Sandra L. Venegoni.
   p. cm.
Includes bibliographical references and index.
ISBN 0-397-55180-0
1. Nurse practitioners. 2. Primary care (Medicine) 3. Nurse practitioners--United States. 4. Primary care (Medicine)--United States. I. Hickey, Joanne V.
II. Ouimette, Ruth M. III. Venegoni, Sandra L.
  [DNLM: 1. Nurse Clinicians. 2. Nurse Practitioners. WY 128
A2443 1996]
RT82.8.A385 1996
610.73'06'92--dc20
DNLM/DLC
for Library of Congress   95-38552
                                             CIP

9 8 7 6 5 4 3 2 1

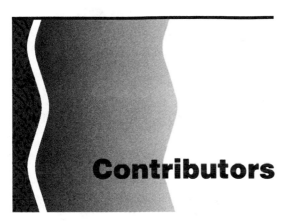

Contributors

Kristie Asimos, MSN, RN, CRNP
Part-Time Clinical Lecturer
School of Nursing
University of Pennsylvania
Philadelphia, PA

Judith G. Baggs, PhD, RN
Assistant Professor
School of Nursing
University of Rochester
Rochester, NY

Cynthia A. Bennett, MBA, RRA
Administrative Director
Clinical Decision Support Services
Hospital Administration
Duke University Medical Center
Durham, NC

Peter I. Buerhaus, PhD, RN, FAAN
Assistant Professor
Harvard School of Public Health
Department of Health Policy and
    Management
    and
Director
Harvard Nursing Research Institute
1991–1994 Robert Wood Johnson
    Foundation
Faculty Fellow in Health Care Finance
Harvard School of Public Health
Boston, MA

Catherine Borkowski Benoit, MSN, RN,C
Nurse Practitioner/Neurosurgery
Beth Israel Hospital
Boston, MA

Susan Burns-Tisdale, MPH, RN
Director of Community and Continuing
    Care Nursing
Beth Israel Hospital
Boston, MA

Angeline Bushy, PhD, RN, CS
Associate Professor
College of Nursing
University of Utah
Salt Lake City, UT

Jimmie K. Butts, RN, CS
Family Nurse Practitioner
SAS Institute: Retired
Cary, NC

Mary T. Champagne, PhD, RN
Dean and Associate Professor
Senior Fellow, Center for Aging and
    Human Development
Duke University School of Nursing
Durham, NC

Colleen Conway-Welch, PhD, RN, FAAN
Professor and Dean
Vanderbilt University School of Nursing
Vanderbilt University
Nashville, TN

Karen L. Dick, MS, RN,C, PhD (Candidate)
Nurse Manager, Home Care
Program Coordinator, Gerontological Nursing
Beth Israel Hospital
Boston, MA

Barbara H. Dunn, PhD, RN, CPNP
Clinical Associate Professor and
Coordinator of At-Risk Populations
School of Nursing
Medical College of Virginia
Virginia Commonwealth University
Richmond, VA

Shotsy C. Faust, MN, RN, FNP
Associate Clinical Professor
University of California at San Francisco Medical Center
San Francisco, CA

Bonnie Jones Friedman, PhD, RN, FNP
Associate Clinical Professor
School of Nursing
Duke University Medical Center
Durham, NC

Sandra G. Funk, PhD
Professor and Associate Dean for Research
School of Nursing
The University of North Carolina at Chapel Hill
Chapel Hill, NC

Catherine L. Gilliss, DNSc, RN, CS, FAAN
Professor and Chair of the Department of Family Health Care Nursing
School of Nursing
University of California at San Francisco
San Francisco, CA

Jean Goeppinger, PhD, RN
Chair of the Department of Psychiatric and Community Mental Health
School of Nursing
University of North Carolina at Chapel Hill
Chapel Hill, NC

Sandra L. Graves, MS, RN, CS, FNP
Clinical Instructor and
Coordinator of Homeless Healthcare
School of Nursing
Medical College of Virginia
Virginia Commonwealth University
Richmond, VA

Mary Wachter Gulbrandsen, RN, MSN, CPNP
Associate Professor
School of Nursing
University of Rochester
Rochester, NY

Joan P. Gurvis, MSN, RN
Clinical Nurse Educator
Moses Cone Health System
Greensboro, NC

Charlene M. Hanson, EdD, FNP-CS, FAAN
Director of Center for Rural Health and Research
Georgia Southern University
Statesboro, GA

Martha L. Henderson, DMin, MSN
Clinical Assistant Professor
School of Nursing
University of North Carolina at Chapel
 Hill
Chapel Hill, NC

M. Elizabeth Hixon, MSN, RN, A/GNP, CS
Clinical Associate
Duke University Medical Center
Durham, NC

Anne Keane, EdD, MSN, FAAN
Associate Professor
School of Nursing
University of Pennsylvania
Philadelphia, PA

Kathleen B. King, PhD, RN
Associate Professor of Nursing
University of Rochester
Rochester, NY

Susan Koesters, BSN, RN, CS, FNP
Family Nurse Practitioner
Mountain Area Hospice
Asheville, NC

Patricia C. Murphy, MSN, FNP, PNP
Captain, Nurse Corps,
U.S. Navy
Pearl Harbor, HI

Kathleen M. Parrinello, PhD, RN
Clinical Chief for Surgical Nursing
Strong Memorial Hospital
 and
Assistant Professor of Clinical Nursing
School of Nursing
University of Rochester
Rochester, NY

Frances K. Porcher, EdD, RN, CPNP
Private Pediatric Practice
Bountiful, UT

Therese S. Richmond, PhD, FAAN, CCRN
Research Assistant
School of Nursing
University of Pennsylvania
Philadelphia, PA

Valinda R. Rutledge, MSN, MBA, RN
Assistant Chief Operating
 Officer–Medicine
Hospital Administration
Duke University Medical Center
Durham, NC

Marjorie A. Satinsky, MBA, FACHE
Director, Managed Care Contracting and
 Operations
Duke Health Network
Duke University Medical Center
Durham, NC

Neville E. Strumpf, PhD, RN,C, FAAN
Doris Schwartz Term Associate Professor
 and
Director, Gerontological Nurse Practitioner
 Program
School of Nursing
University of Pennsylvania
Philadelphia, PA

Elizabeth M. Tornquist, MA
Lecturer and Editor-in-Residence
School of Nursing and Curriculum of
 Public Health Nursing
The University of North Carolina at
 Chapel Hill
Chapel Hill, NC

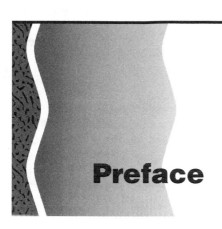

Preface

Promise of sweeping healthcare reform in the United States suggests unprecedented change in the structure and focus of the healthcare system. The evolution of a new healthcare system is paralleled by the redesign and development of new healthcare professional practice roles and models of care that are dramatically changing the way physicians, nurses, and other health professionals practice. In nursing, the clinical nurse specialist (CNS) and the nurse practitioner (NP) have evolved along different professional paths, each with its own focus and practice model to provide care for patients and their families. Graduate nursing education, in preparing for the future healthcare needs of society, is also changing in ways that spark differences of opinion among nurse educators. Some nurses advocate the continuation of separate NP and CNS tracks, whereas others strongly support blending the skills of the CNS and the NP roles into a nursing professional called the advanced practice nurse (APN). This evolution combines the strengths of each of the roles into the APN, who possesses advanced assessment skills with the community based primary care focus of the NP and the hospital-based acute illness management strength of the CNS. The result is an APN who is well prepared to provide comprehensive primary care and illness management in a variety of settings and transitional points of illness, and who works with physicians and other health professionals in expanded collaborative relationships. New models of care will make important contributions to achieving the goal of access to quality, cost-effective care for all people, especially underserved and vulnerable populations that have either been completely excluded from healthcare or that have been recipients of fragmented poor quality care. APNs can be instrumental participants in achieving the goals of a healthier American society for the 21st century.

We have undertaken the writing of **Advanced Practice Nursing: Changing Roles and Clinical Applications** because we have not found a suitable text for use in our program to prepare advanced practice nurses. As we talked to colleagues throughout the country, we learned that they, too, are rethinking their curricula and revising their programs to better meet the needs of students and society. The purpose of this text is to provide a comprehensive resource for APN faculty, students, and practitioners. The text addresses the evolution, issues, and scope of advanced practice nursing, and presents exemplars of innovative practices of nurses who provide care for underserved, vulnerable, or special patient populations in a variety of settings. In a sense, it is a celebration of what nurses have accomplished and also provides stimulation and helps to create a vision of what can be as we continue to meet the healthcare needs of society in creative new ways.

This text is intended both for graduate nursing students and faculty, who are creating the future of professional nursing and healthcare for society, and for nurses engaged in practice, who have been actively creating the infrastructure for the new breed of professional nurses. It is also for dreamers who pursue and practice excellence every day through their influence in providing care for patients and their families. We all share visions of what care can be. We hope that this text will energize and inspire nurses to envision new and exciting possibilities for the care of patients, their families, and society.

The scope of the text is a comprehensive presentation of content related to the roles, issues, and clinical applications of advanced practice nursing. This is accomplished through the organization and format of chapters. The content is organized into four sections:

Section I presents the background and trends related to advanced practice nursing. We begin with a discussion of healthcare reform and the need to redesign nursing practice to be congruent with the needs and goals of the reformation. The remaining chapters examine education for preparing advanced practice nursing to be competitive in the 21st century, including the key role of preceptors, professional development, and the process of socialization. The last chapter in the section examines the renaissance of primary care and opportunities for APNs.

Section II focuses on the changing environments of healthcare delivery and new models of care. The focus of care is rapidly changing from hospital-based to community-based care. Patients are going home "quicker and sicker," and they often need high-tech care in the community. The concept of "hospital without walls" suggests continuity of care that transcends environments and phases of illness. More and more rehabilitative care and management of patients with chronic illness is being provided in the community. Cost considerations, and the demand from consumers for more humanistic care as well as more control over their healthcare, are fueling this trend. As a result, there is phenomenal growth occurring in the ambulatory and home healthcare industries. Rural and inner city areas have historically been underserved, and there is a renewed commitment to meet the care needs of culturally diverse populations. Meeting these needs requires substantive changes in environments and models of care.

The section begins with an examination of the changing environments of care and how APNs can develop adaptive skills to survive ongoing changes. Cultural competence and cultural diversity are explored, along with approaches to creating environments and dimensions for healthcare that will more effectively meet the needs of multicultural populations. Case management and managed care environments, two areas in which APNs are currently practicing, are discussed in some detail. The final chapter in the section examines interdisciplinary collaboration, the key word in models of care for the 21st century, and presents collaborative models of practice in primary and acute-care settings.

The six chapters of **Section III** address issues related to advanced nursing practice, such as accountability for quality care, ethical-legal dimensions of care, and healthcare economics and reimbursement. The complex maze of licensure, credentialing, and certification is addressed. Professional activism, empowerment, and research-based practice complete the discussion of issues that control and shape the way the professional nurse practices.

The last section, **Section IV,** presents ten exemplars in which innovative and visionary nurses describe creative models of providing care to a variety of patient populations and their families. The format used to present the exemplars includes: identification of the focus of care (population, health problems, setting); how care is provided and why care is necessary; identification of specific care needs and outcome-related services; interventions and available services including nursing management, collaborative care, and referrals to other healthcare providers; outcomes of care; and cost/reimbursement mechanisms. We have selected exemplars to give the reader a sample of diverse and innovative advanced practice nursing. The final chapter provides a perspective about the promising future for APNs as key participants in meeting the healthcare agenda for a healthy society through practice, education, and research. It also sets the stage for the evolving role of professional nursing and prepares nurses to become the role models and nursing leaders for the 21st century.

Without the contributions of nurses throughout the country who took time from their busy schedules to write chapters and exemplars, this book would not be possible. It is their collective visionary thinking about advanced nursing practice that the reader will find within the pages of this text.

J.V.H., R.M.O. and S.L.V.

Acknowledgments

This book grew out of a need to provide a textbook for graduate nursing students preparing to become Advanced Practice Nurses. Because there was no textbook available to meet this need, a collaborative effort was initiated to write one.

There are many people to be thanked for their role in its completion. First, we thank our many contributing authors who shared their expertise and talents with this project: Each was selected for the unique piece they could contribute from their individual perspective and range of experiences. Because of the in-depth presentation of their topics, the chapters can stand alone as well as contribute a critical component to the integrated whole.

We thank our publication colleagues at Lippincott-Raven for their encouragement and support throughout the project: Diana Intenzo, whose vision and discussion about the role of the APN first encouraged us to start the book; Donna Hilton, who took over when Diana retired, and who carried on the project with sustained dedication; Margaret Belcher, Senior Nursing Editor, for her ability to join us mid-stream; and, lastly, Erika Kors, our friendly and dedicated project editor, who kept us on schedule and became a familiar member of our electronic mail network.

We thank our family, friends, and colleagues, without whose support, understanding, and encouragement this textbook may never have reached completion. We sincerely appreciate all you did with and for us.

And lastly, we thank our students—past, present, and future—whose presence reminds us of why we started the book. We dedicate this book to each of you. It is the famous line from the play "The King and I" that we understand so well in our interactions with you: "If you become a teacher, by your students you'll be taught." Thank you for continuing to teach us while we are teaching you. May this textbook help you in your lifelong journey of learning. If it succeeds in doing that, we will have successfully completed our mission.

J.V.H, R.M.O. and S.L.V.

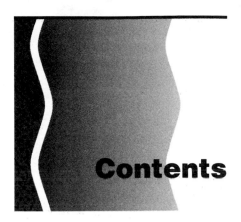

Contents

SECTION

Background and Trends

Introduction: Ruth M. Ouimette

The Pew Health Professions Commission report (O'Neil, 1993) has set a direction and provided recommendations for how academic health professional schools can prepare to meet the population's healthcare needs by the year 2005. Inherent in part of the recommendations is the requirement that each health professional school reexamine its mission and implement strategies that link the schools more closely to other professional schools and to the community. The recent Institute of Medicine interim report *Defining Primary Care* (Donaldson, Yourdy, Vanselow, 1994) set forth a provisional definition of primary care. The definition is an expansion of that developed by the Institute of Medicine in 1978. The revised definition incorporates many of the Pew Commission report recommendations.

The chapters in Section I provide a conceptual understanding of the forces driving healthcare reform. These forces are the education of advanced practice nurses (APNs) to meet the challenges of reform, the complexity of the socialization and resocialization processes, and a proposed "new" primary care that provides opportunity for nursing.

In Chapter 1, Reformation of Healthcare and Implications for Advanced Nursing Practice, Hickey provides a comprehensive overview of the political and economic forces that have contributed to the reformation of the U.S. healthcare system, such as the profound implications of societal demographics and the increase in immigrant populations. Hickey also describes a proposed method of restructuring, reengineering, and redesigning healthcare, with implications for the providers of care, specifically APNs.

In Chapter 2, Education for Advanced Practice Nursing, Gilliss addresses the complex issues associated with the academic preparation of APNs. She identifies the trends associated with where and how healthcare will be delivered, and draws on the work of the American Nurses' Association's former Council of Nurses in Advanced Practice and the Pew Commission report to formulate the competencies APNs must have to practice in the emerging healthcare environment. Gilliss also describes how the clinical nurse specialist and the nurse practitioner have traditionally been educated and offers the insight that the core curriculum for both APNs is not that dissimilar. She presents a curricular exemplar that emphasizes the knowledge and credentials required for advanced practice. She discusses the possibility of merging the strong characteristics of the clinical nurse specialist and the nurse practitioner. Gilliss states, "In developing practitioners for the future, the nursing profession must distill the best features of each traditional role [clinical nurse specialist and nurse practitioner] and work to create new role possibilities. Using past stereotypes will limit success . . ." (p. 27).

In Chapter 3, Professional Development: Socialization in Advanced Practice Nursing, Hixon discusses the socialization process of APNs. She puts into context three interrelated dimensions: (1) professional socialization, (2) organizational socialization, and (3) role socialization of the APN. She describes the complexity of socializing and resocializing APNs, the organizational milieu in which the APN will practice.

In Chapter 4, Preceptorship in Primary Care, Gurvis, Ouimette, and Friedman address the complementary and important role of the preceptor in the education and socialization of students in advanced practice nursing. The authors incorporate Benner's (1984) conceptual framework with their approach to the clinical component of student learning. The authors suggest that the development of partnerships between schools of nursing and clinical agencies will create the most dynamic learning environment for students, faculty, and preceptors.

In Chapter 5, Renaissance of Primary Care: An Opportunity for Nursing, Goeppinger gives a historical overview of several primary-care practice models. She further develops an excellent comparison of the models using seven characteristics common to each. Goeppinger challenges practitioners to address practice variables common to primary-care practice settings thoughtfully and systematically. Citing the Pew Commission report, Goeppinger suggests "that the 'new' primary care will take a broad view of both the patient and the goals of healthcare" (p. 71). Consistent with the Institute of Medicine interim report *Defining Primary Care* (Donaldson, Yourdy, Vanselow, 1994), she advocates partnerships between the provider and the patient in decision making regarding healthcare. In addition, Goeppinger says the new direction for primary care also includes the "development of partnerships between health professional faculty and students and between health professional schools and the communities they serve."(p. 72).

References

Benner, P. E. (1984). *From novice to expert: Excellence and power in clinical nursing practice.* Menlo Park, CA: Addison-Wesley.

Donaldson, M., Yourdy, K., & Vanselow, N. (Eds.). (1994). *Defining primary care: An interim report.* Washington, DC: National Academy Press.

O'Neil, E. H. (1993). *Health professions education for the future:* Schools in service to the nation. San Francisco: Pew Health Professins Commission.

1

Reformation of Healthcare and Implications for Advanced Nursing Practice

Joanne V. Hickey

The 1990s was forecast to be the decade of national healthcare reform legislated by the federal government. But, while the turbulent winds of debate in healthcare have been stalling in Washington, DC, the gentler breezes of change have been wafting through the countryside, reordering the healthcare delivery system. From the nervous third-party payers attempting to control cost and profit to Wall Street investors trying to read the tea leaves, change has been occurring in the trial-and-error manner that has always characterized the American democratic process. Viewed on a long-range basis and from a systems theory perspective, what happens in healthcare—a major segment of the U.S. economy—has far-reaching implications for all segments and institutions of society, including healthcare recipients and providers. In response to the forces driving healthcare, professional nursing practice, like all other healthcare professions, is being redesigned.

The fundamental force driving change in the U.S. healthcare system is cost. The present system is an unruly, cost-ravenous giant that must be tamed to become a more controlled, cost-effective, and efficient servant to our population. There is little debate about the need to pursue this broad objective. The more contentious issues surround the questions of how to make the giant more docile and responsive and who will bear the brunt of the sacrifices necessary to win the battle. It is interesting that one does not hear or read about *changing* the healthcare system but, rather, about *reform* or *reformation* of the healthcare system. *Webster's Collegiate Dictionary* (7th edition) defines *reform* as (1) amending or improving by change of form or removal of faults or abuses; (2) putting an end to an evil by enforcing or introducing a better method or course of action; and (3) inducing or causing to abandon evil ways. The common thread in all three variants of the definition is removal of evil, faults, or abuses. If the current healthcare system is intrinsically evil, how can an exorcism be orchestrated? Among all the competing demands for change, which should become the hallmarks of a new healthcare system?

Hickey JV: ADVANCED PRACTICE NURSING: Changing Roles and Clinical Applications © 1996 Lippincott–Raven Publishers

ACCESS–COST–QUALITY TRIAD

The healthcare debate can be viewed from the perspective of an access–cost–quality triad. This popular relational model for the forces affecting healthcare delivery emphasizes a zero-sum interplay among the three components at a given level of system funding. The quality of the U.S. healthcare system is often touted as "the best in the world," although some have challenged that assertion, citing indices of health status such as high infant mortality rates and low average life expectancy in certain segments of the population. Challengers also have cited the lack of emphasis on preventive care in the United States as compared with other industrialized countries. Owing to the lack of validated research linking indicators of quality to measurable outcomes, perceptions and claims in this regard continue to be suspect. Despite a certain amount of ambiguity and exceptions, the quality of healthcare for the bulk of the U.S. population is generally recognized as good, and there is great concern that so-called reform may negatively affect quality. On the positive side, a research agenda directed at stimulating and supporting outcome research is a national priority at the National Institutes of Health.

Just as quality is generally recognized as good, a consensus considers the cost of U.S. healthcare too high. Furthermore, the percentage of the population covered by health cost-reimbursement insurance—the de facto definition of access—is too low. An estimated 37 million Americans do not receive some level of health benefits as a condition of employment or through a government subsidy program. This includes those described as the "working poor," who cannot afford to pay out of pocket for healthcare insurance. The working poor population does receive healthcare, however, albeit not necessarily optimum healthcare, mostly through hospital emergency rooms and government-subsidized clinics. The cost of this care is absorbed by the system through higher insurance premiums for insured parties and through state and federal taxes for targeted health services (e.g., Indian Health Service, Frontier Nursing Service, veterans' health services). The estimate of 37 million Americans also includes people who choose not to buy healthcare insurance, although they could afford it. These are often young and healthy people who expect to stay healthy and are willing to pay for whatever healthcare they may need on a pay-as-you-go basis (Monheit, 1994).

As a result of the rising percentage of the gross national product (GNP) devoted to healthcare and escalating healthcare costs, which increasingly are being blamed for the failure to control the budget deficit, healthcare providers are compelled to do a better job of controlling costs through schemes for managing the type and amount of care a subscriber receives. However, the concept that cost is directly linked to quality has become ingrained; a discussion of cost-effective care inevitably involves the assumption that quality is compromised by managing or controlling cost.

Access is inversely related to quality at a fixed level of total revenue. If one increases the number of participants in the system while simultaneously holding the available revenue constant in real terms or decreasing revenue, then quality is doubly affected. This is the outcome unless one postulates that the system is riddled with waste, inefficiency, and fraud that can easily be eliminated to reduce cost—the contention of the reform minded. Waste and inefficiency, however demonized by the reformers, nevertheless translate mostly into jobs of one type or another, not profits, for the largely nonprofit healthcare system. Elimination of waste, therefore, often results in unemployment, or at the very least dislocation, which only contributes to the growing uninsured segment of the population. This reinforces the widespread belief that if one attempts to lower cost while increasing access, the effect on quality will inevitably be greater than predicted, at least in the short term. Consumers and healthcare providers do not want to see quality affected. Patients and their families want access to high-tech treatment modalities and services when they are sick. If a provider offers every available treatment modality and service, however, the cost of healthcare will skyrocket. Increased access means increased cost.

Two unpredictable factors may severely affect the cost of providing healthcare. The first factor is the controversy over the provision of preventive health services as part of basic coverage. One argument holds that preventive health services will decrease the need for expensive modalities because potentially costly medical problems will be detected at an early stage when they can be treated less expensively. Another argument predicts skyrocketing cost increases as the result of a growing volume of routine screening tests that identify conditions requiring follow-up or treatment. The second factor impinging on cost projections is demographics. Baby boomers—an estimated 76 million Americans born between 1946 and 1964—are now entering middle age and about to reach the age when the need for medical care becomes much more prevalent. Even with successful measures to address cost containment, these factors alone could defeat any chance of keeping the overall cost of healthcare in check.

The term quality, when applied to healthcare, not only refers to traditional measures of quality, such as the competence of practitioners and the accuracy of testing results, but has come to include quantity of healthcare—*how many procedures, medications, and so forth are covered by a benefits package*. The egalitarian model of healthcare argues that everyone should have the same level of care—meaning quantity—regardless of ability to pay. Proponents of this philosophical position seek to change the existing system of healthcare coverage in which employers and Medicare provide a basic level of care and more extensive healthcare benefits are available at personal cost. The system of variations in healthcare coverage has been in effect for years. Insurers such as Blue Cross offer basic to deluxe healthcare coverage, with the cost of the policy reflecting the value of the benefits included in the package. Presumably, employees receiving a higher level of benefits forgo some salary or other benefits to obtain the more desirable coverage or make higher copayments, as is increasingly the case.

Higher levels of care are available for additional cost even in socialized healthcare systems in other areas of the world. For example, a new privately owned state-of-the-art medical facility in the United Kingdom provides high-level care outside the national system. Here privileged and wealthy patrons from the United Kingdom, Europe, and the Middle East can receive the timely and state-of-the-art care unavailable in their own countries.

Inequity in access, quality, and quantity of care has been a part of civilization since the beginning of care. Every nation, in accordance with its social conscience, must determine what amount and type of care the government (i.e. taxpayers) should and can provide and to which citizens it should be provided. Support for the traditional healthcare payment schema in the United States—as a benefit through one's employer—has eroded as a result of escalating costs, but there is also great resistance to change. Unemployed segments of society are covered mostly by governmental programs. The problem of healthcare coverage relates not only to the provision of adequate healthcare to citizens without coverage, but also to the continuing provision of meaningful healthcare to the many citizens who already have coverage. How can the access–cost–quality triad be fairly balanced for a nation of people without bankrupting the nation in the process?

HISTORY OF HEALTHCARE AND COST ESCALATION

The healthcare system of a country is a unique reflection of its political, social, economic, cultural, and demographic characteristics. As these characteristics change over time, the system evolves in an attempt to respond to newly perceived needs and attitudes and also to accommodate new technological and economic realities. The following discussion highlights selected historical influences on the economics of healthcare in the United States (refer to other sources for a more detailed review of the U.S. healthcare system).

During the middle and latter parts of the 19th century, hospitals in the United States became the sites of healthcare delivery. However, healthcare or *sick care*—a more accurate term—was not always provided in hospitals. In the late 1800s, hospitals were dirty, unsanitary, disease-infested, deplorable institutions intended more to isolate the poor and the seriously diseased than to provide real care. Communicable diseases were the major cause of morbidity and mortality. People avoided hospitals, and ill people generally were cared for in their homes by their families. Families of means employed professional nurses as private duty nurses to care for their ill family member at home.

This situation began to change with a key scientific breakthrough in healthcare in the 1860s and 1870s as a result of the work of Pasteur and Koch (Starr, 1982, p. 135). The 1880s was a time of diffusion of knowledge based on applications of Pasteur's work on the germ theory of disease and Koch's work in bacteriology. An understanding of sanitation and its relationship to disease emerged, and medical science developed. By 1890, the impact of Pasteur and Koch's work was evident in practice. It was not until after hospital reform that sanitation and cleanliness became the hallmarks of hospitals. The influence of Florence Nightingale on nursing and the development of professional nursing in the United States promoted standards of care in hospitals. Hospitals became the desired environment for the care of ill people. Still, few hospitals existed and the quality of care they provided varied greatly. The best hospitals were located in the larger cities and had schools of medicine and nursing. These hospitals became centers for the development of medical science, quality care, and, eventually, healthcare technology.

Until relatively recently, healthcare was a scarce resource available to few. The widespread suffering that came with the Great Depression of the 1930s accentuated the need for basic healthcare for the masses. There was a public outcry for more hospitals to provide that care. The Depression came in the midst of a period of increased industrialization in which a growing number of people abandoned farming and moved to the city to work in industry. The social and family supports available during times of illness, the fiber of rural farm communities, were left behind. Independent, self-sufficient farmers were becoming employees who would now look to their employers to provide for their healthcare and other social needs. Some level of care, although not optimal, was provided through this system of corporate paternalism.

The Depression and its widespread unemployment exposed the vulnerability of these workers and led to the demand for federal government involvement in social programs. The inexorable and growing involvement of federal and state governments in the provision of basic necessities including healthcare began with the Social Security Act of 1934, enacted to assist people temporarily during times of unemployment. People now looked both to their employers and to the government to provide basic needs.

A historical review of the role of federal and state governments in healthcare provides a perspective from which to appreciate the escalation of healthcare costs over the past 40 to 50 years. With the social changes brought about by the increasing industrialization, people flocked to the cities to live and work. Communicable disease control became the focus of the federal, state, and local governments. Programs were developed for infants and children. Workers came to expect healthcare benefits from their employers. Blue Cross and healthcare insurance were born.

In response to the public demand for hospital care, the Hill-Burton legislation was enacted in late 1946. It provided federal funds for the construction of hospitals, increasing the number of hospitals exponentially. The huge Veterans' Administration hospital system was established to respond to the needs of returning World War II veterans. After a period of national reflection about the role of government during the Eisenhower years, the Kennedy administration put forth a large-scale social and civil rights agenda with mixed success due to lack of congressional support.

Following the assassination of President Kennedy, this mood changed, and the Great Society programs of the Johnson administration, including Medicare and Medicaid created in 1965, were enacted with only mild resistance. Medicare increased access to healthcare for the elderly by providing basic coverage for hospitalization. In 1965, people aged 65 years and older accounted for only 10% of the population. Most coverage was for hospital-based care only; reimbursement for home- or community-based care was not covered. Thus, Medicare promoted the use of more expensive hospital care. Medicare also created a new bureaucracy to administer the complex rules and regulations of this massive program. With Medicare, the federal government took charge of healthcare by mandating the components of coverage and setting reimbursements rates for providers. Fees for the bulk of both Medicare and private services were now a matter of public record, giving government regulators the data with which to control reimbursement rates. The predominant governmental presence in healthcare was expanded through Medicaid, a state-implemented program that parallels the federally sponsored Medicare program and provides care for the poor. Medicaid includes many federally mandated state regulations that set standards for eligibility and reimbursement schedules.

Medicare/Medicaid programs did not cure all the ills of society, however. An increasing number of taxpayer-funded programs were enacted to provide entitlement programs for multiple purposes, such as welfare, housing, and education, as well as to provide expanded healthcare to special groups. The cost of financing these programs was sorely underestimated. Healthcare costs in particular were rising rapidly, consuming a larger percentage of the GNP each year. As concern over costs and access grew, the federal government mandated state health planning, requiring each state to develop an overall comprehensive health plan.

Among the services to be included in state health planning was the allocation of beds for people with chronic illnesses, a facet of medicine that was beginning to receive attention. With the advent of antibiotics and identification and control of communicable diseases, people were living longer and developing chronic illnesses. Chronic illnesses began to escalate rapidly during the 1950s. Expensive, high-tech diagnostic tools and therapeutic interventions became available at an increasing rate. A costly phenomenon was the need to replace expensive equipment every few years to take advantage of the latest improvements. Healthcare planners were considering the implications of increasingly expensive modalities for chronic illness. Certificate of need was instituted; it was designed to address the growing problem of expensive services or resources duplicated in the same service area. A certificate of need required a provider to obtain approval by a government agency before purchasing expensive equipment, beginning construction, or initiating or expanding programs. This attempt to harness the escalating costs of healthcare met with spotty results, because providers exerted political pressure and took advantage of loopholes to frustrate program objectives.

The next major approach to cost containment was introduced in the early 1980s: diagnosis related groups (DRGs). Under this system, each admission diagnosis and surgical procedure is assigned a designated length of stay. Based on this measure of reimbursement, the hospital receives a prospective payment for the hospitalization rather than a retrospective payment based on individualized lengths of stay judged appropriate by a provider. Because the hospital receives a flat rate for the hospitalization, it is to its advantage to be efficient in providing care within the same or in a shorter time frame than that allocated by DRGs. If the patient exceeds the length of stay, the hospital must absorb the additional cost. In essence, the DRG concept is a form of managed care adopted by the federal government for all Medicare admissions.

Since the beginning of the 1990s, the federal government has continued to have a major presence in healthcare as a provider, consumer, and regulator. The healthcare industry is ranked as the fourth major industry in the United States. Control of healthcare costs continues to be a national priority; the "beast" continues to resist change.

SOCIETAL FORCES AND TRENDS INFLUENCING HEALTHCARE

Several key societal forces and trends, many of which are interrelated, are influencing the design and cost of the American healthcare system. These interrelated trends include the increased demand for healthcare and wellness tied to scientific and technological advances; the computer and telecommunication revolution; the demographic trends of aging and multi-culturalism; and the rise in attention to women's issues. The demands imposed on the U.S. healthcare system include the need not only for increased healthcare, but also for redesigned healthcare to better meet the changing needs of a diverse population.

Demand for Healthcare and Wellness

There is a seemingly inexhaustible demand for healthcare and a concomitant unrealistic expecta-tion of wellness in the United States. In 1946, the World Health Organization defined *health* as "a state of complete physical, mental, and social well being, and not merely the absence of dis-ease or infirmity." In a recent *New England Journal of Medicine* article, Fitzgerald (1994) point-ed out that this state of complete and absolute wellness is a highly desirable state, but not a real-istic expectation of the healthcare system, healthcare professionals, or life on this planet. Preventive care, health promotion, and healthy lifestyles, according to Fitzgerald, should be encouraged and undertaken; however, these measures will not completely eradicate disease, ill-ness, or prevent ultimate death. Most Americans believe in the right to healthcare for all, but the issues of how much and what kinds of healthcare each person is entitled to remain unresolved. The more components included in the "basic package" for each person, the higher the cost of healthcare. This significant increase in expectations in one sense is a result of an explosion in the demand for new rights fostered by a generation of entitlement politics, a trend that has brought about a crisis in governmental financing. In another sense, it is a result of the amazing progress that has been made and continues to be made in diagnosing and treating illness, a trend that most people would agree is a positive aspect of the U.S. healthcare system. However, along with this progress has come the wholesale demand for organ transplants, joint replacements, autologous bone marrow replacement, care for very low–birth weight babies, and many other expensive but life-sustaining interventions.

People concerned with medical ethics are struggling as never before to balance the cost of and demand for this increasing array of high-priced procedures, which, as already demonstrated in some notable studies, may turn out to be no more efficacious than less expensive traditional procedures or simple symptomatic management. Or, as some studies with very low–birth weight infants have suggested, serious life-diminishing disabilities may result later in life. Rationing of healthcare, many have argued, offers a possible answer to the cost–demand dilemma and is already a reality for those who are inadequately insured. In 1993, following the passage of a popular referendum, Oregon became the first state to eliminate certain medical procedures from reimbursement through programs supported by state taxes. Oregon has also taken steps toward discouraging the use of expensive procedures to prolong life for people characterized as hope-lessly terminally ill. Despite resistance primarily from religious groups, the trend toward official-ly sanctioned rationing in healthcare, especially with regard to marginally effective or unproven procedures, seems likely to grow. The ethical dilemma in medicine of establishing criteria for choosing who lives and who dies can only become more difficult as the anticipated era of biotechnology and gene-based intervention merges with the present high-tech era to provide ever more miraculous and expensive roads to wellness.

In the effort to cut costs, concern has been expressed that healthcare reform will discourage financial support of biomedical research (Kirschner, Marincola, & Teisberg, 1994). Kirschner et al. have suggested that research cutbacks would be shortsighted, citing past achievements from biomedical innovations as substantial in both cost savings and improved quality of life. For example, since the introduction of lithium for the treatment of manic depression, an estimated savings of more than $145 billion in hospitalization costs have been reported. Healthcare reformers should recognize, Kirschner et al. have argued, that biomedical innovation can reduce healthcare costs in the long term, just as other industries have recognized the long-term role of research and development in cost containment and improved quality. The goals of biomedical research are disease prevention, health promotion, and health maintenance, which are often achieved only after long-term investment. Failures along with successes must be expected and accepted. The payback comes when the results produce an effective way of managing a particular disease that greatly reduces cost from what it otherwise would be, as was the case with lithium. It is shortsighted, although sometimes politically popular, to advocate curtailing support of biomedical research as a means of saving money. However, available funds could be more effectively targeted to research projects that have the potential to make major contributions to improving outcomes while concurrently reducing cost.

Computer and Telecommunication Revolution

Extraordinary developments in computer technology and telecommunications networks are having a profound impact on civilization. Improvements in the memory capacity and processing speed of computer hardware have been nothing short of amazing in recent years and apparently will continue at a rapid pace. Constant technological progress in computer hardware has made possible the creation of more complex software with applications to most aspects of our lives. This improves the way we manipulate and analyze information and the way we control, with more precision, complex electromechanical equipment. One problem created by this rapid development rate, however, is that current technology is obsolete almost immediately, and unless people continuously upgrade—often at great expense—they will quickly fall behind.

An equally impressive revolution in methods of communication has been underway—a revolution directly related to the computer revolution. Space satellites have made instant worldwide communication a reality. For example, people can watch fighting in the Middle East or an earthquake in India while in progress and see the devastating results. The Internet is an example of a communication system available by way of a worldwide computer network that provides anyone with a personal computer and a modem access to a vast array of information. People can gain access to research in progress and expert commentary as well as engage in personal networking.

Application of these technologies has had a profound effect on the diagnosis and treatment of illnesses as well as the processing of medical and business information. For example, some programs provide expert consultation from a distance using specialized two-way video equipment for examining patients and transmitting high-quality radiographic and other test data. Digital acquisition of information and computer enhancement of images have vastly improved the ability of radiologists and surgeons to distinguish and precisely locate pathologic conditions. Virtual reality systems, whereby patients can be physically examined by remote control, are under development and not beyond the capabilities of current technology.

Old means of communicating, such as through the postal service and ordinary voice telephone, are no longer satisfactory for other than low priority and personal communications. Confidentiality, integrity, and security of data systems are increasingly threatened as data systems become interlinked and, hence, more vulnerable. Practitioners (many of whom are influential) who view their functions as being displaced rather than enhanced or who would rather not learn the new skills required by changing technology represent a barrier to progress in some settings. However, such attitudes will give way as patients migrate to those settings where progressive practitioners have taken advantage of the potential for higher quality diagnoses and treatments as well as the potential for reducing errors and administrative cost through more efficient information management. This trend offers hope for ameliorating the effects of other trends that are reducing quality and increasing costs.

Demographic Trends

Like the demands for healthcare, the need for healthcare is expected to increase. Some people believe that the changing demographic profile of America is the greatest force shaping healthcare, at least for the next 40 years. The nation's baby boomers will drive the nation's health-care consumption curve up steeply as they enter the age bracket when the manifestations of chronic illness predominate. By the year 2000, an estimated 36 million Americans will be in the 45- to 54-year-old age group and the onslaught of their increased healthcare needs should be well underway. Recall the disruptions this segment caused in the education sphere in the 1970s. First there was a wholesale opening of new schools and then a wholesale closing of the same schools.

By 2030, those 65 years old and older will account for 20% of the population, a percentage greater than that for children (Kennedy, 1993, p. 311). The fastest growing segment of the population is the age group 85 years and older. These segments are growing not only because the absolute numbers entering these age groups are growing, but also because a larger percentage is surviving to an older age. This longevity is a result of an improved economic condition for older Americans, together with improved access to affordable quality healthcare; advances in the treatment of many diseases of old age, especially cancer and heart disease, that have extended life significantly; and a new appreciation for the benefits of a healthy lifestyle, including diet, personal habits, exercise, and stress reduction. Nevertheless, with aging eventually comes an overall increase in chronic illnesses such as coronary artery disease and chronic obstructive pulmonary disease, an increase that can be projected with certainty. Treatment of these chronic illnesses will require an increased allocation of scarce societal resources. At some point, the common good may require that some of the resources devoted to elder care be allocated to other more critical purposes such as maintaining an infrastructure to sustain the productive elements of society.

Ethical decision making in these matters is likely to focus on the care provided for the growing number of chronically ill elderly people who have a substantially decreased quality of life. On average, a person's use of healthcare resources is the highest during the last year of life, and these resources are often expended with the expectation of no gain in quality or quantity of life. The underdevelopment of less costly community-based care and support services to assist elderly people and their families in managing their needs in their homes has led to use of the high-cost alternative—hospital care. At the same time, many healthy, vibrant, active, and independent elderly people need help with continued health promotion and preventive measures to keep them healthy. There is a special urgency to address through comprehensive planning the extraordinary stress about to be placed on the healthcare system and the country's economic resources by the graying of America.

The other major demographic trend likely to increase the need for healthcare into the twenty-first century is the increased infusion of multiple ethnic and culturally diverse groups into the United States. The primary migration from Western Europe in the first half of the 20th century has been replaced by an influx of people from Asia, Africa, and Central and South America. Smaller but growing numbers are coming from the Muslim countries of the Middle East and the newly structured countries of the former Soviet Union. Many immigrants come through special immigration programs such as the resettlement of Southeast Asians after the fall of South Vietnam and as the result of government policies regarding the relocation of political refugees.

A relatively small number of immigrants come through the traditional and legal immigration channels. The problems accompanying the illegal influx of millions of uneducated and poor immigrants from Mexico and Central and Latin American countries have become a source of great political and economic stress in the border states affected. Taxpayers who live in these areas have become intolerant of this influx, arguing that it is overburdening schools, healthcare facilities, and other institutions while placing an unfair tax burden on state and local taxpayers. Large numbers of women immigrate illegally to the United States during pregnancy because they have immediate access to prenatal and delivery care unavailable in their home countries. Moreover, babies born in the United States to illegal aliens become citizens immediately and are thereby eligible for healthcare, education, welfare, food stamps, and various other social benefits. Illegal aliens impose an enormous burden on state welfare and healthcare systems, and the federal government, which has been unsuccessful in curbing the illegal migration, is under increasing pressure to absorb the cost of these services.

Immigrant groups bring with them ethnic and cultural values that include belief about health and illness throughout the life cycle. This reality is changing the economics, process, and structure of healthcare delivery in many communities because immigrants from non-Western cultures are finding traditional Western healthcare values and rituals strange and suspect. Immigrants may reject Western healthcare in favor of their own ethnic and folk medicine. Healthcare professionals, whose attitudes can be influenced by the politics of blaming immigrants, must nevertheless understand and respect immigrants' cultural values and strive to become competent in developing and implementing culturally sensitive and effective programs. Healthcare professionals must blend different, sometimes clashing, values about healthcare. Education of both health providers and health recipients, with the goal of easing the transition from native culture to American culture, is indicated if mutual needs are to be addressed.

It has been repeatedly demonstrated that immigration has been the real American success story. With the established trend in the birth rate of middle-class Americans at less than replacement levels and with the percentage of younger middle-class Americans declining, the future health of our aging society depends more than ever on the revitalization and economic strength provided by new waves of immigrants. All disciplines, including healthcare, are gradually incorporating practitioners from a wide variety of cultural backgrounds to assist in the assimilation process. To ease the stress, we need to find ways to moderate the pace of immigration and to facilitate a more rapid transition to the best of American life while preserving the ethnic and cultural heritage of people.

Attention to Women's Issues

A remarkably important social and political trend labeled feminism or equal rights for women has been steadily growing in the United States since the 1960s and has gradually changed the role of women in society. The choice between working for an income outside the home, working for an income from a home-based office, or working without an income in the home as a full-time homemaker or mother is a difficult one. An increasing number of women have joined the workforce because of financial need imposed by being a single parent or having a single lifestyle, or because their family needs two incomes to make ends meet. Intermingled with financial need is the desire of some women to have careers. Fewer women are choosing traditional women's careers of teachers, nurses, and secretaries and are entering occupations previously dominated by men. With new confidence, status, and expectations, women refuse to be treated differently from men and are influencing the policies and behavior of all types of institutions.

Healthcare has been changing along with all other segments of society, both in regard to how women are treated as patients and to how women's healthcare practitioners are regarded. For example, many medical school graduating classes are now more than 50% female. Women's health programs designed to meet the special health needs of women across the life cycle are being established. Women's health is being recognized as a legitimate specialty practice, and more health providers are practicing in this area. In addition, research funds are being earmarked to support women's health issues. Breast cancer research, screening, and treatment are now receiving increased funding for research and care. Coronary artery disease in women, previously neglected because of a gender bias in medical thinking, is now receiving the attention it deserves on the basis of the prevalence and severity of the disease in women. Most women would agree that this trend, although promising, is long overdue, and still has a long way to go to before gender equity is achieved. However, this is also a trend that increases healthcare costs.

Epidemiologists have observed negative lifestyle changes that tend to increase disease frequency among women. For example, smoking has recently been increasing in certain segments of the female population after many years of steady decline. With so many serious chronic diseases associated with smoking, this is an ominous trend for women. Also, most other negative lifestyle factors, such as poor diet, infrequent exercise, and increased stress, seem to be afflicting women as grievously as they have been afflicting men. It is not known how this cultural phenomenon will affect the access–cost–quality triad. However, it will affect many practice settings.

IDEOLOGY AND POLITICS OF HEALTHCARE

In recent years, there has been a keen philosophical debate among those seeking to influence the soul of healthcare delivery in the United States. Like any important area of human concern, the details of proposals regarding healthcare issues have evolved based on a theoretical framework that makes assumptions about good and evil as they relate to long-term goals and solutions to perceived problems. The most influential writers and speakers tend to be academics specializing in healthcare policy, health planning, and hospital administration. Planners and bureaucrats in state and federal agencies eventually forge and implement public policy on healthcare; their actions are heavily influenced by their academic experiences and contacts. It is from these bureaucrats and academics that special interest groups, lobbyists, and legislative committee staffs derive theories, data, and arguments to support their special outlook on the advantages or disadvantages of legislative proposals for changes in healthcare delivery. These academics and their followers tend to fall into the two broad philosophical camps that characterize the body of politics: liberal and conservative. Liberal proposals draw their support from champions of the lower economic strata who tend to be less concerned with outcome-based planning and more concerned with expanding coverage and access through increased governmental funding of healthcare. Conservative proposals, which draw support from the private sector establishment and institutional sphere (e.g., insurance companies, drug companies, and the American Medical Association) tend to emphasize outcome-based planning, choice of provider, and individual responsibility for healthcare costs. Conservative proposals, however, deemphasize expanding coverage and access through government funding and control.

The mood of the electorate tends to vacillate between these two philosophical goalposts as the economic realities and political sentiment swing from election to election. The established long-term trend in legislation seems to favor a slow incremental approach toward a moderately liberal approach, that is, more governmental involvement, rather than a quick wholesale overhaul of the payment system, as some prominent liberal advocates favor. At the same time, the de facto influence of economic realities in healthcare continues to remake the system based on a lower cost, rather than a higher quality, increased access model.

HOSPITALS AND INSTITUTIONAL CARE

There is a parable about hospitals and trains, two seemingly unrelated concepts. Morrison (1994) wrote that, in the late 19th century, railroads were at the center of the industrial economy, the key part of the transportation industry. The owners, operators, and financiers of this industry were influential players in the national economy. Now in the postindustrial economy of the late 20th century, hospitals play a similar role as the key part of healthcare—the fourth major industry in the United States. Likewise hospital owners, administrators, and financiers have become key players in the national economy. Today, the railroads are no longer top dogs in either transportation or the national economy. The railroads died not because of interstate highways, airplanes, trucks, or buses, but because the people who ran them really liked "choo-choos"! These people forgot they were in the transportation business and not the choo-choo business. By analogy, hospitals are operated by people who are fascinated with huge white buildings and all they contain, says Morrison. They seem to have forgotten that they are in the healthcare business and not in the business of building and expanding more impressive hospitals. The mission of the healthcare industry is to provide comprehensive healthcare to people across a continuum of care that spans settings from tertiary centers to community-based care. To narrowly focus on one aspect of care—hospital care—is to lose sight of the comprehensive needs of society and the big picture.

People want healthcare from sensitive, caring, and competent health providers. Most hospitals, and especially medical centers, are intimidating to patients and their families. Patients often feel they have lost personal control and choice at the admissions office door. In many hospitals, patients feel like inmates, following hospital rules and regulations regardless of how impractical or severe the hardships imposed on them and their families. Patients admitted to hospitals far from home must leave most support systems behind. The vulnerability of being ill is compounded by the strangeness of the hospital culture. Families who wish to visit must sometimes travel long distances or subject themselves to heavy traffic and to high-crime areas. People prefer care in the community in which they live and in friendly and home-like environments. Many community hospitals, using media advertisement and public relations professionals, have trumpeted their friendly atmosphere and attention to the special comfort needs of patients and families as selling points. They also boast of the latest technology and the finest staff of health professionals. These approaches have had some degree of success. But community hospitals and medical centers have been feeling the pinch of fewer patients. In addition hospitalized patients are more seriously ill than in previous times and are limited by their managed care contract to stays of fewer days.

Part of the crisis in healthcare relates to the large number of empty beds in hospitals. Consequently, hospitals nationwide are closing or being taken over by private healthcare corporations. Those that are surviving are undergoing major restructuring, downsizing, and changes in institutional culture. Hotel services are appearing on organizational charts with the sole purpose of providing services that cater to the comfort and individual needs of hospital "guests," formerly known as patients. The biggest change is the development of health networks centered at hospitals that include ambulatory care services, outpatient surgery, short-stay protocols, and community-based care such as home healthcare programs. The growth in these services is fueled by patient demand and third-party reimbursement policies through managed care. Change in the focus of hospital care from specialty-driven services to primary care is also apparent. The concept of primary care itself is changing, placing internists and pediatricians as gatekeepers for referral to specialized care and emphasizing wellness, disease prevention, and health promotion. For chronically ill patients, symptom management and interventions to control or retard the progress of the illness is becoming the goal. There is also a new commitment to patient education, multidisciplinary management of care, and the forging of partnerships among the patient, family, and health providers to achieve optimal outcomes while being cost conscious. Regardless of an emphasis on prevention and wellness, people become seriously ill and require hospitalization. Hospitals, although fewer and smaller in size, are rapidly becoming giant intensive care facilities complete with high-tech equipment and interventions, reserved for truly critically ill patients.

NATIONAL AGENDA TO FOSTER QUALITY HEALTHCARE

A number of initiatives have been undertaken by governmental, private, and professional organizations in an attempt to influence the direction of U.S. healthcare. Three of the more ambitious and promising initiatives are *Healthy People 2000: National Health Promotion and Disease Prevention Objectives*, Patient Outcomes Research Teams (PORTs), and prevention guidelines.

Healthy People 2000

The quintessential document outlining a comprehensive plan for U.S. healthcare is *Healthy People 2000: National Health Promotion and Disease Prevention Objectives* (U.S. Department of Health and Human Services [DHHS], 1990). This unprecedented cooperative effort brings together a wide spectrum of interests including government and business, voluntary and professional organizations, and private individuals. The report urged the following three broad public health goals: (1) increase the span of healthy life for Americans; (2) reduce health disparities among Americans; and (3) achieve access to preventive services for all Americans. The report identified 300 specific objectives organized around 22 priority areas to meet these goals by the year 2000. Measurable targets were set for improvements in health status, risk reduction, and service delivery. The national objectives are organized under the broad categories of health promotion, health protection, and preventive services (p. 6). An additional priority, surveillance and data systems, addresses the need for systematic collection, analysis, interpretation, dissemination, and use of health data to understand health status of the nation and to plan effective prevention programs (p. 79).

The challenge of *Healthy People 2000* is

> to use the combined strength of scientific knowledge, professional skill, individual commitment, community support, and political will to enable people to achieve their potential to live full, active lives. It means preventing premature death and preventing disability, preserving a physical environment that supports human life, cultivating family and community support, enhancing each individual's inherent abilities to respond and to act, and assuring that all Americans achieve and maintain a maximum level of functioning. (DHHS, 1990, p. 6)

The reader is encouraged to review the entire publication to appreciate the magnitude of this national health agenda. Individuals, organizations, and communities are responsible for determining how they will work singularly and collectively to achieve the goals by the year 2000.

Patient Outcomes Research Teams (PORTs)

Medically effective research relating clinical practices and their costs to measurable improvements in patients' health is a mandate of the Agency for Health Care Policy and Research (AHCPR). This mandate is being accomplished through patient outcome research teams (PORTs). The purpose of the PORTs program is to fund multidisciplinary teams of investigators to identify effective care for a variety of common medical and surgical health problems (Greene, Maklan, & Bondy, 1994). The ultimate goal of this program is to disseminate the findings of the studies to the clinical community in the form of clinical practice guidelines as a means of establishing effective standards of care (Greenfield et al., 1994). Examples of topics that have been the focus of PORTs studies are non–insulin-dependent diabetes (type II diabetes mellitus), management of cancer pain, and unstable angina. Once clinical practice guidelines are made available through the AHCPR Publications Clearinghouse, they become the standards of care for health professionals' routine health practices. These guidelines are exceptional resources for advanced practice nurses (APNs) to incorporate into their practices.

Prevention Guidelines

The U.S. Public Health Service has taken a major step in enhancing the delivery of preventive care in primary-care practice through the campaign "Put Prevention into Practice." The *Clinician's Handbook of Preventive Services: Put Prevention Into Practice,* published by the American Nurses' Association (1994), is part of a set of published materials created for dissemination to primary-care clinicians as a practical and comprehensive reference on clinical preventive services. Included are health screening schedules for the early detection of disease, immunizations and prophylaxis to prevent disease, and counseling to modify risk factors that lead to disease. The book provides concise, brief descriptions of current, targeted, age-specific preventive interventions and strategies recommended by major authorities on preventive care. This outstanding up-to-date reference, which also lists educational resources on preventive care for health professionals, patients, and their families (p. xi), is now the gold standard for preventive care in the United States.

Primary care has become a central component of many federal, state, local, and private initiatives to reorganize healthcare, highlighting preventive care as a component within the context of primary care. The term *primary care* was introduced in the 1960s from Europe at a time of alarming decline of family physicians in the United States (Starfield, 1994). Starfield has pointed out that the original definition of primary care specified the following main components: the provision of first-contact care, person-focused care over time, comprehensive care, and coordinated care. In the 1990s, the traditional definition has seemed inadequate for the contemporary complexities in healthcare delivery and the more interdependent and collaborative models of practice among health professionals. As a result, the Institute of Medicine refined the definition of primary care in a report entitled *Defining Primary Care: An Interim Report* (Donaldson, Yourdy, & Vanselow, 1994). In that report, primary care is defined as "the provision of integrated, accessible healthcare services by clinicians who are accountable for addressing a large majority of personal healthcare needs, developing a sustained partnership with patients and practicing in the context of family and community." The *American Nurse* (1994) noted in an editorial that the new definition "stresses the importance of the patient and family, the community, an integrated delivery system, and the relationship between patient and primary care provider" (p. 32). The refined definition provides a context for evaluating primary-care strategies. The full Institute of Medicine report on the future of primary care is expected in 1996.

Three key initiatives are part of the agenda for a healthy nation. There is broad consensus regarding the priority of comprehensive preventive care for the nation, the need to set measurable objectives for care and the need to disseminate clinical guidelines for the most cost effective and efficacious interventions. Other important broad consensus projects are sure to follow as the healthcare needs of all Americans are addressed within a cost-efficient and outcome-oriented framework. Central to the refocusing of healthcare to a primary-care model is the shifting of emphasis from solo clinician practice to integrated health delivery systems comprising teams of clinicians working collaboratively to meet patient needs. These are the enormous challenges involved in meaningful healthcare reform.

WHERE IS HEALTHCARE HEADING?

The more things change, the more they remain the same. This dependable adage is often forgotten in the throes of the seemingly high level of political dissatisfaction extant in the United States. As we listen to debate between those who predict the destruction of the American healthcare system and those who predict the bankrupting of America by healthcare costs, we should remember that, short of an economic collapse or a violent change in the political form of our government, we are likely to continue to have a healthcare system that will gradually improve in some aspects and deteriorate in others. The healthcare system will change at a pace that is readily absorbed by the resources and capabilities of the time. However, this does not mean that the forces and trends, both political and professional, are not having a major effect on the structure and processes of healthcare. To the contrary, these changes undoubtedly seem drastic to those healthcare professionals who had envisioned a different future and had planned accordingly. More than 80% of U.S. residents are happy with their own healthcare and are unlikely to condone drastic and unpredictable remedies for an unperceived problem. Therein lies the reason for the defeat of the Comprehensive Health Care Reform Act of 1994.

Unquestionably the U.S. healthcare system is undergoing fundamental changes in structure and processes. One can argue, however, that these changes are driven by a consensus of the healthcare establishment and are a normal evolutionary response to ongoing forces and trends in society that have been evident for some time. Certainly, the concern about cost is valid and the trend in governmental funding of healthcare is disturbing. More than 90% of the federal budget is devoted to entitlement programs (e.g., Medicare, Medicaid, or Social Security), interest on the national debt, and defense spending, leaving a small percentage for discretionary funding of all other federal government activities. Thus, a gradual shift toward more direct individual and employer responsibility for healthcare costs seems inevitable, as does pressure on third-party payers to reduce administrative paperwork and adopt uniform standards for reimbursement. This shift will likely lead to a more user-friendly system in which competition is based more on the price of coverage and less on the arcane details of coverage or the reputation of providers and insurers.

The demographic trends of a large aging population along with an increasingly numerous and diverse ethnic population mean that the mix of modalities of care will be changing to meet a new mix of needs. With longevity comes increased chronic illness and the need for social programs to support elderly residents of a community. Home care, including house calls, may come back into fashion for physicians and APNs. Home healthcare is a rapidly developing area of practice. The solo physician's office may become a relatively rare artifact of affluent areas as more efficient, targeted primary-care clinics affiliated with publicly and privately owned hospitals assume the bulk of routine care in white middle-class as well as ethnic communities. While this increase in emphasis on primary care proceeds, there will also be an increased demand for access to the life-enhancing benefits of secondary and tertiary care. The population likely is unwilling to return to the "dark ages" of medicine, and the popular media have become healthcare's willing arm for the encouragement and dissemination of every new "medical breakthrough." In addition to this demand for care requiring specialized staff and facilities, there is a keen appreciation among the populace and politicians alike for the benefits of medical research and the need to train new practitioners. For this reason, academic medical centers are likely to continue to enjoy support while constantly struggling to ferret out new cost centers in an attempt to sustain their burdensome overhead costs.

What is in store for practitioners in the new world of healthcare? Pollsters have become the soothsayers of our time and, at their best, can be devastatingly accurate in predicting trends in public sentiment. With regard to healthcare, they have said for a long time that people rate access to high-quality healthcare as a basic need, on a par with food, clothing, and shelter. Also, healthcare professionals continuously rank among the professions enjoying the highest respect from average citizens. It is a mistake to judge the current displeasure with the healthcare system as a lack of appreciation for the worth of healthcare or a lack of respect for healthcare practitioners. The future holds promise for continued political support for healthcare spending.

Can a reformed healthcare system provide everything that everyone wants and do so in a cost-effective way while staying within the constraints of the federal budget? This, of course, is an impossibility. The healthcare reform measures proposed by the Clinton administration in 1994 failed for many reasons, but mainly because these reform proposals attempted to do too much too fast. Small-scale demonstration projects involving insurance reform, increased access, cost containment, and measurements of quality are expected to be funded to test the effectiveness of various ideas that have been prominent in the healthcare reform debate. The national agendas for the health of the nation and outcome research programs already in progress will be instrumental in identifying what is cost-effective care not only on a short-term but also on a long-term basis. The stakes are high, and business as usual is not an option. What must occur is a paradigmatic shift in the healthcare system that will set new priorities and include restructuring, reengineering, and redesigning of healthcare for the 21st century.

OVERHAULING HEALTHCARE

Healthcare practitioners certainly know that fundamental change is happening, but many are uncertain about the nature of these changes. To provide context for the changing healthcare scene, it is important to understand the meaning of three basic terms relating to how change is implemented in institutions. *Restructuring* means rebuilding, reorganizing, reconfiguring, reconstructing, or changing the structure of an organization or system. In healthcare, restructuring refers to the reconfiguring of the organization or institution and is usually diagrammatically recorded on the organization chart. *Reengineering* is the fundamental rethinking and radical redesign of *processes* to achieve dramatic improvements in critical, contemporary measures of performance such as cost, quality, service, and speed (Hammer & Champy, 1993, p. 32). In healthcare, it means the rethinking all of the processes involved in providing care. *Redesigning* focuses on the revision in appearance, function, or content of what people in an organization do. In healthcare, it means redesigning who does what in providing care and services to patients; redesigning of practice has the utmost effect on nurses and nursing practice.

Restructuring Healthcare

Dramatic and innovative changes are underway in the structuring of healthcare facilities as they attempt to respond to marketplace forces and trends. Some hospitals have closed after realizing that they could not offer quality care amidst the new economic realities. Most are either downsizing, often called "rightsizing," or merging with other healthcare organizations. Mergers allow independent facilities to work collaboratively to capture a mutually profitable market share of patients rather than compete on an independent basis for a limited pool of patients. In many mergers, services that were previously duplicated in the independent facilities are consolidated or reapportioned to eliminate duplication. This is true not only for medical services but also for administrative, purchasing, janitorial, and other nonmedical functions. Some mergers and buyouts are designed to create major comprehensive regional networks of healthcare providing a continuum of care from primary preventive care through centralized tertiary care. Large regional networks are forming to serve both rural and urban areas. These networks use sophisticated systems of communication and transportation for consultations and referrals to health providers who schedule periodic clinics in facilities near where the patients live. Comprehensive care networks also offer community-based care (e.g., home care or hospice care), ambulatory clinics, short-stay hospitalization, and tertiary care centers.

Restructuring is apparent in the changed mix of facilities and services being offered by providers; it is also evident in their altered organizational charts. Decentralization, begun in the 1980s, continues, and the business concepts of a matrix structure and product lines are being added to better delineate responsibility and accountability for managers. New product line categories, such as hotel services, are now included in the organizational structure reflecting the new emphasis on creature comforts of patients and their families. Healthcare facilities are striving to become user-friendly, comfortable environments that meet the needs of their patients, rather than inflexible structures requiring conformity of patients and their families.

Reengineering Healthcare

Reengineering, as it pertains to healthcare, focuses on the processes involved in providing care and services to patients and their families. According to Hammer and Champy (1993), reengineering begins with asking, "Why do we do what we do? and why do we do it in the way we do?" (p. 32). Particularly in healthcare, the answer is often "that's the way we have always done it here, or that's our policy." One can identify countless ways of conducting business that appear mindless and idiotic, yet the traditions live on. How we as healthcare professionals develop standards of care or care maps, how we develop and regulate visiting hours, admissions, discharges, and transfers, and how we teach patients and families are examples of processes that can be conducted in many ways—some more reasonable, sensible, and successful than others.

Many of the confusing and imprecise terms used to describe healthcare reform refer to new processes in the delivery of care intended to increase efficiency through coordination and collaboration, control cost, and improve whatever measurable outcomes seem appropriate at the time. Managed care, a key concept in healthcare reform, is an example. Other process-focused reengineering initiatives intended to control cost are managed competition, health alliances, and capitation. One could argue that health alliances are also new structures within healthcare and therefore are examples of restructuring. Although they may be viewed as conceptual structures, the primary purpose of alliances is to reengineer business processes; for that reason, they should be considered a reengineering rather than a restructuring initiative.

Redesigning Healthcare

Another important term in understanding the changes occurring in healthcare—redesigning—is people oriented. Redesigning means redefining who does what. The optimum staff mix for a unit providing healthcare has been a matter of debate for many years, regardless of whether the unit is within a hospital, clinic, or community-based program. From a nursing perspective, we saw the trend to an all–registered nurse (RN) staff in the 1980s intermingled with the optimistic goal of requiring a bachelor's degree in nursing for all nursing staff. As cost-conscious eyes scrutinized operating budgets and it became apparent that a substantial portion of a facility's operating budget was devoted to RN salaries, the following question arose: Does one need a person prepared as a professional nurse to do all of the activities that are commonly performed directly and indirectly for patients? The informal communication network of nurses, as well as the nursing literature, had long been discussing the inappropriate use of professional nurses and the need to assign tasks based on educational preparation.

Inappropriate assignment of lower-skill activities to more costly staff is considered to be a significant source of unnecessary costs in the healthcare system. With the new focus on redesign, many healthcare organizations have engaged consultants to examine which types of activities professional nurses and other staff conduct and how much time they spend performing each activity. Activities such as transporting some patients, finding and restocking equipment, and answering the telephone can be assumed safely by nonlicensed personnel at a savings of salary. It is the data from these consultations that are being used as the basis for proposed changes of the staff mix on units and for the redesign of roles and responsibilities. Proponents of redesign also have argued that redistributing nonnursing functions to nonlicensed personnel will improve nurses' job satisfaction. Many healthcare organizations begin redesign of staff by changing it to a nurse/nonnurse mix of 70:30. The typical goal of redesign is to arrive at a mix of at least 50:50. The effects of this effort in redesign are apparent nationwide; many new graduates and experienced nurses are unable to find nursing positions.

Embedded within the redesign process is the unresolved issue of what is the appropriate differential practice for nurses educationally prepared at the associate, baccalaureate, and graduate levels. Integrative trilevel models of professional practice have been proposed (Newman, 1990), but there has been little success over the years in clearly differentiating roles in nursing practice based on educational preparedness. Moreover, both nurses with master's degrees and those with doctorates have traditionally been lumped together for purposes of describing nurses with graduate education. Much of current discussion on redesign centers on the need for graduate preparation of nurse practitioners and on the appropriate role for clinical nurse specialists, who have been traditionally prepared at the master's level. The debate seeks to resolve the issues surrounding educational preparation and the clinical roles of those nurses considered APNs. Should the roles of clinical nurse specialists and nurse practitioners be blended into one role, or should any nurse who holds a graduate degree in nursing be considered an APN? Preparation for advanced practice is discussed in Chapter 2.

Development of advanced practice nursing has many barriers. In hospital-based practice, for example, the stifling of innovation and creativity that nurtures full actualization of advanced practice nursing is common. Aiken (1990) has advocated the role of attending nurse for APNs, a role that has similarities to the attending physician. She has proposed reorganizing senior nurse clinicians into attending nurse services and integrating those services into the existing medical staff organization so that each clinical service would consist of a nurse/physician group practice. Attending nurses would assume 24-hour responsibility for patients on their service and would make clinical decisions about nursing care for all patients on the service, regardless of location in the hospital (Aiken, 1990, pp. 76–77). A few nurses have taken on the challenge of developing the attending nurse role. The attending nurse concept may provide an alternative model that is both cost effective and improves patient outcomes.

A relatively new phenomenon in nursing practice concerns the appropriate role for the increasing number of nurses with doctorates who continue to see patients clinically as part of their professional responsibilities. The major goal of doctoral nursing education has been to increase the number of nurses prepared to conduct research and teach. *Practice-based research* has been loosely defined to include almost anything that remotely relates to a patient. Much of nursing research has had limited application to improving care or outcomes for patients and their families. An increasing number of clinical nurse specialists are joining the ranks of nurses with doctorates, and some are using their expertise in clinical practice to increase practice-based research (Collins, 1992). However, nurses with doctorates who wish to blend an academic career that includes direct patient care with the traditional roles of teaching and research may find themselves without an identity, mentors, role models, or career paths. Riesch (1987) proposed the academic clinician role for those nurses who hold a doctoral degree and wish to maintain their direct clinical involvement. The academic clinician is an expert practitioner of a scientific discipline, prepared to teach the principles of that discipline to others, and is a researcher working to expand the knowledge that makes up that discipline (p. 583).

Physicians are also feeling the impact of redesign changes imposed on their practice in a capitated environment. Solo practice is a thing of the past and collaborative interdisciplinary models of practice are considered the only way to survive. In the redistribution of who does what, APNs are assuming responsibility and accountability for care that was once the physician's domain. Physicians, in turn, are taking on other responsibilities, particularly if they are in high-tech practice environments. These transitions and renegotiations of practice boundaries within collaborative models need to be developed with care and sensitivity so that the roles are truly complementary and collaborative and not adversarial. For a win–win outcome for APNs, physicians, other health providers, and patients, everyone must work together. The key word for the 1990s and the 21st century is *collaboration*. This requires excellent communications skills, respect, and mutual commitment to a common goal.

One of the results of the ongoing redesign of healthcare is the appearance of a larger number of *middle-level provider* positions. Although probably not the term that APNs nurses would choose, it nevertheless is a broad classification, common in the literature, that includes physicians' assistants and APNs—principally nurse practitioners and some clinical nurse specialists. As redesign moves forward, opportunities for APNs are becoming exciting, numerous, and diverse. Subsequent chapters address advanced practice nursing issues in detail and provide exemplars of exciting innovative practice.

IMPLICATIONS OF HEALTHCARE REFORM AND ADVANCED PRACTICE NURSING

As we contemplate the effect of healthcare changes on advanced practice nursing, the complexities and interrelatedness of the multiple systems that form the fiber of healthcare delivery are both immobilizing and empowering. The restructuring, reengineering, and redesigning of healthcare is occurring around us; it cannot be stopped, nor are we foolhardy enough to try to stop the inevitability of change. Nurses cannot passively let healthcare reform and the redesign of practice happen without a strong, active, and collective voice in shaping our own destiny. These are times of unprecedented opportunities for nursing; they are also times of risk and perils. What is needed are leaders—not any kind, but transformational leaders (Marriner-Tomey, 1993) who envision what advanced nursing practice can be, not only for nurses but also for a nation in need of healthcare. Transformational leaders empower others to attain the vision; they create a culture in which success is possible and expected. Also needed are APNs who are excellent critical thinkers and who can optimize advanced practice within the context of collaborative practice models.

Nurses must be risk takers and be actively involved, because the stakes are high. Remember the parable of the choo-choos and hospitals? Nursing does not have a narrow focus; rather, nursing and nurses are broadly focused on the healthcare needs of all people regardless of age, lifestyle, ethnicity, economic status, or residency in rural or urban setting. Nurses are well prepared to assist patients and their families across the continuum of health-care needs, from the tertiary setting to community-based care as well as the transitional care needed to progress from one level of care to the next. Nurses are exquisitely prepared to manage chronic illness, a major focus in U.S. healthcare. Nursing has been an enduring, respected profession because nurses have stayed close to the core of our being: the patients and their families whom we serve. It is for the patients and their families as well as for professional nursing that we continue to be actively involved in healthcare reform to shape our destiny. To not be involved is to ignore the covenant that nursing has with society. Perhaps the words of Jack London capture the imperative for nursing to be actively involved:

> I would rather be ashes than dust!
> I would rather that my spark should burn out in a brilliant blaze than
> it should be stifled by dryrot.
> I would rather be a superb meteor, every atom of me in magnificent glow,
> than a sleepy and permanent planet.
> The proper function of man is to live, not to exist.
> I shall not waste my days in trying to prolong them.
> I shall use my time.

(Jack London 1876–1916)

References

Aiken, L. H. (1990). Charting the future of hospital nursing. *Image: The Journal of Nursing Scholarship, 22*(2), 72–78.

American Nurses' Association. (1994). *Clinician's handbook of preventive services: Put prevention into practice.* Washington, DC: Author.

Collins, E. G. (1992). Increasing practice based-research: Doctorally prepared clinical nurse specialists may be the answer. *Clinical Nurse Specialist, 6*(4), 6–200.

Donaldson, M., Yourdy, K., & Vanselow, N. (Eds.). (1994). *Defining primary care: An interim report.* Washington, DC: National Academy Press.

Fitzgerald, F. T. (1994). The tyranny of health care. *New England Journal of Medicine, 331*(3), 196–198.

Greene, R., Maklan, C. W., & Bondy, P. K. (1994). The national medical effectiveness research initiative. *Diabetic Care, 17*(Suppl. 1), 45–49.

Greenfield, S., Kaplan, S. H., Sillman, R. A., Sullivan, L., Manning, W., D'Agostino, R., Singer, D. E., & Nathan, D. M. (1994). The uses of outcomes research for medical effectiveness, quality of care, and reimbursement in type II diabetes. *Diabetes Care, 17*(Suppl. 1), 32–39.

Hammer, M., & Champy, J. (1993). *Reengineering the corporation.* New York: HarperBusiness.

Kennedy, P. (1993). *Preparing for the twenty-first century.* New York: Random House.

Kirschner, M. W., Marincola, E., & Teisberg, E. O. (1994, October 7). The role of biomedical research in health care reform. *Science, 266,* 49–51.

Marriner-Tomey, A. (1993). *Transformational leadership in nursing.* St. Louis, MO: C.V. Mosby.

Monheit, A. C. (1994). Uninsured Americans: A review. *Annual Review of Public Health, 15,* 461–485.

Morrison, J. I. (1994). Railways of the nineties. *Healthcare Forum Journal, 37*(2), 30–34.

Newman, M. A. (1990). Toward an integrative model of professional practice. *Journal of Professional Nursing, 6*(3), 167–173.

Riesch, S. K. (1987). Academic clinician: A new role for nursing's future. *Nursing and Health Care, 8*(10), 583–586.

Starfield, B. (1994). Primary care participants or gatekeepers? *Diabetes Care, 17*(Suppl. 1), 12–17.

Starr, P. (1982). *The social transformation of American medicine.* New York: Basic Books.

U.S. Department of Health and Human Services, U. S. Public Health Service (1990). *Healthy people 2000: National health promotion and disease prevention objectives* (DHHS Publication No. PHS 91-50212). Washington, DC: U.S. Government Printing Office.

World Health Organization. (1979). Constitution of the World Health Organization. In T.L. Beauchamp & J.F. Childress (Eds.), *Principles of biomedical ethics* (pp. 284-285). New York: Oxford University Press.

2

Education for Advanced Practice Nursing

Catherine L. Gilliss

As indicated in Chapter 1, significant changes in healthcare problems, their treatment, and the proposed reformation of the care and payment structure have significantly altered the demand for nurses. Although the need for staff nurses has declined, hospitals now are seeking more advanced practice nurses (APNs). Healthcare problems are more complex, and more knowledge and creative problem solving are expected of care providers. Thus, as the demand for APNs grows, the profession must develop a clear understanding of what is required to prepare nurses for advanced practice. This chapter describes advanced practice nursing, identifies areas for potential growth or opportunity in advanced practice and identifies the needed knowledge and skills for advanced practice in nursing. It also recommends one curricular approach to preparing APNs and suggests priority areas for resource allocation for APN education.

ADVANCED PRACTICE NURSING

What is advanced practice nursing? As described by the American Nurses' Association's former Council of Nurses in Advanced Practice (cited in Pokorny & Barnard, 1992),

> nurses in advanced clinical practice have a graduate degree in nursing. They conduct comprehensive health assessments, demonstrate a high level of autonomy and expert skill in the diagnosis and treatment of complex responses of individuals, families, and communities to actual or potential health problems. They formulate clinical decisions to manage acute and chronic illness and promote wellness. Nurses in advanced practice integrate education, research, management, leadership, and consultation into their clinical role and function in collegial relationships with nursing peers, physicians and others who influence the health environment. (p. 6)

According to the American Nurses' Association (Nursing Facts from the ANA, 1993), nurses in advanced clinical practice fall into four principal groups:

Hickey JV: ADVANCED PRACTICE NURSING: Changing Roles
and Clinical Applications © 1996 Lippincott–Raven Publishers

1. *nurse practitioners*—currently, there are approximately 25,000 to 30,000 practicing in the United States; their annual salary is estimated at $35,000 to $40,000
2. *certified nurse midwives*—currently, there are approximately 5000 midwives practicing in the Unites States; their annual salary is estimated at $45,000
3. *clinical nurse specialists*—currently, there are approximately 40,000 in the United States; their annual salary ranges from $30,000 to $80,000
4. *certified registered nurse anesthetists*—currently, there are approximately 25,000 practicing in the United States; their annual salary is estimated at $78,000.

Similar figures have been reported from a 1992 survey of nurse practitioners and certified nurse midwives conducted by the Washington Consulting Group (1994). Numerous reports have indicated that these advanced practice nurses are accessible and cost effective; although they are not doctor substitutes, they are capable of addressing health problems in a satisfying and qualified way (Brown & Grimes, 1992; Office of Technology Assessment, 1986; Safriet, 1992).

What are the common goals of nurses in advanced practice nursing? According to Barnsteiner, Deatrick, Grey, Hayman, and O'Sullivan (1993), the common goals of nurses in advanced pediatric nursing include:

• improved access to care
• increased interdisciplinary and intradisciplinary collaboration within the healthcare system between providers delivering primary and specialized care for children and their families
• an expanded knowledge base for clinical decision making, including health assessment, clinical judgment, health and social policy, scholarly inquiry, and leadership activities
• the provision of services in new arenas
• increased professional autonomy and eligibility for reimbursement by various payment mechanisms.

The Pew Health Professions Commission reports have described the directions to be taken by all professions, including nursing, to meet the challenges of the year 2005 (O'Neil, 1993). Based on the Commission's projected vision of the emerging healthcare system as one in which the orientation shifts toward health and uses a population perspective, there will be more limited resources. However, these resources will address coordinated services focused on the consumer and, in particular, on treatment outcomes. Expectations for provider account ability will increase, as will the need for the integration of domestic and global concerns for health, education, and public safety (O'Neil, 1993).

Practitioners for this emerging system must be prepared with appropriate competencies, including a focus on the community, current clinical skills, expanded accountability, the ability to use costly technology appropriately, knowledge of health promotion, and the skill to involve patients and families in decision making (O'Neil, 1993).

For nursing education, the Commission identified six specific strategies to address these changes:

1. changing licensing and care delivery regulations to ensure that nurses are employed in positions for which they were trained
2. restructuring faculty positions in schools of nursing to directly involve more faculty in patient care and nursing practice
3. developing interdisciplinary education, research, and service programs for the maintenance of chronic patient populations
4. redirecting resources toward the health needs of community-based populations
5. continuing to develop graduate-level clinical training programs to prepare nurses to deliver services that reduce costs and improve quality and access to care
6. conducting comprehensive and ongoing programs of strategic planning within each nursing school.

Clearly, change is needed, and specific directions have been offered. Beyond the world of the contemplative task force, change is occurring in the healthcare system.

McFadden and Miller (1994) surveyed 288 master's-prepared clinical nurse specialists (CNSs) regarding the implementation of their clinical practice roles and how they viewed the healthcare system changes affecting those roles. The CNSs indicated that their most important—and most time-consuming—responsibility was patient care and consultation, which includes clinical practice; case management; patient advocacy; consulting; role modeling for staff nurses; and development of patient care standards, policies, and procedures. Four additional sets of responsibility followed: education (e.g., of staff, patients, and students) and program development; administration (e.g., general, committee work, budget, documentation, and quality assurance); research (e.g., consumer, identification of problems, collaboration, and nursing research committees); and professional development (e.g., continuing education, marketing, networking, and publishing). The factor reported as most responsible for changes in the implementation of the CNS role was cost containment. Participants also acknowledged the changes in length of stay, changes in reimbursement mechanisms, and patient acuity as influences to role implementation. However, the data collected in this survey suggested that the CNS's role, as currently implemented, was not viewed as cost effective.

New roles are emerging, roles that combine the best of the specialty knowledge and indirect practice skills of the CNS with the primary care knowledge and direct care skills of the nurse practitioner (NP). Taking over house staff responsibilities (Mallison, 1993), serving as "attending nurses" (Aiken, 1990), expanding care (and collaborative) roles in critical care (Dracup & Bryan-Brown 1993), and implementing the role of tertiary care NPs (Keane & Richmond, 1993) are among the proposed changes for institutionally based nurses.

A quiet revolution has been underway. In 1992, 2219 nurses reported that they were certified as both NPs and CNSs. Most of these nurses were educated in NP programs. Moreover, the nurses who held both NP and CNS certifications had the highest rates of full-time employment (Washington Consulting Group, 1994). What are the practice challenges that have led these nurses toward combining the credentials of NP and CNS?

HEALTHCARE REFORM: WHAT LIES AHEAD?

Although the exact form of the expected reforms is still unknown, there is little doubt that significant changes will occur by the year 2000. Certain principles as follows will undergird any particular reform package:

- coverage for the uninsured
- reduction in healthcare costs
- limitations in coverage breaks for people who have changed their employment status
- better support for illness prevention/health promotion services
- improved physical access to healthcare
- creation of partnerships between care recipients and care providers to more clearly respond to the needs of particular peoples and communities
- elimination of barriers to full scope of professional practice
- reduction of reimbursement bias to qualified providers of healthcare.

The failed 1993 Health Security Act, as proposed by President Clinton, included a minimum benefit package covering the following: Clinical preventive services; family planning, pregnancy-related services; hospitalization and emergency treatment; hospice care for the terminally ill (which includes registered nurse care or registered nurse–supervised care, family counseling, and social services); home healthcare as a hospital alternative; extended care after acute illness or injury or as an alternative to hospital care; mental health and substance abuse treatment; vision and hearing for children younger than age 18 years; dental care for children younger than age 18 years; and health education to reduce risk and improve health.

Given the principles embedded in the Health Security Act and embraced by others, certain trends can be expected in healthcare. We should expect to see the locus of care move from high-cost centers to low-cost centers (e.g., from hospital to home or nursing homes). Given that patients who can move from costly hospital beds will go to less costly centers, hospitals then will be left to care for more acutely ill patients. Despite the increase in acuity, the actual number of hospitalized patients can be expected to decrease, resulting in the continued downsizing of hospital nursing staffs and further development of differentiated staffing models. Hospitals will require highly skilled clinicians who are able to address patient needs during and after hospitalization. There will be more continuity in the monitoring of patient recovery after discharge.

Because more patients will be cared for in settings other than the acute-care hospital, we can expect new and growing opportunities in extended care facilities and home health. These opportunities will include caring for patients who use life-support technology in the home and caring for their families.

Better funding for preventive and primary care can be anticipated. The number of health education, wellness, and fitness centers will increase. Based on a personalized assessment of individual risk (i.e., genetic, familial, or individual), dedicated centers may address the prevention of specific diseases. Consistent with current government initiatives, physician practice patterns will shift. Fewer specialists will be needed to serve the population's needs; an enlarged primary care work force will be developed.

To better meet the needs of an increasingly diverse population, efforts will be made to diversify the caring professions to match the diversity in the population. Workers who are well known and influential in a community will become important allies to healthcare providers who wish to plan healthcare programs to address the community's needs. In the interest of economy and effectiveness, outcomes of intervention will be critically evaluated; professionals able to evaluate the outcomes of care will be in demand.

Applying this forecast specifically to nursing, several predictions can be made. The CNS, traditionally employed in the hospital to deliver direct care and consult with the staff in the development of care plans, will accept more responsibility for direct care delivery. Given the high acuity and long-term needs of the hospitalized population, the APN in this setting will need to develop a more comprehensive array of direct practice skills and knowledge of patients and their families' concerns about homecoming or recovery. The hospital-based APN will develop a continuity relationship with patients and follow patients' needs in and out of illness episodes.

Another developing area involves providing primary care to specialty populations or providing continuity for specialty populations who suffer from functional disability or are managing difficult symptoms. Provision of such care requires care provider expertise in the special problem as well as expanded skills to manage common problems. An example of an expert care provider would be a diabetes expert who provides for the primary care needs of a group of patients with insulin-dependent (type I) diabetes, or a renal specialist who sees patients both in and outside of the hospital and tends to their various needs, including for healthcare maintenance.

In some institutions, the APN may substitute for physicians in well-baby nurseries, admissions, and emergency areas. In addition, highly skilled nurses working in critical care and trauma units will perhaps assume even more responsibility for patient management. They will work closely with others in planning and implementing extremely sophisticated treatments.

Nurses will be well positioned to own and operate home health and extended care facilities. Because nurses have skills to help people stay healthy, contracts with large managed care organizations should be available to nurses for health promotion and illness treatment for elderly people and others.

As the United States moves toward placing priority on preventive services and primary care, nursing can expect its roles in those areas to grow. More NPs, nurse midwives, community health nurses, and health educators will be needed. The need for primary care providers to live and work in health professional shortage areas will lead to even greater incentives for geographic disbursement. Educators in the health professions will be needed. The need for faculty to expand primary care NP programs is already critical.

The future of community health nursing is bright, but only if nursing leaders in community health will assist in the massive education program that the public health system must develop and conduct. Few government officials or citizens seem to realize that the proposed reforms of the healthcare system will free the public health sector for exciting new roles. The public health sector might be charged with assisting communities to identify their health needs and developing approaches to measuring outcomes of care (Pestronk, Oxman, Gilliss, et al., 1993). In addition, the nursing profession needs to prepare administrators and researchers who can evaluate costs and outcomes of care. The politics of this responsibility cannot be underestimated. Nurses with an intimate knowledge of nursing practice and its intended outcomes will be critical to documenting the value of advanced nursing practice within the healthcare system.

WHAT KNOWLEDGE AND CREDENTIALS ARE REQUIRED FOR ADVANCED PRACTICE?

Currently, advanced practice in nursing is assumed to require particular credentials and skills. Given the proposed healthcare reforms, other skills will be needed. The nursing profession must consider educating advanced practitioners for the future.

Advanced nursing practice commonly requires the following credentials: basic nursing education, basic licensure, graduate degree in nursing, and experience in the specialization (National Council of State Boards of Nursing, 1992). Generally, the following are assumed to comprise the skill base of nurses in advanced nursing practice: comprehensive assessment, diagnostic ability, management of health and illness problems, assessment and intervention of complex systems, the ability to critically analyze research findings, leadership in healthcare, cooperation and collaboration skills, and autonomy and the ability to make critical, independent judgments. The degree to which these abilities have been developed in traditional CNS and NP programs varies. Perhaps there is a difference in the core competencies needed to perform each of the traditional roles (Anderson, 1994).

A careful examination of the traditional approach to CNS and NP curricula reveals differences. Table 2-1 lists the skills identified as necessary for advanced practice and shows how these skills have been developed in traditional curricula. Research, which generally receives equivalent coverage, has been omitted from the table.

Each curriculum has different strengths. The physical assessment or health assessment skills taught in CNS programs have often been limited to a particular system, whereas the

TABLE 2-1 **Contrasting CNS and NP Curricula for APN Preparation**

Skills	CNS Curriculum	NP Curriculum
Physical assessment	Often limited to particular system	Comprehensive
Diagnostic reasoning	Limited	Curricular thread
Management of health problems	Limited, requiring approval of others	Comprehensive
Systems focus	Generally strong; addresses consultation	Often focused on individual; limited focus on context
Leadership	Strong focus	Variable
Interdisciplinary approach	Nurse to nurse	Nurse to physician
Autonomy	Limited	Essential; contributes to role crisis

NP curricula have taught comprehensive assessment skills and encouraged efficient, integrated practice of those skills. The ability to develop sound clinical reasoning skills and differentiate a diagnosis is critical to NP education, because NPs are expected to diagnose and treat previously undiagnosed conditions. Clinical nurse specialist education has not exposed nurses to the rigors of diagnostic reasoning. Clinical nurse specialists rely on the nursing process and sound scientific reasoning to make clinical judgments. By the nature of their work, the scope of concern of CNSs and NPs differs. Clinical nurse specialists generally work with a specialty population under a somewhat circumscribed set of conditions. Although able to initiate management actions in dealing with some patient problems, much of the management authority continues to rest with physicians. In contrast, NPs have developed an autonomous role in which collaboration is encouraged. The scope of practice is wide and the legal authority to implement management actions is generally present. Thus, the educational program includes opportunities to develop a fund of knowledge on a range of problems and their treatment as well as practice opportunities to diagnose and manage patient problems.

With respect to understanding larger systems and developing leadership abilities, traditional CNS curricula have provided more content and practical experience. The CNS has been expected to implement a role characterized by five components: (1) direct care, (2) consultation to others, (3) education, (4) research, and (5) leadership. The NP curriculum has encouraged the development of the direct care component, usually focused on the individual. Often the focus on direct care has overwhelmed the development of leadership abilities in the NP. Fenton and Brykczynski (1993) have made similar observations.

Consistent with the expectation that the CNS will develop consultation skills as one component of the advanced practice role, the CNS generally learns how to supervise and collaborate with other nurses. Nurse practitioners, in contrast, generally work with physicians as practice partners. As a result, the NP and CNS often have different views of their relationships with other nurses and with physicians.

The development of autonomy is essential to the successful implementation of the NP role. This shift in behavior represents a significant divergence from basic education in nursing and, for most NP students, creates a frightening role crisis. Nurse practitioner trainees fear they will kill patients or they will never know enough to practice. Once comfortable that they are able to recognize a particular condition, they panic at the prospect of selecting the treatment and a date for the patient's return visit. The practice of the CNS, like that of the nurse with basic preparation, is generally far more consultative. Applicants to NP programs have identified autonomy as one of the most attractive aspects of the NP role.

Whereas most CNS graduates once worked in hospitals and NPs practiced in ambulatory care, there is now considerable crossover. Nurse practitioners are employed in hospitals to deliver primary care to specialized groups or as physician "substitutes." Clinical nurse specialists are seen in group practices in which their continuous care of groups with special needs complements the care offered by physicians and surgeons.

Although traditionally different in areas of emphasis, the curricula preparing CNSs and NPs include considerable common ground. A fundamental assumption underlying the discussion of educational programs in this chapter is that preparation for advanced practice, across areas of specialization, is more similar than different. An efficient and practical curriculum should be easy to teach, allow nurses to further develop their common knowledge base while permitting the development of specialty-based knowledge, and facilitate the socialization of nurses for advanced practice roles. Furthermore, moving forward in new and creative ways demands that nurses develop a language to describe nursing roles that is free of the heavily charged politics of the past. The terms *NP* and *CNS* have become codified to mean something rather distinctive within the profession. In developing practitioners for the future, the nursing profession must distill the best features of each traditional role ... and work to create new role possibilities. Using past stereotypes will limit success.

Fenton and Brykczynski (1993) have described three ideologies for the preparation of NPs and CNSs: (1) merge the two roles into one, (2) keep the two roles separate, and (3) identify a common core for the two roles, to which specialty content can be added. Based on Fenton and Brykczynski's analysis of the similarities and differences between the two roles, this author proposes a curriculum approach based on a common core.

EDUCATIONAL APPROACH TO THE PREPARATION OF ADVANCED PRACTICE NURSES

Despite its reputation for lagging behind the healthcare system, nursing education has already begun the changes necessary for the future. The changes proposed for advanced nursing practice are targeted at the graduate level at which beginning specialists are prepared.

The first generation of curricular change involved consolidation within NP programs. Schools that offered more than one NP specialization developed a core primary care curriculum, supplemented by specialty seminar sessions. Such consolidations provided economy of scale and often enabled programs to enroll more applicants. These programs have been implemented at the University of Washington, St. Louis, MO; Oregon Health Sciences University, Portland; and the University of California, San Francisco.

The second generation of changes, still underway in many places, involved the development of acute-care NP roles. Motivated by changes in the healthcare system and declining applicant pools, programs have been developed to prepare NPs for secondary and tertiary care. At the University of Pennsylvania, Philadelphia, tertiary care NPs practice in cardiovascular, neuroscience, renal–metabolic, and surgical care. Whatever their specialty areas, all practitioners are qualified for admission into the American Nurses' Association adult NP exam. In addition, the pediatric faculties at the University of Pennsylvania and the University of California, San Francisco, have developed a curricular plan that is built on the strong clinical assessment base of the NP but prepares nurses for the care of children with acute or chronic illnesses, or for critical care.

Case Western Reserve University in Cleveland began a program in 1992 to prepare NPs to offer a full range of NP services plus coordinate patient care in hospitals and clinics. The role is similar to that of a case manager. Neonatal NP programs are also changing the face of specialization in nursing. In addition to meeting the needs of hospitalized infants, these neonatal NPs continue to help with the multiple demands imposed on families during the baby's first year of life—a role that incorporates features of the case manager.

In California, the title *NP* is reserved for primary care practice. Hence, California programs have moved beyond the acute-care NP toward what may be viewed as the third wave of change: the development of the advanced practice curriculum. This curriculum includes the elements that all APNs require. Topic areas may be divided into the following three core areas: (1) graduate-level core (e.g., research, theory, ethics, leadership, and sociocultural contexts for care); (2) advanced practice core (e.g., health assessment, physiology, pharmacology, health promotion, management of health problems, and nutrition); and (3) specialty content (e.g., family assessment and intervention for family NPs, child development for pediatric NPs, epidemiology for community health nurses, special topics in family primary care for family NPs, and advanced pathophysiology for trauma CNSs).

To develop a plan or even an example requires that assumptions be made. The proposed plan assumes full-time study for two academic years, using a trimester structure. No academic credits have been assigned in this plan. Obviously, converting the model to a semester structure would require some consolidations and reorganizations. (Full-time study is still possible for students when tuition costs are reasonable and courses are scheduled into a full 2-day block of time.)

Table 2-2 sets forth one example of an approach to organizing a curriculum for the preparation of APNs. The completed program would include core content required of all mas-

TABLE 2-2 **Example of an Approach to Organizing an FNP Curriculum**

	Trimester		
	Fall	*Winter*	*Spring*
Year 1			
	Research	Research	Pharmacology
	Health Assessment Clinical Lab	Health Promotion/ Disease Prevention	Management I
		Clinical Practicum	Clinical Practicum
	Psychiatric Symptoms and Management	Family Intervention	Family Nurse Practitioner Seminar
	Family Theory	Leadership	Pediatrics Seminar
Year 2			
	Health Care Policy and Economics	Nutrition	
	Management II	Family Nurse Practitioner Management III	Comprehensive Exam or Thesis
	Clinical Residency	Clinical Residency	Clinical Residency
	Family Nurse Practitioner Seminar		
	Pediatrics Seminar		

ter's-level students, core advanced practice content for students preparing for direct care roles, advanced practice, and the content of the chosen specialty. The plan shown in Table 2-2 was developed specifically for family NPs.

The sample plan begins in the fall of year 1 with a combination of master's core courses, advanced practice core courses, and specialization courses. Research represents content intended for inclusion in the master's core curriculum; all students who are studying for direct care advanced practice specializations would select Health Assessment and Psychiatric Symptoms and Management; and Family Theory represents a course that would be taken only by students in the specialty or a subgroup of specialties.

In the winter of year 1, Research would continue. The master's core curriculum would also include Leadership. All students in the advanced practice core would begin a course on Health Promotion. In addition, a supplemental seminar would be scheduled, to be directed by faculty from the specialty. Clinical Practice would also begin, under the supervision of specialty faculty. Family Intervention, a course specifically for practitioners who care for the family, would be included as a course for the specialty.

In the spring of year 1, the advanced practice core would include Pharmacology and Management I (the management of common health problems). These courses would be supplemented by Clinical Practice, which the specialty faculty would supervise, and specialty seminars on the management of health problems common for children and across the life cycle for families.

The fall of year 2 would begin with another master's core course: Healthcare Policy and Economics. In addition, the advanced practice core would address assessment and the management of complex health problems. The specialty faculty, in addition to supervising the clinical residency, would conduct case-based seminars on the management of the complex health problems of children and families.

In the winter of year 2, the advanced practice core would continue with Nutrition. At this point, specialty content comes into sharper focus, with a course on the management of complex problems in family primary care and the supervised Clinical Residency.

In the spring of year 2, the exit assignment (Comprehensive Exam or Thesis) would be completed, as well as more specialty-focused Clinical Residency hours.

In addition to explicit courses mentioned, several topics would be threaded throughout the curriculum for all APNs. These would include clinical problem solving and decision making, collaboration in practice, communication, ethics in clinical decision making and professional behavior, sociocultural variation and cultural competency, and personal self-evaluation. Each would be addressed in each trimester in a deliberate fashion, building on previous exposure to the topic.

HOW DO WE PRIORITIZE RESOURCE ALLOCATION IN THE PREPARATION OF ADVANCED PRACTICE NURSES?

A strategic approach to allocating resources for the development and redevelopment of APNs will facilitate the development of a workforce that is able to meet the population's needs. Faculty development must be viewed as a top priority. Currently, many schools are recruiting doctorally prepared NPs or other clinically competent practitioners. The demand is greater than the supply. In response, many schools are supporting the reentry of their existing faculty for the development of clinical practice competencies. Because many of these faculty were originally prepared for CNS roles, most are entering programs that prepare NPs. Through the combination of the existing knowledge of an area within nursing and the expanded practice skills, many faculty are able to develop clinical practices that enrich and enliven their teaching and research contributions.

Similarly, nurses with master's degrees, who have been practicing in traditional CNS roles, are returning for post-master's preparation as NPs. For many of these nurses, the underlying interest is not to become a primary care provider but to expand the scope of practice to include health promotion and to create new opportunities. Supporting the reeducation of returning nurses should be viewed as a priority for three reasons. First, they generally reenter the workforce within 1 year, rather than the 2 years required for master's study. Second, they are important consultants to faculty in the development and implementation of educational programs. Their current clinical practice informs the curriculum and influences the relevance of what is taught. Third, post-master's programs facilitate the creation of a community of APNs who can advise on curricular matters and serve as preceptors to master's students.

Nursing education must address the curricular redundancy that currently exists. The resources of the past are no longer available to support small, identical class offerings. Where opportunities exist to combine classes and co- or team- teach, faculty should consider creating offerings that combine students from multiple advanced practice specialties (core classes). That is not to say that small class offerings are not an important part of the curriculum; seminar work is fundamental to graduate education because it allows for the development of critical thinking and communication skills. The development of core offerings will create economies, share the work, and aid APNs in understanding the overlap and complementarity of their roles.

Redundancy must be addressed on a regional level as well. The need for duplication of programs within a region should be challenged. Incentives should be developed for programs to cooperate in the sharing of resources and faculty. "New" programs should be encouraged to work with existing ones in the development of complementary programs and experiences. When possible, broadcast and interactive technologies must be used to facilitate collaboration among programs and to improve the availability of programs to Health Professional Shortage Areas.

Although caution must be used in applying the old terminology of *NP* and *CNS* to future roles, scope of practice opportunities in many states is broader for nurses referred to as *NPs*. Consequently, APNs should be encouraged to meet the requirements that would enable them to use the NP title. The public and legislators have come to understand the functions of an NP. Given these advantages, more APNs should be prepared to use the NP title, even when they are not employed in primary care. An alternative to this strategy is to work with state boards of nursing to enlarge the scope of practice for appropriately prepared CNSs. The curricular changes implemented to prepare APNs must be recognized in the practice settings and the roles must be readily enacted.

The need for an enlarged primary care workforce has already been acknowledged. It has been proposed that primary care programs be expanded radically to double the number of primary care NPs by the year 2000. Until faculty become available to teach in these enlarged programs and funds are found to support expansions, qualified applicants will wait and the population's primary care needs will go unserved.

Research training for nurses on the costs and outcomes of care must be a high priority. Health services research has been dominated by population-based scientists and economists. Nurse scientists with an understanding of care systems and the health problems of individuals, families, and communities must be prepared to participate fully in research on healthcare delivery and outcomes. Postdoctoral programs and sabbatical leaves are one route to preparation until doctoral programs can more fully address this area.

Finally, faculty clinical practice must be supported. These practice ventures should be viewed as important opportunities for teaching and the development of clinical research programs, not merely a place to "keep skills up." Faculty practices demonstrate excellence to students and the community. They ground clinical research questions and provide the opportunity for evaluation of practice outcomes. Furthermore, they provide opportunities to generate revenue to support the faculty and educational programs.

We sit on the edge of some of the greatest opportunities that the nursing profession has ever faced. Education has often been the tool of disfranchised groups for self-improvement and social ascension. This is true in nursing, but our diverse educational pathways defy public understanding. As public understanding of NPs and CNSs grows, it is important to maintain continuity in the public understanding. Thus far, the public seems to understand and accept advanced practice nursing. It is important to prepare nursing practitioners who can maintain the public trust through the competence and relevance of their practice.

Acknowledgment: The author wishes to acknowledge that interactions with several groups of colleagues have influenced her thoughts on the subject of this chapter. Notably, she is grateful to her faculty colleagues at the School of Nursing, University of California, San Francisco, and the faculty of the College of Nursing, Arizona State University, Tempe.

References

Aiken, L. (1990). Charting the future of hospital nursing. *Image: The Journal of Nursing Scholarship, 22*(2), 72–78.

American Nurses Association. (1993). *Nursing facts from the ANA.* Washington, DC: Author.

Anderson, C. (1994). Graduate education in primary care: The challenge. *Nursing Outlook, 42*(3), 101–102.

Barnsteiner, J., Deatrick, J., Grey, M., Hayman, L., & O'Sullivan, A. (1993). Future of pediatric advanced practice nursing. *Journal of Pediatric Nursing, 19*(2), 196–197.

Brown, S., & Grimes, D. (1992). *Meta-analysis of process of care, clinical outcomes and cost effectiveness of nurses in primary care roles: Nurse practitioners and nurse–midwives.* Kansas City, MO: American Nurses' Association.

Dracup, K., & Bryan-Brown, C. (1993). Critical care and healthcare reform. *American Journal of Critical Care, 2*(5), 351–353.

Fenton, M., & Brykczynski, K. (1993). Qualitative distinctions and similarities in the practice of clinical nurse specialists and nurse practitioners. *Journal of Professional Nursing, 9*(6), 313–326.

Keane, A., & Richmond, T. (1993). Tertiary nurse practitioners. *Image: The Journal of Nursing Scholarship, 25*(4), 281–284.

Mallison, M. (1993). Nurses as house staff. *American Journal of Nursing, 93*(3), 7.

McFadden, E., & Miller, M. (1994). Clinical nurse specialist practice: Facilitators and barriers. *Clinical Nurse Specialist, 8*(1), 27–33.

National Council of State Boards of Nursing. (1992). *Position paper on the licensure of advanced practice nursing.* Chicago: Author.

Office of Technology Assessment. (1986). *Nurse practitioners, physician's assistants, and certified nurse-midwives: A policy analysis.* Washington, DC: U.S. Government Printing Office.

O'Neil, E. H. (1993). *Health professions education for the future: Schools in service to the nation.* San Francisco: Pew Health Professions Commission.

Pestronk, R., Oxman, G., Gilliss, C., Dempster, J., Badgett, J., Garrett, E., Parham, D., & Toro-Alphonso, J. (1993). Managed outcomes: A strategy to improve the nation's health. *Journal of the American Academy of Nurse Practitioners, 6*(3), 121–124.

Pokorny, B., & Barnard, K. (1992). ANA to revise nursing statement. *American Nurse,* 6.

Safriet, B. J. (1992). Health care dollars and regulatory sense: The role of advanced practice nursing. *Yale Journal on Regulation, 9*(2), 417–487.

Washington Consulting Group. (1994). *Survey of certified nurse practitioners and clinical specialists: December 1992* (Prepared for the Division of Nursing, Bureau of Health Professions, HRSA No. 240-91-0055). Washington, DC: Author.

3

Professional Development: Socialization in Advanced Practice Nursing

M. Elizabeth Hixon

Socialization is the lifelong process of acquiring the knowledge, skills, and values necessary to function effectively as a member of a group or society (Kozier, Erb, & Blais, 1992; Laing, 1993; Oermann, 1991). *Occupational socialization,* a significant portion of adult socialization, is the process through which an individual learns the skills, knowledge, and behavior of the professional role and internalizes the values, attitudes, and goals integral to the profession. Socialization in advanced practice nursing can be conceptualized as three, interrelated dimensions: professional socialization, organizational socialization, and role socialization. The development of the personal self, an essential element in the socialization of advanced practice nurses (APNs), underpins these dimensions of socialization. It is the driving force behind the synthesis of all socialization experiences in advanced practice nursing. Maximum effectiveness for APNs thus hinges on the development of the personal self.

Given the emerging number of master's-prepared APNs and the considerable experience with the role, it is important to rethink how professional development can be pruned, shaped, and nourished. Shifting societal needs, increasingly complex patients, cost-constraints, as well as actual and potential changes in healthcare delivery demand that APNs continually grow and integrate both the direct and the indirect care aspects of the role. Clinical expertise alone, although central to advanced practice nursing, is insufficient. Nursing's future healthcare delivery role in an increasingly competitive healthcare arena may well depend on the ongoing socialization of APNs.

The purpose of this chapter is to examine the three dimensions of socialization in advanced practice nursing and the development of the personal self. It includes practical strategies for facilitating the socialization process and explores considerations that may further influence the personal and professional development of APNs.

Hickey JV: ADVANCED PRACTICE NURSING: Changing Roles and Clinical Applications © 1996 Lippincott–Raven Publishers

PROFESSIONAL SOCIALIZATION

Professional (or occupational) socialization is the process by which an individual acquires the skills, content, and sense of occupational identity characteristic of that profession. This process involves the internalization of the profession's values and norms into one's own behavior and self-concept. During professional socialization, novices must learn the technology and language of the profession, internalize the professional culture, find a personally and professionally acceptable version of the role, and integrate the professional role into all other life roles.

It is important to recognize that professional socialization does not begin at entry into a professional school, but has its roots in an individual's earlier experiences that influenced the choice of a particular occupation (Jacox, 1973; Kozier et al., 1992; Watson, 1981). In professional socialization, however, formal education or training may be seen as the building block of all further socialization (Lurie, 1981). It is within one's initial nursing educational program that their basic professional values are developed, clarified, and internalized (Watson, 1981). Watson (1981) outlines four values critical for the profession of nursing: (1) a strong commitment to the service that nursing provides for the public, (2) belief in the dignity and worth of each person, (3) a commitment to education, and (4) autonomy.

Socialization (or perhaps resocialization) at the master's level is crucial to the maintenance and refinement of these professional values for advanced nursing practice. *Resocialization* is a process of reshaping or change (Hinshaw, 1982; Malkemes, 1974) and is central to the graduate curriculum (Keane & Richmond, 1993). It is needed to help the student synthesize the changed theory base and new role expectations reflecting a redefined, internalized professional self-image (Leddy & Pepper, 1993). Resocialization forever alters the APN's sense of "what nursing is. . ." but it contains elements of both the previous and the new conceptions (Leddy & Pepper, 1993).

Defining one's professional identity is a continuous and cumulative process in which interactions with reference groups play an essential part (Campbell-Heider, 1986; Laing, 1993; Lum, 1988; Meleis, 1975). Reference groups provide an individual with a set of norms as well as values and a standard for the proper level of performance in a given role (Lum, 1988). They are "those groups whose perspectives constitute the frame of reference for the individual" (Lum, 1988, p. 257). Nurses within the work environment usually become the principal reference group for novices (Laing, 1993; Lum, 1988; Simpson, 1972). Advanced practice nurses who are geographically isolated from other APNs oftentimes select physicians as their primary reference group. Although a reference group of APNs may become secondary or supplemental for these nurses, it remains essential to both their personal and professional development.

> By expanding into medicine, [APNs] will need, more than ever before, to increase [their] consciousness of what nursing is all about. The values of nursing must not get lost in the dominant medical culture. If they do, [APNs] justly risk the epithet of junior doctor[s]. (Bates, 1990, p. 139)

Review of the Literature

The largest amount of research on the socialization of nurses has focused on examining certain values and attitudes of graduating diploma, associate, and baccalaureate degree students or on measuring these same variables on a sample of nurses practicing in their first position. The professional resocialization of APNs is not as well described. Although much of this research lacks a conceptual base, the advanced practice role itself cannot be overlooked as one specialized aspect of socialization in nursing (Conway, 1983). Due to the lack of studies on the professional resocialization of clinical nurse specialists, however, research and nonresearch literature related chiefly to the nurse practitioner is included in this review.

Nursing advocates have tended to stress that the "right" personal characteristics augmented by the right educational preparation lead to an innovative and effective nurse practitioner with appropriately changed attitudes and knowledge (Davis & Olesen, 1972; Davis, Olesen, & Whittaker, 1966; Lurie, 1981; Malkemes, 1974; Oermann, 1991; Olesen & Whittaker, 1968; Simpson, 1972). Attributes such as assertiveness, independence, and decisiveness have been cited as essential for successful implementation of the nurse practitioner role (B. A. Baker, 1978; Editor, 1975; Moniz, 1978). White (1978) reported that effective nurse practitioners combine empathy, compassion, and assertion, as measured by their scores on Gough's California Psychological Inventory and Adjective Checklist. Nurse practitioners have also been found to be different from their nursing peers in that they are more self-reliant, aggressive, and competitive (Miller, 1977). In addition, "those who advocate placing nurse practitioner preparation at the graduate level emphasize that better educated nurses have different role orientations to their roles than those less well educated"(Lurie, 1981, p. 32). Better educated nurses are less bureaucratic and more professional (Corwin, 1961; Oermann, 1991; Simpson & Simpson, 1969; Whelan, 1984); are better prepared to generalize from scientific bases in making decisions; and are better prepared to cope with uncertainty and to assume responsibility (Bucher & Stelling, 1977; Howell, 1978; Partridge, 1978; Zornow, 1977).

A lack of confidence as well as hesitation in seeking increased responsibility and accountability have been identified as psychological barriers to the full enactment of the nurse practitioner role. The transformation from nurse to nurse practitioner is often associated with insecurity and anxiety (Lukacs, 1982; Sullivan, Dachelet, Sultz, Henry, & Carrol, 1978). New nurse practitioners fear incompetent performance, worry about their relationship with other healthcare providers, and struggle to avoid unconscious participation in "doctor–nurse" games (Katzman & Roberts, 1988; Lukacs, 1982; Stein, Watts, & Howell, 1990; Sullivan et al., 1978). They must also learn to delegate and to feel comfortable in not performing direct patient care. It is a precarious period of uncertain professional identity during which the novice nurse practitioner is particularly vulnerable to role challenges from other nurses, physicians, and patients (Bass, Rabbett, & Siskind, 1993; Hawkins & Thibodeau, 1993; Katzman & Roberts, 1988; Lukacs, 1982; Lurie, 1981; Sullivan et al., 1978). The nurse practitioner, confronted with the psychological barriers instilled and reinforced during past education and practice experience, must overcome nonassertive behaviors to assume the role of a decision-maker and diagnostician and to become an autonomous, capable, responsible, and accountable professional (B.A. Baker, 1978; Katzman & Roberts, 1988; Lukacs, 1982; Sullivan et al., 1978).

Perhaps the most challenging psychological barrier facing the nurse practitioner is the insecurity that inevitably accompanies a major role change. It appears that nurse practitioners are meeting this challenge (Sullivan et al., 1978). In a national longitudinal cohort study of 497 primary-care nurse practitioners and 407 of their employers, Sullivan et al. found that only 11.3% of the nurse practitioners and 10.3% of the employers identified "lack of confidence/willingness in taking on the responsibilities of the new role" (p.1101) as a barrier to nurse practitioner role development. Furthermore, the reasons most frequently cited by nurse practitioners for selecting their present positions—role autonomy and a perception that the new setting offered a creative approach to healthcare delivery (Sultz, Zielenzy, Gentry, & Kinyon, 1978; 1980)—reflected a desire to maximize the potential of the new role. This finding is consistent with that of Lukacs (1982).

A study of 127 graduate students enrolled in a short-term medical nurse practitioner program between 1972 and 1976 and 31 of their physician counterparts also lends support to the assertion that nurse practitioners are overcoming psychological barriers to the role (Sullivan, 1978). Using the Edwards Personal Preference Schedule, Sullivan reported that the medical nurse practitioner students showed a noteworthy shift in identified personality needs. Whereas nurses have traditionally scored high on "order," "deference," and "endurance," the medical nurse practitioner students scored highest in the needs of "heterosexuality," "dominance," "intraception"(the need to examine one's own and others' motives), "change," and "achievement"(Sullivan, 1978, pp. 257–258). White (1975) has documented similar findings.

More recent studies of the professional socialization of APNs are noticeably absent; information about this process is needed because record numbers of baccalaureate-degree nurses are returning for advanced degrees. Longitudinal studies focusing on resocialization or attitude formation and change also need to extend beyond the graduate curriculum. Cutting off studies of resocialization at the point when APNs graduate from their educational programs is an arbitrary endpoint and neglects that professional socialization is a continuing, interactive, lifelong process. Resocialization is only begun in the graduate educational program and to study it only within those boundaries is inappropriate (Lynn et al., 1989).

Professional socialization is the internalization of the professional identity. It is "the development of a professional soul" (Styles, 1978, p. 29). Baccalaureate education has the difficult task of socializing the student to competent practice as well as providing the basis for the process of continuing professional resocialization (Leddy & Pepper, 1993). "Without this initial socialization, there would be no professional at all" (Lurie, 1981, p. 46).

ORGANIZATIONAL SOCIALIZATION

When the new professional enters the work setting, another dimension of socialization occurs—organizational socialization (Kozier et al., 1992; Leddy & Pepper, 1993; Laing, 1993; Lum, 1988; Lurie, 1981; Oermann, 1991). *Organizational socialization* is the process of learning what is important in an organization or a subsystem of that organization (Krcmar, 1991; Schein, 1968). The focus of this process is the interaction between a stable social system and the novice who enters the system (Krcmar, 1991). The organizational socialization new nurses and employees undergo forms the foundation for personal satisfaction and later allegiance to bureaucratic and professional standards (Ahmadi, Speedling, & Kuhn-Weissman, 1987).

On entering the work setting, novices must integrate professional beliefs acquired through education into a primarily bureaucratic setting (Hinshaw, 1982; Laing, 1993; Leddy & Pepper, 1993; Oermann, 1991). Because bureaucratic values are frequently inconsistent with professional ideals (Conway, 1983; Laing, 1993; Leddy & Pepper, 1993; Oermann, 1991), organizational socialization can result in "reality shock" (Ahmadi et al., 1987; Kramer, 1974; Olsson & Gullberg, 1988). However, work setting is a powerful determinant of socialization because it is the source of one's income and social identity (Kozier et al., 1992; Laing, 1993; Lum, 1988; Lurie, 1981).

Organizational socialization also recurs with entry into each new position or organization. Because APNs traditionally enact their role as employees in organized work settings, they are also faced with how to operationalize professional values in these settings and how to integrate into their behavior and values certain role expectations of the organizations. This issue has been labeled *the professional–bureaucratic conflict* (Ahmadi et al., 1987; Hinshaw, 1982). The label acknowledges the existence of two dominant value systems that may require the APN to have two sets of behaviors (Hinshaw, 1982; Nyberg, 1994).

"It is not the expectation or the desire of either the profession or the work setting that professional values be changed to work–bureaucratic values" (Hinshaw, 1982, p. 31). Organizations employ APNs to use their acquired professional behaviors and standards. Concurrently, the nursing profession assures quality by requiring that APNs have a commitment to the delivery of patient care based on its values and standards (Hinshaw, 1982; Nyberg, 1994). Thus, transition to one set of values is not a desired or an expected goal in the organizational socialization process. Resolution of value and role conflict instead must encompass an integration or adaptation of the professional and the bureaucratic value systems (Hinshaw, 1982; Nyberg, 1994).

The bureaucratic nature of work settings, however, has not always allowed nurses the opportunity or autonomy to maximize their impact on the system (Nyberg, 1994).

Organizations must provide the potential for both autonomy and accountability to allow APNs to actualize their full potential. Autonomy implies independence and self-direction that will enable APNs to be accountable to both themselves and their patients without an intermediary (Conway, 1988; Hawkins & Thibodeau, 1993). Autonomy does not mean that APNs work in isolation without the benefit of consultation and collaboration from other healthcare professionals; rather, it means that they have the freedom to practice at the maximum potential permitted legally within the scope of their defined role (Conway, 1988; Hawkins & Thibodeau, 1993). Therefore, "[advanced practice] nursing's maximum contribution . . . is dependent on . . . the organizational, legal, economic, social, and political arrangements that enable the full and proper expression of nursing values and expertise" (Styles, 1982, p. 213).

Review of the Literature

Most information on organizational socialization derives from studies of baccalaureate nursing graduates. There is, however, a dearth of literature on the organizational socialization of APNs. Some of these studies have identified organizational and structural characteristics of the practice setting that oppose maximum implementation of the advanced practice nursing role. Thus, this review primarily reflects the existing literature on variables in the practice setting that influence advanced nursing practice.

A major issue surrounding the optimum performance of the clinical nurse specialist is placement in the employing agency's organizational structure. Variations of staff, line, project, and matrix placements have been described in the literature (Baird & Prouty, 1989; Blount, Burge, Crigler, Finkelmeier, & Sanborn, 1981; Crabtree, 1979; Fox, 1982). Although no consensus exists, authors seem to agree that the crucial point is whatever model is used must be congruent with the goals of the organizational structure in which it is implemented but must allow the clinical nurse specialist to move across traditional organizational lines.

Elements of the organization and structure of the healthcare system are also determinants of the employment and use of nurse practitioners. Bicknell, Walsh, and Tanner (1974) doubted whether physician assistants or nurse practitioners (terms they use interchangeably) could make a substantial contribution unless fundamental changes were made in the U.S. medical care system. Specific features of the American healthcare system, such as the fee-for-service payment structure, the emphasis on inpatient care, and the content of training programs, would militate against the effective use of nurse practitioners (Bicknell et al., 1974). Berki (1972) also stated that "If there is any one issue relating to the introduction of [new types of health manpower] on which there is a degree of consensus, it is that both the mode of delivery and the organizational structure within which it takes place need to be altered if [new types of health manpower] are to be successfully integrated into [the practice setting]" (p. 118). The specific structural and organizational characteristics of individual delivery sites have also been recognized as critical factors in determining the ultimate success of the integration of the nurse practitioner role into a particular practice setting. Availability of examining rooms, clerical assistance, support personnel, office space, diagnostic and treatment equipment, colleague interaction, physician backup, and, of course, access to patients are required if the nurse practitioner is to practice efficiently and competently (Lewis, 1975; Sullivan et al., 1978).

"Of all the changes that must occur before the system fully incorporates the nurse practitioner, perhaps the most obvious will be the ones in the structure and organization of individual practice settings within the healthcare system"(Sullivan et al., 1978, p. 1102). In a study of barriers to the development of the nurse practitioner role in primary care, Sullivan et al. (1978) found that legal restrictions, limitations of space and facilities, and resistance from other providers were identified as barriers by 20% or more of the 497 nurse practitioners and 407 of their employers. Furthermore, 7 of the 15 specific barriers identified by nurse practitioners and employers were to some extent related to the physical structure or organization of the practice setting. Of these, "limitations of space and/or facilities" was the most frequently reported barrier by both the primary care nurse practitioners and their employers (Sullivan et al., 1978, p.1100). Sullivan et al. (1978) asserted that, in general, nurse practitioners more frequently cited specific barriers within this group because their practices are most directly thwarted by these particular structural or organizational inadequacies.

Lurie (1981) examined the relationship of socialization to role content, change in role attitudes and role behaviors over time, and working relationships for non-master's graduates of the University of California Adult Health Nurse Practitioner Program. She found that the socialization in training and that occurring in the work setting in enactment of the nurse practitioner role resulted in the practice of clinical assessment and management skills on which both agents of socialization were consistent. But in regard to other skills, attitudes, and expectations (e.g., patient education and counseling, expectations for collegial relations with physicians, supportive behaviors from other nurses and healthcare professionals), the socialization received in training conflicted with socialization in the work setting (Lurie, 1981). In the areas of patient education and counseling, Lurie reported that the nurse practitioners could negotiate to practice in accord with their earlier socialization. "But practitioners were not able to change the work setting sufficiently to replicate the socialization model of their training" (p. 31). She concluded that professional socialization is therefore a two-step process in which the skills and values acquired in training must be adjusted to the demands of the work setting.

In addition, organizational socialization and role development are enhanced if role models are available and if the APN seeks out and uses these resources (Krcmar, 1991). "The period of organizational entry [a stage of organizational socialization] takes longer, involves more negatives of organizational socialization, and has a greater impact on role development for the new clinical nurse specialist than for an experienced clinical nurse specialist entering a new organization"(Krcmar, 1991, p. 38). Learning the politics of the system, having an administrator willing to share knowledge of the system, and peer support have been noted as facilitators to role development for both novices and experienced clinical nurse specialists (Hamric & Taylor, 1989).

The organizational socialization of APNs has received little research consideration, but has significant relevance to further development of the APN role. Attention has been directed to such influential factors as the history of the practice unit, scope of the extended role, patient load, nature of physician backup, and levels of satisfaction with the nurse practitioner as the primary provider. Although other factors thought to affect APN performance such as organizational structures and barriers, economic issues in primary care, and psychological variables have been touched on in the literature, they continue to warrant further investigation.

Organizational socialization is the process of operationalizing or integrating the values and behaviors of both the professional and the bureaucratic work systems (Hinshaw, 1982). It is a specific dimension of socialization, distinct from but not independent of socialization in general. Today, APNs function in complex systems dealing with social, economic, ethical, professional, legal, and regulatory incentives and constraints. Each of these forces can become an obstacle to fully actualizing the APN role.

> We must now systematically begin to address those barriers in our system[s] that have hindered both the training and the autonomous practice of [APNs]. We must strive to provide appropriate regulatory flexibility to ensure that those professionals who desire to practice autonomously, whether in hospitals or birthing centers, or on an out-patient basis, can in fact do so. We must ensure that those [APNs] . . . possess viable career and reimbursement mechanisms to enhance their productivity and professionalism. (Kalisch & Kalisch, 1982, p. ix)

ROLE SOCIALIZATION

It is through yet another dimension of socialization that one learns how to perform in a certain role, be it marital, parental, or occupational (Hurley-Wilson, 1988; Laing, 1993). *Role social-*

ization is described as "the training and preparation for the performance of specific tasks"(Hurley-Wilson, 1988, p. 107). It occurs through two simultaneous interactional and learning processes (Cason & Beck, 1982; Hurley-Wilson, 1988; Laing, 1993; Oermann, 1991). These processes involve multiple agents of socialization, such as one's family, peers, school, and the media (Hurley-Wilson, 1988; Lum, 1988; Oermann, 1991).

The role socialization or role development of APNs occurs in two phases. Initial role socialization occurs during graduate nursing education and is followed by role socialization in the practice setting (Holt, 1984; Laing, 1993). Indeed, role socialization may occur more through "tacit knowledge" assimilated through work experience than through formal training (Olsson & Gullberg, 1987, 1988). V. E. Baker (1971) has identified the importance of learning the role of the APN through socialization and emphasized the need to interact with a role model in the work environment to enhance role development.

Review of the Literature

The role socialization of APNs has been the theme of little research. Information, however, has been generated related to the role and function of APNs. Thus, due to space limitation, this review comprises only the most recent literature on the role socialization of APNs and the perceptions of the role.

A number of investigators have examined what perceptions clinical nurse specialists, nurse educators, and administrators have of the role and its components. In a study examining the role expectations of students and nursing colleagues, Cason and Beck (1982) surveyed 18 practicing clinical nurse specialists, 29 graduate students, 11 faculty members, and 22 nursing service administrators for their perceptions of the role. They found that the dimensions of the role deemed important by these groups were: acting from a knowledge base in a clinical specialty area; performing clinical skills competently; using a systematic approach to problem solving; promoting self-care through patient education; and collaborating with others to provide quality care. Cason and Beck also noted that there was a greater level of agreement regarding perceptions of the role between practicing clinical nurse specialists and nursing service administrators than between clinical nurse specialists and graduate faculty who were preparing students for this role.

Tarsitano, Brophy, and Snyder (1986) investigated the similarities and differences between nurse administrators and clinical nurse specialists regarding the importance of four components (clinical practice, education, administration, and research) of the clinical nurse specialist role. Using the Clifford Clinical Specialist Functions Inventory, they surveyed 54 nurse administrators and 35 clinical nurse specialists from a large metropolitan area and reported that both groups agreed on the relative importance of the components, except for research. The nurse administrators placed a higher value on the research component than did the clinical nurse specialists. Although the nurse administrators and clinical nurse specialists valued the administration role component least, both groups highly valued the education and clinical practice components. The clinical nurse specialists, however, tended to see themselves as more heavily committed to direct specialized patient care than did the nurse administrators. In addition, the consultant function received the highest rating of all the functions surveyed (Tarsitano et al., 1986).

Wyers, Grove, and Pastorino (1985) conducted a descriptive survey to determine the essential competency behaviors for the clinical nurse specialist role as perceived by nurse administrators, graduate nurse educators, and clinical nurse specialists. They reported that developing an in-depth knowledge base, serving as a role model, and demonstrating clinical expertise in a selected area of clinical practice were considered the most important behaviors in the clinical nurse specialist role by all three groups. In an ethnographic study to identify the common clinical competencies and skilled performance of master's-prepared clinical nurse specialists, Fenton (1985) interviewed and observed 30 clinical nurse specialists functioning in the role. She found that the clinical nurse specialists reported and demonstrated activities in all of Benner's (1984) areas of skilled performance as well as additional clinical, educational, and consultative competencies specific to the role (Fenton, 1985). Fenton asserted that the major role competencies were building and maintaining a therapeutic team, providing emotional and situational support, making the bureaucracy responsive to patient and family needs, monitoring the quality of healthcare policies, and consultation.

In addition, "the role of a master's-prepared nurse practitioner includes not only the technical/medical role, but also involves those activities which reflect master's-level education" (Hupcey, 1990, p. 197). Six role behaviors dominate the literature as those possessed by master's-prepared nurse practitioners The role behaviors are (1) change agent, (2) researcher, (3) leader, (4) educator, (5) evaluator, and (6) user of nursing theory (Billingsley & Harper, 1982; Booth, 1981; Hsiao & Edmunds, 1982; Hupcey, 1990).

A national survey of 94 graduate-level adult nurse practitioner students in their final semester was undertaken to determine if they were being socialized into the role of a master's-prepared nurse practitioner and to identify factors that may influence this socialization process (Hupcey, 1990). This study revealed that factors relating to the students' backgrounds (e.g., gender, age, highest nursing degree, years of nursing experience) did not significantly influence the students' expectations of nurse practitioner role behaviors. Lurie's (1981) study of non-master's nurse practitioner students also documented similar findings. The educational factor "opportunity to practice role behaviors," however, statistically increased the expectations for selected master's role behaviors, suggesting that students need the opportunity to practice role behaviors to enhance the socialization process (Hupcey, 1990, p. 196). Furthermore, the students placed significantly greater importance on technical instead of master's role behaviors. Hupcey (1990) thus concluded that graduate students may be inadequately socialized into the master's-prepared nurse practitioner role.

Investigators have recently determined that the clinical nurse specialist and the nurse practitioner roles are more similar than they are different (Elder & Bullough, 1990; Forbes, Rafson, Spross, & Kozlowski, 1990). Elder and Bullough (1990) surveyed graduates from a master of science program in the School of Nursing, State University of New York at Buffalo. They asked 28 clinical nurse specialist and 46 nurse practitioner alumni of the most recent decade (1977–1987) about their current role functioning, satisfaction with their work and career choice, and opinions about various professional issues, including the merging of the two roles. The most impressive finding was the large number of overlapping activities and opinions of the graduates actually functioning in the clinical role. "Although differences in traditional areas associated with the two groups were noted, they were not nearly as large as the literature suggests" (Elder & Bollough, 1990, p. 78). The majority of the graduates also supported the merging of clinical nurse specialist and nurse practitioner preparation (Elder & Bollough, 1990).

The American Nurses' Association Council of Clinical Nurse Specialists and Council of Primary Health Care Nurse Practitioners conducted a survey of all U.S. graduate nursing programs that prepare clinical nurse specialists or nurse practitioners (Forbes et al., 1990). For the 195 clinical nurse specialist and the 60 nurse practitioner programs analyzed, information was obtained on the following: required courses, mean number of hours of the required courses, students' clinical practicum sites, and graduates' employment settings. Forbes et al. reported a marked similarity between the core curricula of clinical nurse specialist and nurse practitioner graduate programs. The only significant differences found were that nurse practitioner program curricula placed greater emphasis on pharmacology, primary care, physical assessment, health promotion, nutrition, and history taking (Forbes et al., 1990). Furthermore, in both the student clinical sites and the graduate employment settings, nurse practitioners practiced chiefly in primary care settings, whereas clinical nurse specialists practiced mainly in secondary or tertiary care settings (Forbes et al., 1990).

In general, empirical studies on the role of APNs have tended to examine the role behaviors in terms of medical tasks and behaviors. Although the majority of the studies have offered evidence that APNs provide safe and effective healthcare, they have not helped to define advanced nursing practice. Although additional research is needed to demonstrate the effectiveness of the APN, future studies related to the role should focus on the APN's functions (Naylor & Brooten, 1993). This research will play a significant role in distinguishing the unique services provided by APNs to different patient groups as well as the unique knowledge and skills required by APNs to meet the complex needs of vulnerable populations (Naylor & Brooten, 1993).

Model for Advanced Practice Nursing

Implementing the APN role is a formidable challenge. Not only is the role of the nurse in advanced practice not entirely understood, but APNs themselves are not always clear about their role (Editor, 1975). According to the literature, the APN role encompasses a number of direct and indirect care aspects (Hamric, 1989; Price et al., 1992). Identifying the competencies inherent to these care aspects can be helpful in analyzing advanced practice nursing. Although the specific practice setting influences the competencies that the APN must possess, Brykczynski's (1985; 1989) domains and competencies of practice can serve as an organizing framework for advanced practice (Table 3-1).

These domains and competencies were derived from research exploring the clinical practice of experienced nurse practitioners (Brykczynski, 1985; 1989). This naturalistic research was patterned after Benner's (1984) interpretive approach to describing the knowledge embedded in clinical practice. The domains and competencies of nurse practitioner practice were obtained from observations of nurse practitioners in actual clinical situations and from narrative accounts of clinical situations (Brykczynski, 1985; 1989).

Brykczynski's (1985; 1989) study is based on the framework of practical and theoretical knowledge (Kuhn, 1970; Polanyi, 1958). According to this view, clinical knowledge encompasses these two types of knowledge. Because practical knowledge is contextual and transactional, it can only be learned by active involvement in a situation. Theoretical knowledge, however, can be acquired in a decontextualized fashion through reading, observing, or discussing. Advanced nursing practice requires both practical and theoretical knowledge (Brykczynski, 1985; 1989; Faculty, 1993).

Benner's (1984) definitions of domains and competencies guided Brykczynski's (1985; 1989) study. A *domain* is a group of competencies that have similar intentions, functions, and meanings. A *competency* is an interpretively distinguished area of skilled knowledge identified and described by its intent, function, and meanings (Benner, 1984). Through her research, Benner (1984) identified seven domains of nursing practice that describe the clinical judgment process of expert clinicians in acute-care settings (Table 3-2).

Brykczynski's (1985;1989) study constitutes an adaptation of Benner's (1984) research specifically for nurse practitioner practice. She identified one new domain that was interpreted as more characteristic of nurse practitioner practice. The domain, Management of Patient Health/Illness Status in Ambulatory Care Settings, consolidates and replaces two of Benner's (1984) domains that were more typical of hospital nursing practice, namely The Diagnostic and Patient-Monitoring Function and Administering and Monitoring Therapeutic Interventions and Regimens. Four of the seven domains of nursing practice identified by Benner (1984) were interpreted as valid for the practice of nurse practitioners with minimal change: (1) Monitoring and Ensuring the Quality of Health Care Practices, (2) Organizational and Work–Role Competencies, (3) The Helping Role, and (4) The Teaching–Coaching Function (Brykczynski, 1985; 1989; Faculty, 1993). Brykczynski (1985; 1989) also reported that there were limited data relative to the domain Effective Management of Rapidly Changing Situations.

Although Brykczynski's (1985; 1989) domains and competencies were not intended to be either mutually exclusive categories or an exhaustive list of the skilled practices of nurse

TABLE 3-1 **Domains and Competencies of Nurse Practitioner Practice**

Domain	Area of Skilled Practice*
Domain 1: Management of Patient Health/Illness in Ambulatory Care Settings	1. Assessing, monitoring, coordinating, and managing the health status of patients over time: Being a primary care provider† 2. Detecting acute and chronic diseases while attending to the experience of illness† 3. Providing anticipatory guidance for expected changes, potential changes, and situational changes† 4. Building and maintaining a supportive and caring attitude towards patients† 5. Scheduling follow-up visits to closely monitor patients in uncertain situations† 6. Selecting and recommending appropriate diagnostic and therapeutic interventions and regimens with attention to safety, cost, invasiveness, simplicity, acceptability, and efficacy†

Domain 2: Monitoring and Ensuring the Quality of Health Care Practices	1. Providing a back-up system to ensure safe medical and nursing care:
	  · Developing fail-safe strategies when concerns arise over physician consultation†
	
	2. Assessing what can be safely omitted from or added to medical orders
	
	3. Getting appropriate and timely responses from physicians:
	  · Using physician consultation effectively†
	
	4. Self-monitoring and seeking consultation as necessary†
	
	5. Giving constructive feedback to physicians and other care providers to ensure safe care practices†

Domain 3: Organizational and Work-Role Competencies	1. Coordinating, ordering, and meeting multiple patient needs and requests; setting priorities
	
	2. Building and maintaining a therapeutic team to provide optimum therapy
	
	3. Coping with staff shortages and high turnover:
	  · Contingency planning
	  · Anticipating and preventing periods of extreme work overload
	  · Using and maintaining team spirit; gaining social support from other nurses
	  · Maintaining a flexible stance towards patients, technology, and bureaucracy
	
	4. Making the bureaucracy respond to patients' and families' needs§
	
	5. Obtaining specialist care for patients while remaining the primary care provider†

Domain 4: Helping Role of the Nurse	1. Healing relationship: Creating a climate for and establishing a commitment to healing
	
	2. Providing comfort measures and preserving personhood in the face of extreme breakdown
	
	3. Presencing: Being with a patient
	
	4. Maximizing the patient's participation and control in his or her own health/illness care‡
	
	5. Interpreting kinds of pain and selecting appropriate strategies for pain management and pain control
	
	6. Providing comfort and communication through touch
	
	7. Providing emotional and informational support to patient's families
	
	8. Guiding a patient through emotional and developmental change:
	  · Providing new options, closing off old ones
	  · Channeling, teaching, mediating
	  · Acting as a psychological and cultural mediator
	  · Using goals therapeutically
	  · Working to build and maintain a therapeutic community

Domain 5: Teaching-Coaching Function of the Nurse	1. Timing: Capturing a patient's readiness to learn: · Motivating a patient to change†

(continued)

TABLE 3-1 **Domains and Competencies of Nurse Practitioner Practice** (Continued)

Domain	Area of Skilled Practice*
	2. Assisting patients to integrate the implications of their illness and recovery into their lifestyle
	3. Assisting patients to alter their lifestyle to meet changing health care needs and capacities: Teaching for self-care†
	4. Eliciting an understanding of the patient's interpretation of his or her illness: • Negotiating agreement about how to proceed when priorities of patient and provider conflict†
	5. Providing an interpretation of the patient's condition and giving a rationale for procedures
	6. Coaching function: Making culturally avoided and uncharted health and illness experiences approachable and understandable‡
Domain 6: Effective Management of Rapidly Changing Situations	1. Skilled performance in extreme life-threatening emergencies: Rapid grasp of a problem
	2. Contingency management: Rapid matching of demands and resources in emergency situations
	3. Identifying and managing a patient crisis until physician assistance is available

Note. *Areas of skilled practice are adapted from Benner (1984) unless otherwise noted. †Domain and competencies identified in Brykczynski (1985). ‡Competency expanded in Brykczynski (1985). §Competency identified by Fenton (1985). Benner, P. (1984). *From novice to expert: Excellence and power in clinical nursing practice.* Menlo Park, CA: Addison-Wesley; Brykczynski, K. A. (1985). Exploring the clinical practice of nurse practitioners (Doctoral dissertation, University of California, San Francisco, 1985). *Dissertation Abstracts International, 46,* 3789B. (University Microfilms No. DA86-00592); Fenton, M. V. (1985). Identifying competencies of clinical nurse specialists. *Journal of Nursing Administration, 15*(12), 31-37. From "An interpretive study describing the clinical judgment of nurse practitioners" by K. A. Brykczynski, 1989, *Scholarly Inquiry for Nursing Practice: An International Journal, 3* (2), pp. 90-91. Copyright 1989 by Springer. Reprinted with permission.

practitioners, they are useful as an organizing framework for advanced nursing practice. Based on the marked similarities between the clinical nurse specialist and nurse practitioner roles, this model is also applicable to the master's-prepared clinical nurse specialist. Advanced practice nurses can further Brykczynski's (1985; 1989) work by identifying as well as validating new domains and competencies and by refining those that have practical worth.

Role Development of Advanced Practice Nurses

Advanced practice nurses prepared at the graduate level provide direct patient care, but, in addition to or instead of direct patient care, also assume indirect roles including those of educator, administrator, consultant, and researcher (Hamric, 1989; Price et al., 1992). Neither a new master's degree graduate nor a new reequipped APN can be expected to have expertise in each of these components (Holt, 1984, p. 447). Graduate nursing education provides the academic preparation and the tools for role development in these areas (Holt, 1984, p. 447). Further development of skill in these role components, however, must also come in the practice setting following graduation (Holt, 1984, p. 447; Ryan-Merritt, Mitchell, & Pagel, 1988; Sparacino, 1990).

Several models have been developed to explain the process of socialization in professional roles. The Dreyfus model of skill acquisition (Dreyfus & Dreyfus, 1980) is based on a study of chess players and airline pilots. Benner (1984) has used this model to describe the progression of skills and the competency of the staff nurse in the clinical setting. The five levels of the Dreyfus model of skill acquisition are (1) novice, (2) advanced beginner, (3) competent, (4) proficient, and (5) expert. Using this model, as applied to the nursing profession by Benner, Table 3-3 explores the transition of the APN from novice to expert practitioner that is based on the chapter author's personal experience.

TABLE 3-2 Domains of Nursing Practice

The Helping Role

The Teaching-Coaching Function

The Diagnostic and Patient-Monitoring Function

Effective Management of Rapidly Changing Situations

Administrating and Monitoring Therapeutic Interventions and Regimens

Monitoring and Ensuring the Quality of Health Care Practices

Organizational and Work-Role Competencies

Note. From *From novice to expert: Excellence and power in clinical nursing practice* (p. 46), by P. Benner, 1984, Menlo Park, CA: Addison-Wesley. Copyright 1984 by Addison-Wesley. Reprinted with permission.

Movement through the five levels of skill acquisition for the APN occurs at varying rates (Arena & Page, 1992; Bass et al., 1993; Hamric & Taylor, 1989; Lukacs, 1982). Individual differences in the potential and the experiential background of APNs, as well as the uniqueness of each practice setting, will affect their developmental patterns (Holt, 1984). Because experienced and new reequipped APNs possess a repertoire of clinical paradigms, their transition from novice to expert practitioner may indeed be expedited. In addition, changing positions or areas of specialization returns even an experienced APN to an apprentice level (Arena & Page, 1992). Nevertheless, no one prevents APNs from reaching the expert level of development except themselves (Christman, 1987).

TABLE 3-3 Characteristics of Performance from Novice to Expert Practitioner

Novice	Advanced Beginner	Competent	Proficient	Expert
Has a narrow scope of practice	Enhances clinical competence in weak areas	Has an expanded scope of practice	Incorporates direct and indirect roles into daily practice	Has a global scope of practice
Develops technical skills	Enhances diagnostic reasoning and clinical decision-making skills	Feels competent in diagnostic reasoning and clinical decision-making skills	Enhances clinical expertise	Cohesively integrates direct and indirect roles
Develops diagnostic reasoning and clinical decision-making skills	Begins to develop the educator and the consultant role	Begins to develop administrator role	Conducts or directs research projects	Has an intuitive grasp
Needs frequent consultation and validation of clinical skills	Incorporates research findings into practice	Develops organizational skills	Is an effective change agent	Has a greater sense of salience
Needs and identifies mentor	Sets priorities	Views situations in multifaceted ways	Uses holistic approach to care	Is a reflective practitioner
Establishes credibility	Develops a reference group	Senses nuances	Interprets nuances	Empowers patients, families, and colleagues
Develops confidence	Enhances credibility	Relies on maxims to guide practice		Is a mentor
	Builds confidence	Feels efficient and organized		
		Networks		

Role socialization, the process of learning specific skills (Hurley-Wilson, 1988), is interdependent on the professional and the organizational dimensions of socialization as well as on the development of the personal self. The socialization or development of the APN role is characterized by continued defining, refining, and refocusing (Hamric & Taylor, 1989). It is imperative that role development be an ongoing, dynamic process for the APN to be fully effective (Hamric & Taylor, 1989, p. 81). Truly, there is no shortcut in role development. By using an organizing framework for advanced practice, however, APNs can locate as well as evaluate where they are in the role development process and readily identify directions for further implementation.

DEVELOPMENT OF THE PERSONAL SELF

The development of the personal self is taking time to "sharpen the saw" (Covey, 1989, p. 287). It is preserving and enhancing the greatest asset one has: one's self (Covey, 1989). The development of the personal self (or self-nurturing) underpins the three dimensions of socialization in advanced practice nursing because it is the driving force that makes all the others possible.

The self is a concept of one's own person as distinguished from other objects in the external world. It is one's concept of self as a separate, whole person. The self includes individuals' appraisals of themselves as well as the appraisals others make of them. The self is never constant; it is forever changing and emerging in new ways. The emergence of self is influenced by interactions with others as well as by interactions with one's environment (Leddy & Pepper, 1993; Stuart & Sundeen, 1995).

The professional self-system emerges from the personal self (Leddy & Pepper, 1993). One's self-concept "results from previous interpersonal relationships" and affects one's future relationships (Simms & Lindberg, 1978, p. 9). "A person's view of self controls the roles he or she will be able to assume" (Simms & Lindberg, 1978, p. 9). One's self-system determines one's personal characteristics, and these personal qualities enable one to carry out professional roles (Leddy & Pepper, 1993). An individual's self-concept can, therefore, serve either as a barrier or a support for his or her professional self.

"Strength derives from a strong self-concept"(Hawkins & Thibodeau, 1993, p. 57). A strong self-concept can be linked to motivation and success in one's career (Hawkins & Thibodeau, 1993). Horner (1975) found that women exhibit a need to avoid success. The most competent women, "when faced with a conflict between their feminine image and expressing their competencies or developing their abilities and interests, adjust their behaviors to their internalized sex–role stereotypes" (Horner, 1975, p. 219). Sex–role stereotypes convey messages that say that women are poor decision-makers and are unable to assume leadership roles (Broverman, Vogel, Broverman, Charkan, & Rosenkrantz, 1975; Edmunds, 1980; Hawkins & Thibodeau, 1993; Katzman & Roberts, 1988; Stein et al., 1990). Such messages weaken women's self-concept, planting seeds of doubt about their ability to use their strength and power (Hawkins & Thibodeau, 1993; Katzman & Roberts, 1988; Stein et al., 1990). Knowledge about sex–role stereotyping and the effects it has on self-concept can assist APNs to develop strategies for gaining influence in their clinical settings.

Simms and Lindberg (1978) validated that the professional self directly reflects the personal self-concept. "Responsibility for our own acts—especially toward others—will flourish in an environment which fosters growth of self and independence" (Simms & Lindberg, 1978, p. 7). "Understanding self and working to view self positively inevitable leads to more productive professional self-concepts. Negative self-concepts are barriers to the effective independent functioning vital to the successful performance of professional roles" (Leddy & Pepper, 1993, p. 67).

Self-nurturing and self-esteem are thus "necessary partners" (Bunkers, 1992, p. 155). "To feel good about themselves, [APNs] need to develop the ability to take care of themselves. At the same time, to take good care of their physical, emotional, mental, and spiritual selves, [APNs] need to feel that they are worthwhile" (p. 155). If self-nurturing is absent or deficient, self-esteem is lowered; if self-nurturing is balanced, self-esteem is raised (Bunkers, 1992, p. 155). Several self-nurturing strategies can help APNs develop both a valuing of and a recommitment to their personal self (Table 3-4).

To a great extent, the kind of professional an individual becomes depends on the individual's self-system (Leddy & Pepper, 1993). The development of the personal self or self-nurturing is the single most powerful investment APNs can ever make in life: investment in themselves (Covey, 1989). "Being able to care for others, to connect with others in a meaningful way, depends fundamentally on caring for one's Self" (Chinn, 1991, p. 255). The things APNs do to "sharpen the saw" will have a positive impact on the professional, organizational, and role dimensions of socialization because they are so highly interrelated. The development of the personal self empowers APNs to move on an upward spiral of growth and change—of continuous improvement (Covey, 1989).

SOCIALIZATION STRATEGIES

Socialization in advanced practice nursing is a continuously evolving process that demands both time and energy. By employing proactive behaviors, APNs can not only enhance this process but can also make it easier and less overwhelming. Thus, some practical strategies for facilitating socialization in advanced practice nursing are included in this summary.

1. *Trust your own intuitive processes.*
2. *Conduct an organizational analysis.* Successful implementation of the advanced practice role is often determined by the practice setting (Bass et al., 1993). An organizational analysis enables you to understand complex systems and gives you the skills necessary to function more effectively within them (Conway, 1988; Reddecliff, Smith, & Ryan-Merritt, 1989). Another benefit of an organizational analysis is its worth as a preemployment screening tool. It can serve as a starting point for establishing the "fit" between your own personal and professional needs and goals and those of the potential employer (Reddecliff et al., 1989, p. 136).
3. *Keep abreast of local, regional, and national legislative, regulatory, and health policy issues.*

TABLE 3-4 Self-Nurturing Strategies

Take care of yourself by trusting your own process.

Be assertive.

Embrace your polarities.

Recognize and deal with your own grief and loss.

Learn to let go.

Choose "nourishing" rather than "toxic" friends.

Deal constructively with your anger.

Take care of your body.

Make your home a haven.

Develop meaning and purpose in life.

Note. From "A strategy for staff development: Self-care and self-esteem as necessary partners" by S. J. Bunkers, 1992, *Clinical Nurse Specialist, 6*(3), p. 155. Copyright 1992 by Williams & Wilkins. Adapted with permission.

4. *Write a position (job) description.* A position description is an appropriate place to define and formalize proposed functions, responsibilities, and role expectations. A position description also helps to decrease potential problems with role ambiguity or role conflict (Ball, 1990). In addition, it may serve as a focus for negotiating specifics in a new job and as a "road map" to guide practice performance (Edmunds, 1979, p. 45).

5. *Continually articulate and clarify your advanced practice role to patients, families, colleagues, and the public.*

6. *Identify a suitable mentor.* Mentorship is a careful, nurturing support system essential to personal and professional development, career success, and satisfaction (Hawkins & Thibodeau, 1993). A mentor can help you recognize strengths and weaknesses, assist with the identification of realistic goals, and guide in the achievement of these goals (Bass et al., 1993). A review of the literature on mentors yields a number of tips that are useful in choosing a mentor (Hawkins & Thibodeau, 1993; Kram, 1984; Phillips-Jones, 1982; Zey, 1984; see Table 3-5). However, if a suitable individual is unavailable, networks and reference groups can also serve as mentors.

7. *Keep the ambiguities of your practice setting in perspective and maintain your sense of humor.*

8. *Maintain a positive self-concept.* A good self-concept and feelings of positive self-esteem enable you to concentrate on successes accomplished (Davidhizar, 1994). Take responsibility, however, for generating satisfaction from your job and actively plan to do so without expecting the job or system to supply it (Fenton, 1985,). Remind yourself daily that your work has made a difference to a patient, family, or colleague (Arena & Page, 1992). Pulling out thank-you notes and letters of recognition can also promote positive self-esteem (Arena & Page, 1992). In addition, feelings of personal worth should precipitate pride and rewards such as vacations, sleeping late on Saturday, buying a new novel and taking the time to read it, buying new clothes, or spending an evening out just for fun (Davidhizar, 1994).

TABLE 3-5 Tips for Choosing a Mentor

A potential mentor should be:

- an individual whose company you enjoy
- an individual who is neither your direct supervisor nor a close friend
- an individual with whom you can communicate
- an individual who is trustworthy
- an individual who has the ability to teach and motivate you
- an individual who is respected in the area of your particular interest and in the organization
- an individual who has proven power and influence
- an individual who has confidence in his or her abilities
- an individual who is happy with his or her own career success
- an individual who is 10 to 20 years older than you
- an individual who is accessible
- an individual with whom you believe you have congruent career and life goals
- an individual who has the ability to role model
- an individual who has organizational savvy
- an individual who is ambitious

9. *Nurture yourself without feeling guilty or selfish.*
10. *"Pace yourself for the long haul"* (Davidhizar, 1994, p. 11).
11. *Use your imagination and take risks.* Imagination precedes doing and is a constructive tool for growth and change (Davidhizar, 1994). Advanced practice nurses who think big and take risks are the ones who make great accomplishments (Christman, 1987; Davidhizar, 1994). However, you must first believe in your own ideas and then take the risk of acting on them (Davidhizar, 1994).
12. *Use "personal planning skills"* (Davidhizar, 1994, p. 11).
13. *Cultivate supportive, collegial relationships.*
14. *Maintain your commitment to lifelong learning.* "When you find yourself no longer worrying about whether you know enough, it is time to worry again" (Bates, 1990, p. 137). Continuous formal or self-education is essential for APNs to maintain and expand their level of competencies, to anticipate their role in healthcare delivery, and to expand the body of professional knowledge. As lifelong learners, APNs ultimately become their own best mentors.
15. *Develop yearly, measurable objectives, including an implementation and an evaluation plan.*
16. *Conduct a periodic self-assessment of your development in the advanced practice role.* Self-assessment can provide information about the types and quality of care provided as well as information for personal and professional growth. In addition, you should have a growth plan to assure continued renewal and to prevent fixation at any developmental stage (Holt, 1984). "I believe in planned professional development for all levels of nurses and that each of us must structure and implement our own professional care plan so that we can reach our highest potential in our own careers" (Holt, 1984, p. 449).
17. *Generate a monthly activity summary.* Socialization in advanced practice nursing can be simultaneously frustrating and rewarding, requiring flexibility as well as determination. This summary outlines some concrete suggestions that can aid in expediting the socialization process. Furthermore, APNs can incorporate these strategies into their practice regardless of their work environment.

CONSIDERATIONS

Advanced practice nurses are facing countless challenges and changes as the 21st century approaches. The utmost challenge for APNs, however, will be to avoid hasty compromises in meeting future needs and to carefully plan as well as design the future role they will play (Hein & Nicholson, 1994; Price et al., 1992). The following considerations, although merely speculative, reflect the chapter author's futuristic view of advanced practice nursing.

Independent, autonomous practice will characterize nursing's role in meeting patients' increasingly complex psychological, physiologic, and social needs. Advanced practice nurses will develop sound interpersonal relationships to successfully negotiate with multidisciplinary team members for collaboration and cooperation in providing healthcare. As they continue to demonstrate their knowledge, competence, and skills, referrals between APNs and other healthcare professionals will increase. In addition, prescriptive authority by APNs will move beyond the currently existing pharmacologic protocols (Keane, Richmond, & Kaiser, 1994).

Nursing will continue to witness a trend toward the granting of hospital privileges to APNs who are functioning as primary healthcare providers in private practice. Privileges will enable them to not only provide clinically expert care in a holistic manner, but to also provide the link of continuity in a system that is often typified by fragmentation and impersonalization (Hayden & Rowell, 1982; Keane & Richmond, 1993). More liberal reimbursement benefits and consumer choice will lead to the spread of APNs into independent entrepreneurships: delivering healthcare to defined populations, operating managed care facilities, consulting, and creating group practice arrangements.

The movement of APNs into acute-care settings will flourish. In light of future predictions for nursing (educational and hospital distribution of nurses), associate degree graduates with an associate's degree will implement the plan of care developed by the APN and the multidisciplinary health team. Although APNs clearly provide quality and cost-effective care in a variety of clinical sites (Aiken et al., 1993; Brooten et al., 1986; Daly, Rudy, Thompson, & Happ, 1991; Naylor, 1990; Office of Technology Assessment, 1986; Safriet, 1992), additional research to evaluate their efficacy and acceptability in specialty areas will be essential (Keane et al., 1994).

The increase in chronic illnesses and an aging population will lead to greater involvement of APNs in the long-term care of older adults in various stages along the health continuum. Advanced practice nurses will care for patients in their homes, businesses, corporations, schools, ambulatory health clinics, nursing homes, hospitals, hospices, health maintenance organizations, planned communities, day care centers, wellness centers, and other extended care facilities. The shifting of more APNs into these practice settings will expand patients' options for care and will also enrich the services they receive (Clochesy, Daly, Idemoto, Steel, & Fitzpatrick, 1994; Keane et al., 1994).

In addition, the importance of research to the practice and to the role of the nurse in advanced practice will become well integrated into the APN's professional value system. Advanced practice nurses will acquire the skills to conduct research through continuance of their formal education and through participation, at some level, in the research process (Hawkins & Thibodeau, 1993). They will also prove to be knowledgeable consumers of the research generated by others and will be leaders in developing innovative ways to provide quality care in restoring, promoting, and maintaining health (Hawkins & Thibodeau, 1993).

Innumerable forces at play are likely to dramatically affect the shape and delivery of healthcare. "Although it is probably presumptuous to offer predictions of nursing's future, [APNs] will be better prepared to move into the next century if [they] are informed about the past, have analyzed the present, and have formed visions for the future" (Chinn, 1991, p. 251; Chinn, 1994, p. 429). Now is the time for APNs to begin to picture what their future in nursing might be like and to begin to make it happen by resolving first to improve their own personal and professional development (Chinn, 1991, p. 256; Chinn, 1994, p. 437)

Overall, socialization is a continuous and cumulative process that has significant implications for the development of APNs. It is essential that preparation for advanced practice nursing be at the master's level, facilitating a professional collegial identity (Billingsley & Harp, 1982). Graduate nursing education provides APNs with a solid foundation for advanced nursing practice. The foundation, although solid, is only a beginning. To be responsive to society's changing needs and to maintain a pivotal role in future healthcare delivery, APNs must continually strive to grow and develop. Graduate curricula can well serve both the public and the profession by instilling in APNs the belief in as well as a desire for constant evolution in all aspects of advanced practice nursing (Keane & Richmond, 1993).

Acknowledgment: The author is sincerely grateful to Joanne V. Hickey, PhD, RN, ANP; Ruth Ouimette, MSN, RN, ANP; Mary H. Hawthorne, PhD, RN, ANP; Robert Waugh, MD; and Barbara Trapp-Moen, MSN, RN, GNP for providing insight and support during the preparation of this manuscript as well as for fostering the author's socialization in advanced practice nursing. The author also expresses her heartfelt appreciation as well as love to John F. Hixon, Jr. and Sylvia A. Hixon, whose beliefs and values helped to shape the author's professional identity, and to Madairy Hixon, who taught the author the essence of professional nursing.

References

Ahmadi, K. S., Speedling, E. J., & Kuhn-Weissman, G. (1987). The newly hired hospital staff nurse's professionalism, satisfaction and alienation. *International Journal of Nursing Studies, 24*(2), 107–121.

Aiken, L. H., Lake, E. T., Semaan, S., Lehman, H. P., O'Hare, P. A., Cole, C. S., Dunbar, D., & Frank, I. (1993). Nurse practitioner managed care for persons with HIV infection. *Image: Journal of Nursing Scholarship, 25*(3), 172–177.

Arena, D. M., & Page, N. E. (1992). The imposter phenomenon in the clinical nurse specialist role. *Image: Journal of Nursing Scholarship, 24*(2), 121–125.

Baird, S. B., & Prouty, M. P. (1989). Administratively enhancing CNS contributions. In A. B. Hamric & J. A. Spross (Eds.), *The clinical nurse specialist in theory and practice* (2nd ed., pp. 261–283). Philadelphia: W.B. Saunders.

Baker, B. A. (1978). The assertive nurse practitioner. *Nurse Practitioner, 3*(2), 23, 45.

Baker, V. E. (1971). Retrospective explorations in role development (G. V. Padilla & G. J. Padilla, eds.). *Nursing Digest, 6*(4), 56–63.

Ball, G. B. (1990). Perspectives on developing, marketing, and implementing a new clinical specialist position. *Clinical Nurse Specialist, 4*(1), 33–36.

Bass, M., Rabbett, P. M., & Siskind, M. M. (1993). Novice CNS and role acquisition. *Clinical Nurse Specialist, 7*(3), 148–152.

Bates, B. (1990). Twelve paradoxes: A message for nurse practitioners. *Journal of the American Academy of Nurse Practitioners, 2*(4), 136–139.

Benner, P. (1984). *From novice to expert: Excellence and power in clinical nursing practice.* Menlo Park, CA: Addison-Wesley.

Berki, S. E. (1972). The economics of new types of health personnel. In V. W. Lippard & E. F. Purcell (Eds.), *Intermediate-level health practitioners* (pp. 104–134). New York: Josiah Macy.

Bicknell, W. J., Walsh, D. C., & Tanner, M. M. (1974). Substantial or decorative? Physicians' assistants and nurse practitioners in the United States. *Lancet, 2*(7891), 1241–1244.

Billingsley, M. C., & Harper, D. C. (1982). The extinction of the nurse practitioner: Threat or reality? *Nurse Practitioner, 7*(9), 22–23, 26–27, 30.

Blount, M., Burge, S., Crigler, L., Finkelmeier, B. A., & Sanborn, C. (1981). Extending the influence of the clinical nurse specialist. *Nursing Administration Quarterly, 6*(1), 53–63.

Booth, R. Z. (1981). The preparation of primary care nurse practitioners. *International Nursing Review, 28*(4), 110–113, 115.

Brooten, D., Kumar, S., Brown, L. P., Butts, P., Finkler, S. A., Bakewell-Sachs, S., Gibbons, A., & Deliovria-Papadopoulous, M. (1986). A randomized clinical trial of early hospital discharge and home follow-up of very low-birthweight infants. *New England Journal of Medicine, 315*(15), 934–939.

Broverman, I. K., Vogel, S. R., Broverman, D. M., Charkan, F. E., & Rosenkrantz, P. S. (1975). Sex–role stereotypes: A current appraisal. In M.T.S. Mednick, S. S. Tangri, & L. W. Hoffman (Eds.), *Women and achievement* (pp. 32–47). New York: John Wiley & Sons.

Brykczynski, K. A. (1985). Exploring the clinical practice of nurse practitioners (Doctoral dissertation, University of California, San Francisco). *Dissertation Abstracts International, 46,* 3789B (University Microfilms No. DA86-00592).

Brykczynski, K. A. (1989). An interpretive study describing the clinical judgment of nurse practitioners. *Scholarly Inquiry for Nursing Practice, 3*(2), 75–104.

Bucher, R., & Stelling, J. G. (1977). *Becoming professional.* Beverly Hills, CA: Sage Publications.

Bunkers, S. J. (1992). A strategy for staff development: Self-care and self-esteem as necessary partners. *Clinical Nurse Specialist, 6*(3), 154–159.

Campbell-Heider, N. (1986). Do nurses need mentors? *Image: Journal of Nursing Scholarship, 18*(3), 110–113.

Cason, C. L., & Beck, C. M. (1982). Clinical nurse specialist role development. *Nursing and Health Care, 3*(1), 25–26, 35–38.

Chinn, P. L. (1991). Looking into the crystal ball: Positioning ourselves for the year 2000. *Nursing Outlook, 39*(6), 251–256.

Chinn, P. L. (1994). Looking into the crystal ball: Positioning ourselves for the year 2000. In E. C. Hein & M. J. Nicholson (Eds.), *Contemporary leadership behavior: Selected readings* (4th ed., pp. 429–437). Philadelphia: J. B. Lippincott.

Christman, L. P. (1987). A view to the future. *Nursing Outlook, 35*(5), 216–218.

Clochesy, J. M., Daly, B. J., Idemoto, B. K., Steel, J., & Fitzpatrick, J. J. (1994). Preparing advanced practice nurses for acute care. *American Journal of Critical Care, 3*(4), 255–259.

Cohen, H. A. (1981). *The nurse's quest for a professional identity.* Menlo Park, CA: Addison-Wesley.

Conway, M. E. (1983). Socialization and roles in nursing. *Annual Review of Nursing Research, 1,* 183–208.

Conway, M. E. (1988). Organizations, professional autonomy, and roles. In M. E. Hardy & M. E. Conway (Eds.), *Role theory: Perspectives for health professionals* (2nd ed., pp. 111–132). Norwalk, CT: Appleton & Lange.

Corwin, R. (1961). The professional employee: A study of conflict in nursing roles. In R. M. Pavalko (Ed.), *Sociological perspectives on occupations* (pp. 261–275). Itasca, IL: F.E. Peacock.

Covey, S. R. (1989). *The seven habits of highly effective people.* New York: Simmon & Schuster.

Crabtree, M. S. (1979). Effective utilization of clinical specialists within the organizational structure of hospital nursing service. *Nursing Administration Quarterly, 4*(1), 1–11.

Daly, B. J., Rudy, E. B., Thompson, K. S., & Happ, M. B. (1991). Development of a special care unit for chronically critically ill patients. *Heart and Lung, 20*(1), 45–51.

Davidhizar, R. (1994, Spring/Summer). Stress can make you or break you. *Advanced Practice Nurse,* pp. 10–11, 17.

Davis, F., & Olesen, V. (1972). Initiation into a women's profession: Identity problems in the status transition of coed to student nurse. In R. M. Pavalko (Ed.), *Sociological perspectives on occupations* (pp. 186–195). Itasca, IL: F. E. Peacock.

Davis, F., Olesen, V.L., & Whittaker, E.W. (1966). Problems and issues in collegiate nursing education. In F. Davis (Ed.), *The nursing profession: Five sociological essays* (pp. 138–175). New York: Wiley.

Dreyfus, S. E., & Dreyfus, H. L. (1980). *A five-stage model of the mental activities involved in directed skill acquisition* (USAF Contract No. F49620-79-C-0063). Berkeley: University of California.

Editor. (1975). An interview with Dr. Loretta Ford. *Nurse Practitioner, 1*(1), 9–12.

Edmunds, M. (1980). Non-clinical problems: Gender and the nurse practitioner role. *Nurse Practitioner, 5*(6), 42–44.

Edmunds, M. W. (1979). The position description. *Nurse Practitioner, 4*(7), 45–47.

Elder, R. G., & Bullough, B. (1990). Nurse practitioners and clinical nurse specialists: Are the roles merging? *Clinical Nurse Specialist, 4*(2), 78–84.

Faculty. (1993). *The status of advanced nursing practice.* Unpublished manuscript, Duke University School of Nursing, Durham, NC.

Fenton, M. V. (1985). Identifying competencies of clinical nurse specialists. *Journal of Nursing Administration, 15*(12), 31–37.

Forbes, K. E., Rafson, J., Spross, J. A., & Kozlowski, D. (1990). Clinical nurse specialist and nurse practitioner core curricula survey results. *Nurse Practitioner, 15*(4), 43, 46–48.

Fox, D. H. (1982). Matrix organizational model broadens clinical nurse specialist's practice. *Hospital Progress, 63*(11), 50–53, 69.

Hamric, A. B. (1989). History and overview of the CNS role. In A. B. Hamric & J. A. Spross (Eds.), *The clinical nurse specialist in theory and practice* (2nd ed., pp. 3–18). Philadelphia: W.B. Saunders.

Hamric, A. B., & Taylor, J. W. (1989). Role development of the CNS. In A. B. Hamric & J. A. Spross (Eds.), *The clinical nurse specialist in theory and practice* (2nd ed., pp. 41–82). Philadelphia: W.B. Saunders.

Hayden, M. L., & Rowell, P. (1982). Non-clinical problems: Hospital privileges: Rationale and process. *Nurse Practitioner, 7*(1), 42–44.

Hawkins, J. W., & Thibodeau, J. A. (1993). *The advanced practitioner: Current practice issues* (3rd ed.). New York: Tiresias Press.

Hein, E. C., & Nicholson, M. J. (Eds.). (1994). *Contemporary leadership behavior: Selected readings* (4th ed.). Philadelphia: J.B. Lippincott.

Hinshaw, A. S. (1982). Socialization and resocialization of nurses for professional nursing practice. In E. C. Hein & M. J. Nicholson (Eds.), *Contemporary leadership behavior: Selected readings. Boston: Little, Brown.*

Holt, F. M. (1984). A theoretical model for clinical specialist practice. *Nursing and Health Care, 5*(8), 445–449.

Horner, M. S. (1975). Toward an understanding of achievement-related conflicts in women. In M.T.S. Mednick, S. S. Tangri, & L. W. Hoffman (Eds.), *Women and achievement* (pp. 206–220). New York: John Wiley & Sons.

Howell, F. J. (1978). Employers' evaluations of new graduates. *Nursing Outlook, 26*(7), 448–451.

Hsiao, V., & Edmunds, M. W. (Eds.). (1982). Non-clinical problems: Master's vs. CE: The debate continues. *Nurse Practitioner, 7*(10), 42–46.

Hupcey, J. E. (1990). The socialization process of master's-level nurse practitioner students. *Journal of Nursing Education, 29*(5), 196–201.

Hurley-Wilson, B. A. (1988). Socialization for roles. In M. E. Hardy & M. E. Conway (Eds.), *Role theory: Perspectives for health professionals* (2nd ed., pp. 73–110). Norwalk, CT: Appleton & Lange.

Jacox, A. (1973). Professional socialization of nurses. *Journal of the New York State Nurses' Association, 4*(4), 6–15.

Kalisch, B., & Kalisch, P. (1982). *Politics in nursing.* Philadelphia: J.B. Lippincott.

Katzman, E. M., & Roberts, J. I. (1988). Nurse–physician conflicts as barriers to the enactment of nursing roles. *Western Journal of Nursing Research, 10*(5), 576–590.

Keane, A., & Richmond, T. (1993). Tertiary nurse practitioners. *Image: The Journal of Nursing Scholarship, 25*(4), 281–284.

Keane, A., Richmond, T., & Kaiser, L. (1994). Critical care nurse practitioners: Evolution of the advanced practice nursing role. *American Journal of Critical Care, 3*(3), 232–237.

Kozier, B., Erb, G., & Blais, K. (1992). *Concepts and issues in nursing practice* (2nd ed.). Reading: MA: Addison-Wesley.

Kram, K. (1984). *Mentoring at work: Developmental relationships in organizational life.* New York: Scott, Foresman.

Kramer, M. E. (1974). *Reality shock: Why nurses leave nursing.* St. Louis, MO: C.V. Mosby.

Kremar, C. R. (1991). Organizational entry: The case of the clinical nurse specialist. *Clinical Nurse Specialist, 5*(1), 38–42.

Kuhn, T. (1970). *The structure of scientific revolutions* (2nd ed.). Chicago: University of Chicago Press.

Laing, M. (1993). Gossip: Does it play a role in the socialization of nurses? *Image: The Journal of Nursing Scholarship, 25*(1), 37–43.

Leddy, S., & Pepper, J. M. (1993). *Conceptual bases of professional nursing* (2nd ed.). Philadelphia: J.B. Lippincott.

Lewis, J. (1975). Structural aspects of the delivery setting and nurse practitioner performance. *Nurse Practitioner, 1*(1), 16–20.

Lukacs, J. L. (1982). Factors in nurse practitioner role adjustment. *Nurse Practitioner, 7*(3), 21–23.

Lum, J.L.J. (1988). Reference groups and professional socialization. In M. E. Hardy & M. E. Conway (Eds.), *Role theory: Perspectives for health professionals* (2nd ed., pp. 137–156). Norwalk, CT: Appleton & Lange.

Lurie, E. E. (1981). Nurse practitioners: Issues in professional socialization. *Journal of Health and Social Behavior, 22*(1), 31–48.

Lynn, M. R., McCain, N. L., & Boss, B. J. (1989). Socialization of RN to BSN. *Image: The Journal of Nursing Scholarship, 21*(4), 232–237.

Malkemes, L. C. (1974). Resocialization: A model for nurse practitioner preparation. *Nursing Outlook, 22*(2), 90–94.

Meleis, A. I. (1975). Role insufficiency and role supplementation: A conceptual framework. *Nursing Research, 24*(4), 264–271.

Miller, M.H. (1977). Self perception of nurse practitioners: Changes in stress, assertiveness, and sex role. *Nurse Practitioner, 2*(5), 26–29.

Moniz, D. (1978). Putting assertiveness techniques into practice. *American Journal of Nursing, 78*(10), 1713.

Naylor, M. D. (1990). Comprehensive discharge planning for hospitalized elderly: A pilot study. *Nursing Research, 39*(3), 156–161.

Naylor, M. D., & Brooten, D. (1993). The roles and functions of clinical nurse specialists. *Image: Journal of Nursing Scholarship, 25*(1), 73–78.

Nyberg, J. (1994). The nurse as professnocrat. In E. C. Hein & M. J. Nicholson (Eds.), *Contemporary leadership behavior: Selected readings* (4th ed., pp. 371–376). Philadelphia: J.B. Lippincott.

Oermann, M. H. (1991). Professional nursing practice. In M. H. Oermann (Ed.), *Professional nursing practice: A conceptual approach* (pp. 1–29). Philadelphia: J.B. Lippincott.

Office of Technology Assessment. (1986). *Nurse practitioners, physician's assistants and certified nurse–midwives: A policy analysis.* Washington, DC.

Olesen, V. L., & Whittaker, E. W. (1968). *The silent dialogue.* San Francisco: Jossey-Bass.

Olsson, H. M., & Gullberg, M. T. (1987). Nursing education and professional role acquisition: Theoretical perspectives. *Nurse Education Today, 7*(4), 171–176.

Olsson, H. M., & Gullberg, M. T. (1988). Nursing education and importance of professional status in the nurse role: Expectations and knowledge of the nurse role. *International Journal of Nursing Studies, 25*(4), 287–293.

Patridge, K. B. (1978). Nursing values in a changing society. *Nursing Outlook, 26*(6), 356–360.

Phillips-Jones, L. (1982). *Mentor and proteges: How to establish, strengthen and get the most from a mentor/protege relationship.* New York: Arbor House.

Polanyi, M. (1958). *Personal knowledge.* Chicago: University of Chicago Press.

Price, M. J., Martin, A. C., Newberry, Y. G., Zimmer, P. A., Brykczynski, K. A., & Warren, B. (1992). Developing national guidelines for nurse practitioner education: An overview of the product and the process. *Journal of Nursing Education, 31*(1), 10–15.

Reddecliff, M., Smith, E. L., Ryan-Merritt, M. (1989). Organizational analysis: Tool for the clinical nurse specialist. *Clinical Nurse Specialist, 3*(3), 133–136.

Ryan-Merritt, M. V., Mitchell, C. A., & Pagel, I. (1988). Clinical nurse specialist role definition and operationalization. *Clinical Nurse Specialist, 2*(3), 132–137.

Safriet, B. J. (1992). Health care dollars and regulatory sense: The role of advanced practice nursing. *Yale Journal on Regulation, 9*(2), 417–488.

Schein, E. H. (1968). Organizational socialization and the profession of management. *Industrial Management Review, 9*(2), 1–6.

Simms, L. M., & Lindberg, J. (1978). *The nurse person: Developing perspectives for contemporary nursing.* New York: Harper & Row.

Simpson, I. H. (1967). Patterns of socialization into professions: The case of student nurses. *Sociological Inquiry, 37*(1), 47–54.

Simpson, I. H. (1972). Patterns of socialization into professions: The case of student nurses. In R. M. Pavalko (Ed.), *Sociological perspectives on occupations* (pp. 169–177). Itasca, IL: F.E. Peacock.

Simpson, R. L., & Simpson, I. H. (1969). Women and bureaucracy in the semi-professions. In A. Etzioni (Ed.), *The semi-professions and their organization* (pp. 196–263). New York: Free Press.

Sparacino, P.S.A. (1990). Strategies for implementing advanced practice. *Clinical Nurse Specialist, 4*(3), 151–152.

Stein, L. I., Watts, D. T., & Howell, T. (1990). The doctor–nurse game revisited. *Nursing Outlook, 38*(6), 264–268.

Stuart, G.W., & Sundeen, S.J. (1995). Self-concept responses and dissociative disorders. In G.W. Stuart & S.J. Sundeen (Eds.), *Principles and practice of psychiatric nursing.* St. Louis, MO: C.V. Mosby.

Styles, M. (1982). *On nursing: Toward a new endowment.* St. Louis, MO: C.V. Mosby.

Styles, M. M. (1978). Why publish? *Image: The Journal of Nursing Scholarship, 10*(2) 28–32.

Sullivan, J. A. (1978). Comparison of manifest needs between nurses and physicians in primary care practice. *Nursing Research, 27*(4), 255–259.

Sullivan, J. A., Dachelet, C. Z., Sultz, H. A., Henry, M., & Carrol, H. D. (1978). Overcoming barriers to the employment and utilization of the nurse practitioner. *American Journal of Public Health, 68*(11), 1097–1103.

Sultz, H. A., Zielenzy, M., & Kinyon, L. (1978). *Longitudinal study of nurse practitioners: Phase II* (DHEW Publication No. HRA 78-92). Washington, DC: Department of Health, Education, and Welfare.

Sultz, H. A., Zielenzy, M., & Kinyon, L. (1980). *Longitudinal study of nurse practitioners: Phase III* (DHEW Publication No. HRA 80-2). Washington, DC: Department of Health, Education, and Welfare.

Tarsitano, B. J., Brophy, E. B., & Snyder, D. J. (1986). A demystification of the clinical nurse specialist role: Perceptions of clinical nurse specialists and nurse administrators. *Journal of Nursing Education, 25*(1), 4–9.

Watson, I. (1981). Socialization of the nursing student in a professional nursing education programme. *Nursing Papers, 13*(2), 19–24.

Whelan, E.G. (1984). Role-orientation change among RNs in an upper-division level baccalaureate program. *Journal of Nursing Education, 23*(4), 151 155.

White, M. S. (1975). Psychological characteristics of the nurse practitioner. *Nursing Outlook, 23*(3), 160–166.

White, M. S. (1978). *Competence and commitment: The making of a nurse practitioner.* San Francisco: University of California.

Williams, C. A. (1982). Nurse practitioner research: Some neglected issues. *Nursing Outlook, 23*(3), 172–177.

Wyers, M.E.A., Grove, S. K., & Pastorino, C. (1985). Clinical nurse specialist: In search of the right role. *Nursing and Health Care, 6*(4), 203–207.

Zey, M. (1984). *The mentor connection.* Homewood, IL: Irwin.

Zornow, R. A. (1977). A curriculum model for the expanded role. *Nursing Outlook, 25*(1), 43 46.

CHAPTER

Preceptorship in Primary Care

Joan P. Gurvis ■ *Ruth M. Ouimette* ■ *Bonnie Jones Friedman*

Graduate nursing education programs are preparing advanced practice nurses (APNs), which is a shift in focus from exclusively preparing clinical nurse specialists (CNSs) or nurse practitioners. The evolving change has implications not only for the academic component of preparing APNs but also for the practitioners who, as *faculty extenders* (i.e., clinical teachers), are assuming responsibility for the *preceptorship* of students in clinical sites.

Nurse practitioner faculty are being challenged to teach a greater number of students; other faculty are retooling to develop practitioner skills and a practitioner identity. Moreover, nurse practitioners in practice are being inundated with requests to act as *preceptors* for students who have differing levels of clinical expertise, based on where they are in the educational program.

The current and anticipated pressure to produce the number of clinically competent nurse practitioners required to meet the primary healthcare needs of our society mandates an examination of the concept of the preceptorship—the relationship cultivated between clinical teacher, student, and academic faculty for the purpose of developing a knowledgeable and competent practitioner. This chapter describes the historical development of the *preceptor* (the primary clinical teacher), and discusses both the vital role of preceptorship in the education of APNs in primary care, and the importance of the roles of preceptor, student, and faculty.

HISTORICAL PERSPECTIVE

Only in the past generation has nursing as a profession been transformed from a feminine duty and obligation to care for the ill in times of need to a theory-based profession grounded in scientific inquiry and clinical practice. The art of nursing loved ones back to health, undertaken primarily by women, has been well documented for centuries. However, not until the latter part of the 18th century did the delivery of nursing care to the sick and afflicted become a respected and learned occupation (Brodie, 1988). Reverby (1987), an eminent historian of nursing, noted that, "at anytime the family's long arm might reach out to a daughter working in a distant city or mill bringing her home to care for the sick, infirm or newborn" (p. 320). Reverby also determined that a mother often taught nursing care to her daughter as part of female apprenticeship, or a domestic servant learned nursing care as an additional responsibility.

In 1860, Florence Nightingale elevated the profession to a respectable status by organizing the St. Thomas Hospital School of Nursing in London. Nightingale's keen observations and establishment of care standards set the stage for the development of the profession as a legitimized and important occupation. To gain acceptance of nursing as a profession, Nightingale placed the nursing school in the hospital system, inextricably linking nursing to medicine and the hospital. Nightingale also applied the concepts of the female apprenticeship model to the nurse training program and stressed the importance of using skilled nurses as role models for novice nurses (Brodie, 1988).

During the years immediately following the Civil War, nurses rapidly improved U.S. hospitals, changing them from "pest houses to benevolent places of healing" (Brodie, 1988, p.323). Physicians and hospital administrators were quick to note these reforms and supported the expansion of hospital-based nursing programs. Soon, many hospitals gained an elevated status and reputation for fine care of the sick as a result of the diligent efforts of "a dedicated, intelligent and obedient work force of women" (Brodie, 1988, p.323). Mortality and morbidity rates dropped at the turn of the century as a result of higher standards of care, advances in infection control, and 24-hour supervision of patients by nursing personnel.

Hospitals became the educational arena for nurse training. Nightingale's concept of apprenticeship as an educational strategy was redefined as nursing students worked long hours to staff the hospital and traded physician mentors and experienced nurses as role models for on-the-job training as the primary mechanism by which to acquire knowledge and skills. At that time, "most nursing students paid for their education through an exchange for the labor apprenticeship system" (Hardy, 1987, p. 8). This model enabled patient revenues to support hospital-affiliated schools of nursing and restrained the growth of privately funded sources for nursing education.

Beginning in the 20th century, changes were made in professional organization and control over education with the eventual establishment of baccalaureate nursing programs. World War II generated both a demand and interest in hospitals and healthcare. Congress, through legislation, supported a dramatic expansion of hospital facilities and the medical and nursing personnel to staff them. In 1941, Congress passed a series of federal laws, including the Nurse Training Act. This federal funding gradually increased the amount of financing available for broad-based nursing education at the undergraduate and graduate levels and set the stage for beginning the separation of nursing education from the hospital system and medical model. To resolve the conflict between the growth of hospital services and the increasing independence of nursing education, service and nursing education became separate units in the 1950s. Once moved into the academic setting of colleges and universities, nursing education flourished.

During this same period, the use of practicing nurses as clinical teachers was minimal. According to Holly (1992), not until the 1960s did the concepts of the mentor and role model again appear in the literature. In response to the nursing shortage and the need to bridge the gap between education and practice, preceptorships were developed for new graduates beginning their first work experience in the acute-care setting.

Early master's-degree programs focused on the traditional clinical areas of medicine–surgery, psychiatry, and public health along with the functional majors of teaching and administration. However, as master's-level graduates assumed roles in hospital-based clinical specialty areas and graduate academic programs identified their role as preparing specialists, the need for expert clinician preceptors was again recognized. The new clinical nurse specialist and faculty with acute-care background and expertise were the identified preceptors in the early clinical specialists programs. However, with the development of the primary-care nurse practitioner programs in the late 1960s, physicians assumed the faculty and preceptor role for students in the programs. They did so primarily because nursing faculty were not formally prepared for this role and the newly developed nurse practitioner specialty included what was traditionally labeled as "medical acts," necessitating the participation of physician faculty. There were strong physician–nurse faculty–student ties in these early days that laid the foundation for the strong collaborative relationship between nurse practitioner and primary-care physician that exists today.

At present, nurse practitioner programs are taught by nurse practitioner faculty and many faculty serve as preceptors for students in their practices. However, because of limited numbers of faculty, especially in practice, physicians and nurse practitioners in practice are the mainstay of clinical teaching contributing to nurse practitioner education.

PRECEPTOR

In general, a *preceptor* can be described as a tutor, teacher, and instructor (Hagopian, Ginette, Ferszt, & McCorkel, 1992). The nursing profession has modified the term to describe a role that a nurse assumes in addition to his or her regular duties: the responsibility for a one-on-one teaching–learning process. Alspach (1988) described the three components of the preceptor role as that of an educator, role model, and socializer. The preceptor is responsible for acquainting the learner with and modeling the roles, responsibilities, formal and informal rules, customs, culture, and norms of the clinical setting and workplace (Alspach, 1988, p.2).

The nurse practitioner preceptor for the advanced practice student in primary care serves as a professional role model who facilitates the student's achievement of learning objectives within the clinical setting. Implicit in the clinical objectives is the development of clinical excellence that requires the preceptor to be an experienced clinician.

Benner (1984) explored the concept of clinical excellence in depth through her adaptation of the Dreyfus model of skill acquisition (Dreyfus & Dreyfus, 1980). "Inherent in practice disciplines such as nursing is knowledge that is embedded in practice itself" (Urden, 1989, p. 20). According to Benner (1984), clinical experience is the essential component for the development of this knowledge. Benner's research revealed that the knowledge embedded in actual nursing practice accrues over time (see Chapter 3). Benner's work also revealed how "nurses change their intellectual orientation, integrate and sort out knowledge, and refocus decision-making based on perceptual awareness rather than on process orientation" (Carlson, Crawford, & Contrades, 1989, p. 188). From her research, Benner (1984) identified five levels of nursing proficiency: novice, advanced beginner, competent, proficient, and expert. Through an analysis of critical incidents and exemplars, Benner documented these proficiency levels in practice settings, and examined the knowledge embedded in each level of nursing practice.

The *novice,* according to Benner (1984), has no experience in the situations in which he or she is expected to perform. The *advanced beginner* is characteristic of the nurse who has been exposed to and has coped with real situations. The *competent* practitioner practices deliberately and consciously and is able to move from the concrete to abstract in learning situations. At the *proficient* and *expert* levels, the practitioner demonstrates clinical assessment and judgment, articulates the distinctions between what can normally be expected and deviations from this norm and, most important, demonstrates critical thinking and competence. Although, in general, there is not a formal method for differentiating the levels of nurse practitioners in practice, it can be expected that nurse practitioner preceptors, depending on educational background, nursing experience, program preparation, and qualitative and quantitative experience as a nurse practitioner, range from competent to expert. For example, most NPs state that they do not feel confident or competent enough with their own knowledge and skills during the first year in practice to be able to extend themselves to learners. They feel like, and are in fact, learners themselves. It is sometime after 6 months to a year in practice when professional identity is such that they are able to see beyond themselves to incorporate teaching into their role.

Although literature exists on preceptor development programs for staff preceptors in acute settings, historically the development of preceptors in primary care has received little attention in the literature. Like the physicians who went before them, present nurse practitioner preceptors were initially recruited by faculty and learned on the job. They reflected on how they were taught and generally patterned themselves after preceptors who met their needs as students. Assuming a preceptorship is not something nurse practitioners do for external rewards. In fact, most practices do not accomodate the preceptor with a lighter appointment schedule, nor do academic institutions offer financial remuneration. External rewards are seldom cited as a reason for taking on this added responsibility.

Nurse practitioners act as preceptors for a variety of reasons; some are related to professional responsibility ("to teach their own"), but most are personal. In general, nurse practitioner preceptors enjoy and value what they do and consequently want to impart this enthusiasm to their students. It is an opportunity to have an impact on the future of the profession through molding future practitioners. They like the challenge of teaching—the process of nurturing student growth and the personal stimulation and learning that come from associating with a learner. It has always been a professional truth that students "keep clinicians on their toes." Also, nursing, like medicine, has traditionally used a mentor system and nurse practitioners often would like to give back what they have received.

STUDENT

The student in the advanced practice nursing curriculum is involved with several modes of learning: the classroom, the skills lab, and a variety of clinical settings. The graduate curriculum of the practitioner student focuses on the development of critical thinking, diagnostic reasoning, and clinical decision making. Although formal, clinically related classroom courses give the student the knowledge and tools for practice, it is through the preceptorship that the synthesis and application of knowledge occur. The student must feel comfortable in the preceptorship, and begin clinical experiences well equipped to negotiate and discuss course and personal learning objectives, time commitment, and educational experiences to meet his or her own learning needs (Hagopian et al., 1992).

To ensure educational outcomes, the student must also be proficient in self-assessment, the most powerful kind of feedback and successful motivator of clinical excellence (Dake & Taylor, 1992). To make the most of the experience of working with a preceptor, the graduate learner must assess his or her own skill level and expertise relevant to the clinical situation. This information can be a valuable tool that enables the preceptor to target learning opportunities and develop outcome measures for evaluation. Through the development of mutually relevant goals, the preceptor and learner enter into a contractual learning experience designed specifically for the learner and learning environment. Self-assessment incorporates principles of adult learning by promoting active participation, relevance, and meaning for the learner. These characteristics distinguish the preceptorship for graduate nurse practitioner students from the clinical learning experiences of undergraduate students.

Early in the curriculum, nurse practitioner students address the internal struggle of nursing versus medicine and how to maintain the integrity of their identity as a nurse while blending new skills into the APN role. Nursing is a caring profession with a holistic approach to the patient in the context of the family and community. It is concerned with wellness, health promotion, and disease prevention. Although the medical profession shares the caring philosophy, it is a profession that has always been focused on curing disease. Therefore, as APN students strive to learn the essentials of the medical model, it is imperative that faculty and nurse practitioner preceptors help them incorporate the new knowledge and skill into the nursing model.

The first clinical rotation for nurse practitioner students is very important to the development of a new identity. During rotation, the nurse practitioner model of care is introduced; the preceptor role is pivotal. In addition, during the first clinical practicum, the preceptor not only helps students learn and apply new skills but also assists students to understand and internalize the role of the nurse practitioner. Students experience new levels of accountability, responsibility, and multidisciplinary communication. Learning to live with ambiguity becomes a reality.

Preceptors expect students to come to the first clinical rotation with the basic skills of history-taking and physical examination. However, the most important element they desire is motivation to learn. Preceptors find satisfaction in teaching when they observe the students actively learning through questioning and problem solving. Although the first rotation is instrumental in role development, preceptors expect to see increasing incorporation of skills and values with greater independence as rotations progress.

PRECEPTORSHIP

The preceptorship, as described by Holly (1992), is a "one on one clinical teaching strategy [which] provides the means for orientation and socialization" (p. 49). The six purposes of the clinical preceptorship most frequently cited in the literature are to (1) assess and validate clinical competence, (2) increase skill performance, (3) create consistency in practice, (4) enhance comfort levels with the workplace and learning environment, (5) assist in the application of theory to practice, and (6) integrate the learner into the norms that constitute the organizational culture (Holly, 1992). The key players in the preceptorship are the preceptor, the student, and the faculty member involved in the clinical course; however, the preceptor, as the primary clinical teacher, plays a pivotal role.

After orientation to the clinical setting, the student commonly shadows the preceptor. Then, as the preceptor gets to know the student through questioning, observation, and follow-up, trust develops and the student gains increased independence in patient assessment, diagnosis, and management. However, experienced preceptors are very attuned to the individuality of each student and will move along at the student's pace, recognizing that students never feel ready and need encouragement to take the next step.

Experience is a requisite for expertise. Critical to the development of clinical excellence is the transition of the nurse through the levels of practice described by Benner (1984). As students advance in learning and competence, they will benefit from pairing not only with *expert* preceptors, who themselves can demonstrate advanced levels of clinical practice, but with *competent* preceptors who provide structure and process. Preceptors often comment that they enjoy beginning students because they feel more instrumental in shaping attitudes and clinical approaches to patients. However, the more experienced *expert* NP who generally is involved in a busy and more complex practice mode appreciates the increased knowledge, critical thinking, and skill level of the more advanced students. In the final clinical rotation, students are apt to be more independent and collegial, and provide care to patients that is complementary to that of the preceptor.

Although there is growing interest in the development of curricula for preceptor programs, little has been done to examine the components of the preceptor–student match. As discussed earlier, based on Benner's (1984) model, the pairing of a *competent* nurse as a preceptor with a beginning student may offer greater opportunities for success. The competent nurse can provide a structured learning environment based on guidelines and expectations and is more likely to focus on the preceptor/student relationship. This match obviously will benefit the beginning student. An *expert* nurse is not always an expert preceptor. Expert nurses typically use maxims or cryptic instructions that make sense only if the person has a deep understanding of the situation. Expert nurses usually rely heavily on intuition and hold a holistic view of the clinical situation. As a result, they often have difficulty explaining the rationale for their practice decisions and interventions to nonexpert peers. Because expert practitioners rely on subtle cues and use anticipatory interventions, the beginning student, if paired with an expert, may often miss the true meaning of the critical incident. As noted earlier, the expert preceptor may be a better match for the more experienced or advanced student.

Ideally, the pairing of students with competent and expert preceptors is a deliberate decision based on the student's level or stage in the educational program and the style of supervision and guidance provided by individual preceptors. Different approaches may be more effective with beginning students, whereas other methods may be more effective with more advanced students.

Another area that has not been explored to any extent is the pairing of the advanced practice masters or post-masters prepared student—seeking preparation as a nurse practitioner—with a preceptor. Without formal evaluation criteria, experience tells us that each student must be independently matched with a preceptor, not unlike other students. It cannot be assumed that all APNs are equal in knowledge, clinical competence, and readiness for primary-care practice. In fact, although these nurses may have enhanced problem-solving skills, they experience the same, if not more, role transition dilemmas as other nurse practitioner students.

The pairing of a competent nurse as a preceptor with an expert nurse can offer opportunities for success. The practice of competent nurses is based on previous experience, making them more likely, as discussed earlier, to provide a structured learning environment based on rules and expectations. This match may be beneficial for the expert nurse who has moved into the learner role in a different environment from that in which he or she currently is practicing.

As we have seen, Benner's (1984) work provides a framework faculty can use to make decisions concerning student placements and to establish a student-preceptor match. Once a preceptorship is created, the development of the relationship between student and preceptor becomes a focal point of the experience.

One approach faculty and preceptor can use to facilitate and monitor the development of student progress is to adapt the model of Situational Leadership II, developed by Ken Blanchard (1985). The model offers a practical, easy to understand approach to motivating learners. While the model was originally designed for use by leaders in business and industry, it can be adapted to the preceptor/student relationship. In order to understand this adaptation, one must assume that a preceptor is an informal leader and therefore influences learner behavior.

According to Blanchard, leadership can be defined as the process of influencing the behavior of another person (p.2). The style of leadership is simply a pattern of behavior used while trying to influence the behavior of others and which is perceived by those being influenced. In other words, a leader's success depends upon the use of leadership styles that match the perceptions of others. The Situational Leadership model is unique in that it reflects a dynamic process between the leader and the learner. In the model there are distinct leadership styles that may be effectively used in different situations or stages during the learning process. An adaptation of the Blanchard model depicts four "preceptor" (leader) styles: (1) telling; (2) coaching; (3) promoting experimentation, and (4) encouraging autonomy (Fig. 4-1).

Leadership styles have traditionally been described, in part, as autocratic (directive) or democratic (supportive). Autocratic leaders use authority and position power to achieve results, while, in contrast, democratic leaders use participative problem solving and decision making and rely on personal power for success. For example, the preceptor whose predominant style is directive relies on one-way or telling communication techniques, structure, control, and constant supervision of the student. This style may be appropriate for students early in their practicum, but may not maximize skill acquisition or critical thinking, which are necessary components of the learning process and NP role. In contrast, the preceptor who primarily uses a supportive style will actively engage the learner in the clinical experience, and promote questioning and risk taking. The use of this style with a novice, however, may create frustration and even limit opportunities for success. The preceptor who is able to combine styles that match the student's need for direction and support, and who can change teaching strategies as the student gains confidence and mastery of clinical skills will most likely be the best match for the NP learner.

The adapted Situational Leadership model can be explained further by viewing preceptor styles as fluid; moving from high to low in both the directive and supportive continuums.

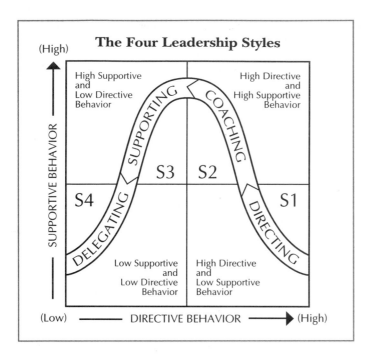

FIGURE 4-1. Situational Leadership II Model: The four leadership styles. (Source: Blanchard, K., Zigarmi, P. & Zigarmi, D. (1985). *Leadership and the one minute manager*. New York: William Morrow)

Taking a closer look, the learning continuum emphasizes competence and begins with high learner needs in task and skill development (on the right side of the bell curve). **Directive (S1)** behaviors by the preceptor support skill development through a "telling" communication style and close supervision. Using the telling style, preceptors define tasks to be learned and often suggest solutions and make decisions for the learner. Emphasis on relationships and social support needs are low in this phase. **Coaching (S2)** behaviors by the preceptor provide continued direction for higher level skill development and address social or supportive needs through coaching or motivational activities. With this style, preceptors often provide creative ideas for learning opportunities, guide goal development, solicit self-evaluation and feedback from NP students, and focus on the learner's socialization and comfort level. Coaching activities motivate and support students as their confidence develops.

In the **Promoting Experimentation (S3)** phase of the learning process, preceptor style is highly supportive and less directive. The locus of control now moves from the preceptor to the student. The preceptor becomes a resource and facilitates critical thinking and problem-solving activities. Recognition for accomplishments is vital to the continued motivation of the learner. In the **Encouraging Autonomy (S4)** phase, the student should be able to move easily into the care provider role with competence. The student completes role-related tasks with ease and demonstrates high levels of critical thinking. The student in this phase actively solves problems and performs advanced assessment, diagnostic, and management skills with minimal direction from the preceptor. By using varied leadership styles, as described, the preceptor can maximize learning in all phases of the curriculum. Critical to the success of any preceptorship is the premise that it is a learning activity for all three—the preceptor, the faculty, and the student. Therefore, the faculty must be able to demonstrate these styles actively as they support and develop preceptors.

A preceptorship is designed to integrate the classroom content with clinical practice and is necessary for all levels of learners (Holly, 1992). A successful preceptorship builds on the partnership that develops between the faculty, student, and preceptor. The preceptor is a facilitator of learning and ideally creates a climate of trust and openness for the student's learning.

A positive preceptor/student relationship incorporates ongoing feedback with oportunities for incremental evaluation, such as weekly learning contracts, written expectations, and evaluation of progress toward meeting the mutually established goals. It is important to note, however, that preceptor evaluation is distinct from faculty evaluation, in that the preceptor works with the student to create a safe and nurturing environment in which the student can practice, apply skills and concepts, and receive information about outcomes. If preceptors were to serve as sole evaluators, the preceptorship would change dramatically. Although preceptors have autonomy in creating the learning environment and developing opportunities to meet curriculum objectives, the role of grading the student is best left to faculty, which allows the preceptor-student relationship to develop to its fullest potential.

FACULTY

There has been rapid development of APN practitioner programs across the United States and increased competition for primary-care sites to provide clinical learning experiences. This has put a great demand on professionals to act as preceptors for primary-care learners. The competition comes not only from graduate nursing programs but also from physician assistant programs and medical schools that are expanding their primary-care curricula. The result is that nurse practitioners at all levels are being asked to take on a greater role as preceptors, a role for which they more than likely have had no preparation except for their own student preceptorship experiences. Therefore, it is a major responsibility of faculty members to identify the learning needs of preceptors and to help them become effective faculty extenders. Teaching the *novice* preceptor should be the role of the faculty. Furthermore, pairing a new preceptor with a more experienced one, thus establishing a communication link, is also a valuable strategy for preceptor development.

Creating partnerships between schools of nursing and clinical sites is essential to the development of close relationships for promoting learning and transferring learning objectives from the academic setting to the clinical environment. Partnerships can be developed and maintained through ongoing communication between faculty and preceptor. Preceptors want and need to feel that the faculty member is available to them and to the student. Although telephone contact is convenient and sometimes the only method of communication with off-campus preceptorships, preceptors generally appreciate planned site visits. These visits allow for exploration of mutual professional backgrounds, interests, and teaching styles. They allow time for discussion of program objectives and preceptor expectations. Partnerships also are strengthened by student-focused clinical site visits, in which faculty members observe students in practice and engage in three-way conferences with student and preceptor regarding the student's objectives and progress.

The preceptorship is a crucial component in the development of student learning and the overall success of a masters program preparing nurses in advanced practice. The vitality and effectiveness of the preceptorship is predicated upon mutual respect and ongoing communication between faculty and preceptor. An important part of the process is the pairing of student and preceptor to maximize student learning. Benner (1984) suggests that this pairing is most effectively done when the preceptor's stage of role development is evaluated and matched with the level of student. A more advanced student may be best placed with an experienced expert practitioner and a beginning student with what Benner describes as a less experienced competent one. With thoughtful matching of preceptor and student it is hoped that the preceptor can then use the proposed adaptation of the Situation Leadership model to guide the student through the evolution of learning.

Acknowledgement: The authors acknowledge the nurse practitioner preceptors who shared their thoughts with the authors and agreed to be represented in the chapter.

References

Alspach, J. (1988). *From staff nurse to preceptor–preceptor training program: Instructor's manual.* Secaucus, NJ: Hospital Publication.

Benner, P. (1984). *From novice to expert: Excellence and power in clinical nursing practice.* Menlo Park, CA: Addison-Wesley.

Blanchard, K. (1985). *A situational approach to managing people.* Escondido: Blanchard Training and Development, Inc.

Blanchard, K., Zigarmi, P., & Zigarmi, D. (1985). *Leadership and the one minute manager.* New York: William Morrow.

Brodie, B. (1988). Voices in distant camps: The gap between nursing research and nursing practice. *Journal of Professional Nursing, 4*(5), 320–328.

Carlson, L., Crawford, N., & Contrades, S. (1989). Nursing student novice to expert: Benner's research applied to education. *Journal of Nursing Education, 28*(4), 188–190.

Dake, S., & Taylor, J. (1992). Motivating adult learners with effective feedback. *Journal of Extra-Corporeal Technology, 24*(2), 64–69.

Dreyfus, S. E., & Dreyfus, H. L. (1980). *A five-stage model of the mental activities involved in directed skill acquisition* (USAF Contract No. F49620-79-C-0063). Berkeley: University of California.

Hagopian, G., Ginette, G., Ferszt, L., & McCorkel, R. (1992). Preparing clinical preceptors to teach master's level students in oncology nursing. *Journal of Professional Nursing, 8*(5), 295–300.

Hardy, M. (1987). The American Nurse's Association influence on federal funding for nursing education, 1941–1984. *Nursing Research, 36*(1), 31–35.

Holly, C. (1992). A program design for preceptor training. *Nursing Connections, 5*(1), 49–59.

Reverby, S. (1987). A caring dilemma: Womanhood & nursing in historical perspective. *Nursing Research, 36*(1), 5–11.

Urden, L. (1989). Knowledge development in clinical practice. *Journal of Continuing Education in Nursing, 20*(1), 18–22.

5

Renaissance of Primary Care: An Opportunity for Nursing

Jean Goeppinger

P*rimary care* is both a familiar term and one with multiple meanings. That it has become a common term reflects the recent resurgence of interest in healthcare, prompted largely by proposals for national healthcare reform. These proposals seek to increase access to healthcare for almost 40 million Americans and, irrespective of the specifics of the proposal, assume that increased access requires an expansion of primary care (Franks, Nutting, & Clancy, 1993, p. 1449). Debates among legislators and the public have focused on how to achieve increased access to healthcare while also controlling escalating costs and maintaining quality. Controversies among healthcare professionals (see, e.g., Capriotti, 1994; Kassirer, 1994; Mundinger, 1994; and Zuger, 1994), however, have also raised questions about the contributions of primary care to healthcare reform and of advanced practice nurses to primary care.

This chapter provides a conceptual foundation for current debates that strengthens the abilities of nurses to respond thoughtfully and proactively to the new opportunities for recognition and reimbursement of advanced practice nurses as primary care providers. The chapter provides a historical overview of the three primary care practice models: Community-Oriented Primary Care, Primary Care, and Primary Healthcare. It discusses the differences and similarities among the models by comparing their characteristics and concludes with a futuristic view of a "new" or revitalized primary care.

PRACTICE MODELS

Practice models represent a perspective or broad approach within which the clinical and population-focused activities of health professionals and their patients can be described. As used in this chapter, they are not an isomorphic representation of the practice world, the sociologist's ideal type, or specific and detailed guidelines for practice. Rather, they are a framework within which practice can be examined. The following sections describe each of the three primary care prac-

Hickey JV: ADVANCED PRACTICE NURSING: Changing Roles and Clinical Applications © 1996 Lippincott–Raven Publishers

tice models. Salient characteristics, or practice parameters, of the models are compared using a modified version of the practice variables delineated by Rothman and Tropman (1987).

Community-Oriented Primary Care

The term *community-oriented primary care (COPC)* was advanced initially to reflect emerging collaborative relationships between epidemiology, a population-based science, and community medicine, the population-oriented clinical practice of medicine (Kark, 1974). The five defining characteristics of COPC are (1) a specified user or target population for which physicians assume responsibility and against which they measure the effect of their services;[1] (2) programs designed to address identified health problems within the target population; (3) participation by the target population in determining the need for health programs; (4) clinical practice that emphasizes a community-based and family-centered approach to patient care, which encompasses disease treatment and prevention as well as health promotion; and (5) accessibility that includes not only geographic accessibility but also the absence of fiscal, social, cultural, and communication barriers (Kark, 1974).

COPC developed internationally, beginning in the 1950s in countries such as South Africa, Israel, and the United Kingdom, with national programs of socialized medicine and capitated healthcare systems. It was subsequently replicated in the United States in ways that reflect our multipayer system. Some well-known examples include the Kaiser-Permanente Medical Care Program of Oregon; the federally funded Montefiore Family Health Center in the Bronx; the Checkerboard Area Health System in rural New Mexico, supported by the Presbyterian Medical Services; the Tarboro-Edgecombe Health Services System of rural North Carolina, a coalition of a private, fee-for-service, multispecialty medical group practice and the county health department (Nutting, Wood, & Conner, 1985); and more recently, the Oregon Basic Services Health Act (Dougherty, 1991).

Primary Care

In March 1982, the Institute of Medicine convened a national conference in the United States on "Community Oriented Primary Care" (Connor & Mullen, 1982). Although conference participants endorsed Kark's perspective on COPC, a more limited concept, generally labeled "primary care," became popular (Nutting, 1985).

In the Primary Care Model (PC Model), care is delivered and success assessed on individual, clinical parameters. The community denominator for impact evaluation was eliminated partly in response to the relative political strength of clinical medicine over public health and partly as a counterweight to the increasing specialization of medicine and health professional education and practice. The emphasis is less on community medicine and care provided to marginal or underserved populations and more on the provision of first-contact and person-centered medical services, that is, primary care, to individual care seekers.

> Primary care provides basic services, including those of an emergency nature, in a holistic fashion. It provides continuing management and coordination of all medical care services with appropriate retention and referral to other levels. It places emphasis, when feasible, on the preventive end of the preventive–curative spectrum of healthcare. Its services are provided equitably in a dignified, personalized, and caring manner (Parker, Walsh, & Coon, 1976, pp. 428-429).

Care provided within this model tends to be responsive to disease, although not disease or organ specific.

---

[1]The *target population* was originally considered a geographic community or neighborhood and later defined as any aggregate group of patients who were users of healthcare.

Primary care has continued to mean a basic level of healthcare, usually provided in an outpatient (or community) setting, that emphasizes a patient's general health needs (Office of Technology Assessment, 1990). The most frequently emphasized aspects are first-contact professional care that is accessible, comprehensive, coordinated, continuous, and accountable (Institute of Medicine, 1978). Primary care advocates have expected that, by improving the quality of the initial contact between a care seeker and professional provider, health would be enhanced, disease would be controlled, illness would be minimized, and the cost-effectiveness of health and illness care would increase. Despite some awareness that these expectations are not necessarily being realized in practice (Franks et al., 1993; Starfield, 1992), and because of the many calls for change in patterns of healthcare delivery, primary care in the United States has continued to emphasize clinical care provided chiefly by medical care professionals who are often referred to as the "usual source of care."

Primary Healthcare

In contrast to primary care, and at about the same time, COPC evolved internationally into primary healthcare (PHC), with a community focus and multilevel, multisectoral approach. The landmark Alma-Ata Conference Joint Report for the World Health Organization (WHO) and UNICEF (UNICEF, 1978) defined *primary healthcare* as

> essential health care based on practical, scientifically sound and socially acceptable methods and technology made universally accessible to individuals and families in the community by means acceptable to them, through their full participation and at a cost that the community and country can afford. It forms an integral part both of the country's health system, of which it is the nucleus, and of the overall social and economic development of the community. . . . It is the first level of contact of individuals, the family and the community with the national health system, bringing health care as close as possible to where people live and work, and constitutes the first element of a continuing health care process. (p.2)

More than 15 years after Alma-Ata and despite uneven progress toward "health for all" (WHO, 1981), the seven basic tenets of PHC remain: (1) PHC is shaped by the life patterns and meets the needs of the community it serves; (2) PHC is supported by the national health system; (3) PHC is fully integrated with the activities of other sectors involved in health and development (i.e., agriculture, education, housing, transportation, and communication); (4) the local population is actively involved in the design, prioritization, and implementation of healthcare services; (5) the healthcare offered places maximum reliance on the available community resources; (6) PHC involves a melding of preventive, promotive, curative, and rehabilitative services for the individual, family, and community; and (7) interventions for health are undertaken at the most peripheral level practicable: the community (WHO, 1975, p. 116). Health workers from multiple disciplines and traditional practitioners cooperate with each other, and with the individuals, families, and communities they serve. The development of self-responsibility for health, at individual and community levels, helps ensure the development of healthcare systems that build on community strengths (Alarcon, 1994; Goeppinger, 1984).

MODEL CHARACTERISTICS

The existence of multiple practice models, together with the similarity of their labels and the liberal mixing of labels and descriptions, is a source of considerable confusion for both emerging practitioners and their teachers. Although the models are not unique representations of different approaches, some clarity can be achieved by examining them using a set of seven characteristics common to all practice models. The COPC, PC, and PHC models each reflects, explicitly or implicitly, orientations toward the (1) goal and (2) scope of practice, (3) client roles, (4) health professional roles, including nursing roles, (5) medium of change or intervention, (6) practice environment or setting, and (7) locus of responsibility for cost. The following sections describe each characteristic and the COPC, PC, and PHC models are compared across each characteristic. The characteristics, that is, practice model variables, are depicted in Table 5-1.

Goals of Practice

The major goals for healthful change are health promotion and disease prevention. Traditionally, health promotion and disease prevention have been distinguished by level of specificity, target of action, and time orientation. Health promotion involves increasing the total well-being of individuals, families, and communities, whereas disease prevention involves altering specific behavior patterns that increase the risk of a particular disease state among identified aggregates (primary prevention); promptly diagnosing and treating diseases (secondary prevention); and rehabilitation to prevent disease progression and disability (tertiary prevention) (Leavall & Clark, 1958).

The Ottawa Charter for Health Promotion, formulated at a WHO meeting in Ottawa, Canada, broadened the definition of *health promotion* from well-being (Leavall & Clark, 1958) to include the "process of enabling people to increase control over, and to improve their health" (WHO, 1986, p. 1). The Ottawa Charter emphasized the following: partnerships between formal and informal as well as professional and indigenous community leaders; partnership defined as lay–professional alliances and shared power between lay and professional participants; social interaction aimed at enhancing problem-solving skills in culturally acceptable ways; and multilevel, multimethod interventions. Health promotion seen as changes in individual lifestyles and health behaviors was broadened to include community development, capacity building, and empowerment.

In the COPC Model, practice goals have generally been described in traditional terms. Care encompasses individual, family, and community-level health promotion activities and disease prevention among aggregates. Disease prevention, particularly primary and secondary prevention, has been emphasized. Exemplars include the CHAD Program in Israel, a program whose acronym represents the "community syndrome of hypertension, atherosclerosis and

TABLE 5-1 Defining Characteristics of Primary Care Practice Models

Characteristic	COPC Model	PC Model	PHC Model
Goals	Primary and secondary disease prevention, health promotion	Secondary disease prevention problem resolution	Health promotion, capacity building
Scope	Population, individual, and environment	Individual	Population, community
Patient roles	Participants, targets	Patients, consumers, recipients, victims	Partners
Professional roles	Participants, collaborators	Provider, program implementor, substantive expert	Enabler, catalyst, teacher of problem-solving skills
Change medium	Small multidisciplinary group, individual	Data	Small multisectoral group, health policymakers, organizations
Change environment	Community based	Healthcare institution	Community
Cost locus	National, federal government	Patient	Unassigned

diabetes," a set of diseases and disease risk factors (Abramson, Gofin, Hopp, Schein, & Naveh, 1994). CHAD was established in 1969 and targets adults at risk for cardiovascular disease who live in an urban neighborhood served by a multidisciplinary family practice group of a local health center. Family conferences, clinic sessions, and health education are used to decrease the behaviors placing community members at risk.

The goals of the PC Model emphasize secondary prevention, the resolution of health problems in their early stages, although primary prevention is also deemed important. Screening for cervical cancer and testing for human immunodeficiency virus among individuals seeking care, vision and hearing screening of elementary school students, and mammograms provided to low-income women at risk through a federally sponsored program are examples of secondary prevention, early diagnosis, and treatment directed toward aggregates defined by age and income status.

In contrast, the goals of the PHC Model relate to health promotion as envisioned by the Ottawa Charter, that is, capacity building and enhanced problem solving at the community level. Some of the clearest examples of healthcare practice directed toward health promotion broadly understood came from activities in developing countries 20 years ago, such as those in Tanzania and Ghana (Bennett, 1979). More recently, the Healthy Cities Movement has reflected use of the PHC Model in industrialized countries such as Canada, England, and the United States, countries where PHC is often referred to as the "New Public Health" (Ashton, Grey, & Barnard, 1986). The Healthy Cities Movement emphasizes city commitment, formation of healthy cities committees, and development of community leadership (Ashton et al., 1986). "Healthy Cities Indiana", for example, used processes aimed at building citizen commitment and developing leadership to address community-level problems related to physical activity and fitness; use of tobacco, alcohol, and other drugs; family planning; violence and abuse; oral health; maternal and infant health; and mental health (Flynn, Rider, & Ray, 1991).

Scope of Practice

Health professionals have targeted their care to individuals, families, communities, and the public. The U.S. public health system has generally provided care judged to contribute to the common good, whereas much of the private healthcare sector has provided care to individuals. As the public health system has recently assumed increased responsibility for providing personal health services to the indigent, uninsured, and underserved populations, the distinction between public and private has blurred. Nevertheless, the public health system remains unique in its orientation to the public and aggregates at risk, and in its use of case-finding strategies. Case-finding rather than care seeking is the hallmark of the public health system.

Both the COPC and PHC models have defined the community or selected populations as their scope of practice. Success is assessed using the population as the denominator; rates and percentages are calculated to express, for instance, the prevalence of cigarette smoking (Abramson et al., 1994). Comparison and control groups are used. COPC also addresses clinical practice objectives and evaluates success in terms of patient outcomes. The PC Model is focused at the level of the active patient—the care seeker; generally, the patient is viewed within his or her family and community environments. This ecological approach to patient care represents the best of individualized primary care practice.

Patient Roles

In the COPC Model, patients are viewed as important data sources for healthcare providers. They may also be seen as targets of change efforts, although the change process is recognized and respected as a collaborative one requiring patient input. The patient's perspective is always sought, irrespective of whether the patient is a single individual or a geographic community. Health surveys, screening programs, and data compiled from the clinical records of a medical practice are epidemiological approaches to gaining this perspective (Abramson et al., 1994). Family health histories, physical assessments of individuals and their work and home environments, and diagnostic reasoning are common approaches when the individual patient is seen within a family-focused, community-based care system.

The PC Model uses the terms "patients," "consumers," or "recipients" of care. Occasionally, patients are seen as victims, such as in the case of stroke and cancer "victims." In any case, the patient role is more passive than in the COPC or PHC models. Health professional care is given to rather than for patients (COPC) or with PHC partners.

Patients in the PHC Model are seen as partners in a common venture, partners whose active, informed contributions are essential to success. Everyone—patient and health professional—participates; everyone is responsible for the outcomes. For instance, in the Healthy Cities Movement, broad-based participatory leadership is seen as critical to goal achievement; health promotion is understood as capacity building (Ashton et al., 1986).

Professional Roles

Professional roles reflect those of patients. In the COPC Model, in which patients are healthcare data sources and targets of care, health professional roles are investigative and collaborative. Professional expertise is recognized, particularly the diagnostic and epidemiological skills necessary to frame a problem, access the "hard to reach," and case-find. In the PC Model, professional roles are more clearly defined on the basis of their substantive expertise; the majority of contemporary health professional education, irrespective of the discipline, is focused on the attainment of this substantive expertise. Professionals are often termed "providers" of healthcare to "consumers." They respond to patients' care-seeking behaviors by gathering data, formulating a diagnosis, and intervening. They may also triage patients using a computerized protocol (Lincoln et al., 1991) and implement a standardized program of health teaching.

The expertise of a health professional working within the rubric of the PHC Model is less dependent on substantive knowledge than process skills. Health professional roles within PHC include those of enabler, mediator, catalyst, and teacher of problem-solving skills, as well as those of a content expert. Professionals assist in coalition building, identification of common interests and reconciliation of differences, and nurturing of productive interpersonal relationships.

Arnstein's (1970) typology of citizen participation, depicted as eight rungs on a ladder ranging from manipulation by the professional, the lowest rung, to citizen control of the professional, the highest rung, has become a classic in the field of community organization. It offers a simple way to summarize patient and professional roles in each of the practice models. Primary care would be placed near the bottom because it engages patients in therapy (rung 2), informs them about alternatives (rung 3), and consults with them about their problems (rung 4). PHC would be placed near the top of the ladder because it strives for full partnership (rung 6), and delegates power and equitable decision making (rung 7) and, ultimately, citizen control (rung 8). It focuses on professional roles that emphasize self-help, involvement of a broad and representative cross section of people, technical assistance, and consensus building. COPC practitioners would be standing on the middle rung, usually involving patients in participative relationships (rung 5), but only sometimes allowing patients to exercise dominance (rung 8).

Nursing roles in these models generally mirror those of other health professionals. In CHAD, an example of COPC, nurses are involved in the planning group and are responsible for community outreach activities as well as physical examinations of individual patients, interviews, and counseling with patients and families, and case management (Abramson et al., 1994). Their principal roles are in intervention, not program design or evaluation. Nurses collaborate with physicians in implementing interventions for the target community's benefit.

Primary care nurses are "midlevel providers," nurse practitioners and certified nurse midwives who provide holistic care including primary and secondary prevention and health promotion services to an aggregate of patients or care seekers defined by age (most nurse practitioners) and gender (certified nurse midwives and women's health nurse practitioners). Some critics (see, e.g., Ulin, 1982) have suggested that the emphasis on nurse practitioner–physician collaboration in the United States has contributed to the neglect of collaboration between patients and nurses and the abrogation of professional responsibility for the healthcare needs of the total community.

In PHC strategies used in developed countries, nurses, as a specific professional group, are not mentioned; in developing countries, nurses often link the lay and professional healthcare systems. In both developed and developing countries, nurses are but one type of community development worker.

Change Medium

The Ottawa Charter for Health Promotion delineated five action strategies for health promotion: (1) building healthy public policy, (2) creating physical and social environments supportive of individual change, (3) strengthening community action, (4) developing personal skills such as increased self efficacy and feelings of empowerment, and (5) reorienting healthcare systems to the population and partnership with patients (WHO, 1986, pp. 1–2). This is the broadest approach to change and reflects precisely the orientation of the PHC Model. PHC change strategies are aimed at individual, family, and community levels, as well as at organizations and public policy. Changes are sought in behaviors, lifestyles, social norms, environments, policies, and resources. Small task-oriented groups, mass organizations, and political processes are all viewed as critical media for introducing and stabilizing broad-level change. Empowerment is a theory supportive of this view of change; its utility is now being subjected to empirical testing in health education and community psychology (Israel, Checkoway, Schulz, & Zimmerman, 1994; Rappaport, 1987).

In the PC Model, change is sought primarily at the individual or care-seeker level; the importance of supportive environments such as the home and workplace is acknowledged, and efforts are made to mobilize and supplement the patient's social support systems. Knowledge, or data, is presumed to alter attitudes, beliefs, and behaviors. The COPC Model uses a blend of change media, primarily individuals and small groups, including interdisciplinary teams of physicians and nurses, epidemiologists, biostatisticians, health educators, and public health nutritionists.

Change Environment or Setting

None of the practice models is setting specific, although patterns are obvious. The PC Model occurs in family health centers, health maintenance organizations, physicians' offices, the workplace, and, increasingly, in community hospitals and homes. Care is community based and not community oriented. The PHC Model is not associated with a setting; it occurs, however, before the public—in community action groups, at foundation board meetings, and at town councils. The practice sites of the COPC Model are similar to those of the PC Model— any healthcare institution that is located where people work, play, attend school, and live out their lives.

Cost Locus

The responsibility for healthcare costs, the last practice model variable, has only recently gained visibility. Its importance continues to vary considerably with the healthcare system endorsed by the country. In the United States, costs for COPC have been assumed, to a limited extent, by federal government programs targeted at specific population groups, such as Medicaid and Medicare recipients, and aggregates at risk, such as military veterans. Costs continue to be assumed by the recipient in the PC Model. Interestingly, in the PHC Model, the issue of costs has not yet been addressed, perhaps because the emphasis of PHC has not been on direct and costly care-giving. Costs in the PHC Model are assigned.

Comparison of Model Characteristics

The preceding comparison of primary care practice models across seven defining characteristics revealed several findings. The COPC Model, an early blend of clinical and community-oriented medical care, has served as the base from which more focused development has occurred nationally and internationally. The PC Model, which emphasizes the individual care seeker as the client and professionally given problem-focused care, represents a clinical perspective, whereas the PHC Model emphasizes the community as the client, health promotion as the practice goal, broad community involvement, and the population perspective.

The models aim to improve the acceptability of care. The COPC Model has also been found effective both in increasing acceptability and accessibility, geographically and fiscally (Connor & Mullen, 1982). Furthermore, evidence has indicated that access to primary care practitioners is linked with improved health outcomes and that patients are satisfied with care (Franks et al., 1993; Safriet, 1992). The COPC Model also offers more comprehensive, continuous care, integrating the clinical and population perspectives and responding to demonstrated health needs. Patients are often included as participants in healthcare, although their roles range from passive data provider (e.g., by way of chart reviews of patients in medical practices) to full participant in problem identification, intervention design and implementation, and outcome evaluation.

It is important for practitioners immersed in the practice world to be able to answer the following questions posed by the practice variables. What are health professionals' views and beliefs about the goals, scope, and setting of their practice? What is the nature of patient and professional roles in healthcare? What are appropriate change or intervention strategies? Who should bear the financial responsibility for care? In this way, practitioners act thoughtfully and systematically. It is also important for practitioners to understand the situational utility of each model and to respond flexibly, as well as thoughtfully, to the challenges of particular patients and healthcare environments. But, it is equally important for practitioners in today's chaotic world of healthcare reform to help shape a "new" primary care.

"NEW" PRIMARY CARE

Much national attention has centered recently on ways of simultaneously improving access to healthcare while controlling costs and preserving quality. Essential to these efforts, although often overlooked in debates increasingly restricted to cost issues, are needs to redefine the client of care and the goals of the healthcare system. As the 1991 (Shugars, O'Neil, & Bader, 1991) and 1993 (O'Neil, 1993) reports of the Pew Health Commission made clear, redefinition requires changes in health professional education and the healthcare system. "Reforming the education of health professionals combined with policies that address their availability, distribution, and utilization is one of the foundations of long-term reform in health care" (O'Neil, 1993, p. 5).

In *Health Professions Education for the Future: Schools in Service to the Nation* (O'Neil, 1993), the Pew Commission describes the "emerging health care system" (p. 6), termed here the *"new" primary care,* as one characterized by its orientation toward health, population perspective, intensive use of information, focus on the consumer, knowledge of treatment outcomes, constrained resources, coordination of services, reconsideration of human values, expectations of accountability, and growing interdependence. The emphasis on a population perspective coupled with the reorientation toward health and a consumer focus suggest that the "new" primary care will take a broad view of both the client and the goals of healthcare. Disease prevention, health promotion, injury prevention, and reduction of environmental hazards are all goals; responsibility for achieving these goals involves the participation of individuals, groups, and communities and changes in public policy. "Patient partnerships in decisions [are stressed]" (O'Neil, 1993, p. 6). By 2005, practitioners will be expected to care for the community's health, practice prevention and promote healthy lifestyles, and involve patients and families in healthcare decision making (Shugars et al., 1991, pp. 17–20).

Two of the most recent illustrations of the "new" primary care (Garr, Rhyne, & Kukulka, 1993; Nutting, Nagle, & Dudley, 1991) reflect changes in the definitions of the patient and the goal of care. They define the *patient* or *target population* as "the [physician's] practice population as a whole" (Garr et al., 1993, p. 1699); they define the *goal of care* as one of meeting identified needs of active patients in the practice. These emphases are similar to elements of the COPC Model.

The Pew Commission reports also called for an emphasis on coordinated care, interdisciplinary teamwork, and cost-effective care. These variables, particularly the link between coordination, interdisciplinary teamwork, and cost-effective care, have not yet been addressed. The most recent presentations of COPC (Garr et al., 1993; Nutting et al., 1991) have failed to reflect the new opportunities for service coordination, teamwork, and improved efficiency and effectiveness. This omission has occurred despite a recognition that nursing has assumed "new responsibilities in the delivery and management of care, particularly in primary care settings" (O'Neil, 1993, p. 83) and that nurse midwives and nurse practitioners "are proving to be important sources for primary health care" (O'Neil, 1993, p. 85). Safriet (1992) noted that the "empowerment" of nurse practitioners and certified nurse midwives "would have the greatest immediate impact on access while preserving quality and reducing costs" (p. 421).

There are, however, two promising examples of innovations designed to foster improved health through collaboration. Both focus on the education of healthcare providers and provide a first step toward testing the cost-effectiveness of an interdisciplinary approach to healthcare. The Pew Charitable Trusts and the Rockefeller Foundation funded the Health of the Public program in 1986 to stimulate academic health centers to develop a population perspective through curricular reform (Showstack et al., 1992). Partnerships with communities and collaboration among health professional schools were required. Today, the program has grown from 6 to 33 participating schools; project directors are faculty in schools of medicine, pharmacy, nursing, dentistry, and public health (Inui & Showstack, 1994).

The ways participating schools educate their students and define their roles in the community have changed. Changes include the student-initiated development of a comprehensive statewide approach to prenatal and postnatal care for pregnant drug abusers; the development of outcome data for health maintenance organization patients with hypertension; the feedback of findings to participating physicians; collaborative teaching and learning activities among faculty and students from the multiple health professional schools in academic health centers; and the teaching of population-level provider roles through partnerships with community-based acquired immunodeficiency syndrome service providers.

A collaborative family-oriented model of providing healthcare to homeless people has been developed in New York, illustrating the promise of collaboration in the practice setting (Morrow, Halbach, Hopkins, Wang, & Shortridge, 1992). The model involves alliances among the nurse-managed clinics in a school of nursing, the family practice department of a medical center, a community hospital, a county health department, and a network of social services for homeless people. The alliances ensure homeless people flexible, responsive community-oriented healthcare beyond the resources of any single partner. Faculty have the opportunity to provide interdisciplinary professional education and training in a population-focused project; the family-oriented care model has a relatively stable base of institutional and fiscal support (Morrow et al., 1992, p. 315).

The development of partnerships between health professional faculty and students and between health professional schools and the communities they serve is an essential step toward demonstrating the cost-effectiveness of the "new" primary care. Once such partnerships are developed, they can be tested to determine the extent to which they represent cost-effective use of healthcare resources. Findings from the "Health of the Public" program (Showstack et al., 1992; Inui & Showstack, 1994) and innovative multidisciplinary practices (Morrow et al., 1992) will help answer questions about the contributions of primary care to healthcare reform and of advanced practice nurses to primary care. Advanced practice nurses have new opportunities to collaborate in the redefinition of the goals and clients of healthcare professionals, to examine the utility of new approaches, and to disseminate their findings to the public and policymakers. Full participation in today's healthcare reform processes is imperative.

References

Abramson, J. H., Gofin, J., Hopp, C., Schein, M. H., & Naveh, P. (1994). The CHAD program for the control of cardiovascular risk factors in a Jerusalem community: A 24-year retrospect. *Israeli Journal of Medical Science, 30,* 108–119.

Alarcon, N. G. (1994). The role of health care professionals in increasing access to primary health care. *Family and Community Health, 17*(2), 15–21.

Arnstein, S. (1970). Eight rungs on the ladder of citizen participation. In E.S. Cahn & B.A.Passett (Eds.), *Citizen participation: A casebook in democracy* (pp. 335–357). Trenton, NJ: Community Action Training Institute.

Ashton, J., Grey, P., & Barnard, K. (1986). Healthy cities: WHO's new public health initiative. *Health Promotion, 1*(3), 319–324.

Bennett, F. J. (1979). Primary health care and developing countries. *Social Science and Medicine, 13A,* 505–514.

Capriotti, T. (1994). [Letter to the editor]. *New England Journal of Medicine, 330*(21), 1538.

Connor, E., & Mullen, F. (Eds.). (1982). In *Conference Proceedings: Community oriented primary care.* Washington, DC: National Academy Press.

Dougherty, C. J. (1991, May–June). Setting health priorities: Oregon's next steps. *Hastings Center Report,* pp. 1–10.

Flynn, B. C., Rider, M., & Ray, D. W. (1991). Healthy cities: The Indiana model of community development in public health. *Health Education Quarterly, 18*(3), 331–347.

Franks, P., Nutting, P. A., & Clancy, C. M. (1993). Health care reform, primary care, and the need for research. *JAMA, 270,* 1449–1453.

Garr, D., Rhyne, R., & Kukulka, G. (1993). Incorporating a community-oriented approach in primary care. *American Family Physician, 47*(8), 1699–1701.

Goeppinger, J. (1984). Primary health care: An answer to the dilemmas of community nursing. *Public Health Nursing, 1*(3), 129–140.

Institute of Medicine. (1978). *A manpower policy for primary health care: Report of a Study.* Washington, DC: National Academy Press.

Inui, T. S., & Showstack, J. (1994). *Health of the public: An academic challenge.* San Francisco: National Program Office, Health of the Public.

Israel, B. A., Checkoway, B., Schulz, A., & Zimmerman, M. (1994). Health education and community empowerment: Conceptualizing and measuring perceptions of individual, organizational, and community control. *Health Education Quarterly, 21*(2), 149–170.

Kark, S. L. (1974). *Epidemiology and community medicine.* New York: Appleton-Century-Crofts.

Kassirer, J. P. (1994). What role for nurse practitioners in primary care? *New England Journal of Medicine, 330*(3), 204–205.

Leavall, H. R., & Clark, E. G. (1958). *Preventive medicine for the doctor in his community.* New York: McGraw-Hill.

Lincoln, M. J., Turner, C. W., Haug, P., Warner, H. R., Williamson, J. W., Bouhaddou, O., Jessen, S., Sorenson, D., Cundick, R., & Grant, M. (1991). Iliad training enhances medical students diagnostic skills. *Journal of Medical Systems, 15,* 93–110.

Morrow, R., Halbach, J. L., Hopkins, C., Wang, C., & Shortridge, L. (1992). A family practice model of health care for homeless people: Collaboration with family nurse practitioners. *Family Medicine, 24,* 312–316.

Mundinger, M. O. (1994). Advanced-practice nursing: Good medicine for physicians? *New England Journal of Medicine, 330*(3), 211–214.

Nutting, P. (1985). Community-oriented primary care: A promising innovation in primary care. *Public Health Reports, 100*(1), 3–4.

Nutting, P. A., Nagle, J., & Dudley, T. (1991). Epidemiology and practice management: An example of community-oriented primary care. *Family Medicine, 23,* 18–226.

Nutting, P., Wood, M., & Conner, E. M. (1985). Community-oriented primary care in the United States: A status report. *JAMA, 253,* 1763–1766.

Office of Technology Assessment, U. S. Congress. (1990). *Health care in rural America 483* (OTA-H-434). Washington, DC: U.S. Government Printing Office.

O'Neil, E. H. (1993). *Health professions education for the future: Schools in service to the nation.* San Francisco: Pew Health Professions Commission.

Parker, A. W., Walsh, J. M., & Coon, M. (1976). A normative approach to the definition of primary health care. *Milbank Memorial Fund Quarterly, 54,* 416–438.

Rappaport, J. (1987). Terms of empowerment/exemplars of prevention: Toward a theory for community psychology. *American Journal of Community Psychology, 15,* 121–144.

Rothman, J., & Tropman, J. E. (1987). Models of community organization and macro practice perspectives: Their mixing and phasing. In F. M. Cox, J. L. Erlich., J. Rothman, & J. E. Tropman (Eds.), *Macropractice: Strategies of community organization* (pp. 3–26). Itasca, IL.: F.E. Peacock.

Safriet, B. J. (1992). Health care dollars and regulatory sense: The role of advanced practice nursing. *Yale Journal of Regulation, 9*(2), 417-487.

Showstack, J., Fein, L., Ford, D., Kaufman, A., Cross, A., Madoff, M., Goldberg, H., O'Neil, E., Moore, G., Schroeder, S., & Inui, T. (1992). Health of the public: The academic response. *JAMA, 267,* 2497–2502.

Shugars, D. A., O'Neil, E. H., & Bader, J. D. (Eds.). (1991). *Healthy America: Practitioners for 2005: An agenda for action for U.S. health professional schools.* Durham, NC: The Pew Health Professions Commission.

Starfield, B. (1992). *Primary care: Concept, evaluation, and policy.* New York: Oxford University Press.

Ulin, P. (1982). International nursing challenges. *Nursing Outlook, 30*(9), 531–535.

UNICEF. (1978). *Primary health care* (Joint Report of the Director General of WHO and the Executive Director of UNICEF). Geneva: World Health Organization/ Author.

World Health Organization. (1975). *Official records no. 226: Twenth-eighth World Health Assembly, part 1.* Geneva: World Health Organization/ Author.

World Health Organization. (1981). *Global strategy for health for all by the year 2000.* Geneva: Author.

World Health Organization. (1986). *Ottawa Charter for Health Promotion.* Copenhagen, Denmark. WHO Regional Office for Europe.

Zuger, A. (1994). [Letter to the editor]. *New England Journal of Medicine, 330*(21), 1539.

Changing Environments and Patient Diversity in Healthcare Delivery

Introduction: Joanne V. Hickey

In Section I, the authors discussed how education and roles for advanced practice nurses (APNs) are changing rapidly to meet the new forces and realities of the marketplace, as we head toward exciting new opportunities for practice in the 21st century. In Section II, the authors take us to some of these changing practice areas, where many of the difficulties accompanying the sea of change in healthcare are being addressed through the use of APNs.

In Chapter 6, Changing Environment of Healthcare, Venegoni provides a framework for considering the changing care environment. Change is inevitable, but the rate of change is accelerating and APNs must not only accept this, but develop strategies to flourish within the changing environment. Venegoni broadly defines the healthcare environment and identifies and describes the five **P**s that are the factors reshaping the healthcare system. They are (1) **p**laces or sites of health delivery; (2) **p**eople receiving care (demographics); (3) **p**reventive model of care, a changing focus; (4) **p**aradigm shift to quality improvement and customer satisfaction; and (5) **p**rocess change, to increasingly sophisticated technology in healthcare. The chapter concludes with practical survival skills for the APN to use to flourish in the changing care environment.

In Chapter 7, Cultural and Ethnic Diversity: Cultural Competence, Bushy focuses attention on the changing profiles of the people receiving healthcare—people whose diverse cultural and ethnic backgrounds influence patient acceptance and modes of care delivery. Cultural competence, the author points out, will be essential for APNs to provide quality care and promote customer satisfaction in the future healthcare environment.

In Chapter 8, Case Management and the Advanced Practice Nurse, Benoit provides an overview of case management that is becoming the universal tool for coordinating patient care in the hospital environment. This trend enhances opportunities for the APN, whose education and expertise are specifically oriented toward assuming the role of case manager in providing care. The processes of care have changed, including the use of care maps driven by complex databases that tell us how to coordinate care and efficiently move a patient through a hospitalization while providing quality care. Care maps guide delivery of care in all environments, from hospital to home. The chapter includes the author's description of her own experiences in developing the case management model with neurosurgical patients.

In Chapter 9, Advanced Practice Nurse in a Managed Care Environment, Satinsky discusses the managed care environment that is coming to dominate the healthcare delivery system. Managed care, of which the health maintenance organization is the principal example, and managed care contracts, with their incentives to keep patients healthy, will be the norm in healthcare. Understanding managed care, both its purposes and its processes, is imperative for the APN, who will be required to work with or within these environments in the future. Managed care proposes to operationalize the paradigm shift of providing improved quality care to increase customer satisfaction. It also recognizes the fundamental importance of the prevention model by emphasizing health promotion and disease prevention in the healthcare provided.

In Chapter 10, Collaboration and Advanced Practice Nursing, King, Parrinello, and Baggs provide a timely discussion of collaboration within the context of primary care and acute-care settings. The models for collaborative practice in primary care and acute care differ. In the primary care model, which is commonly encountered, the APN is often a substitute for the collaborating physician because either could provide competent care. In the acute-care setting, there is a need for ongoing participation of both the physician and the APN to provide quality care for the patient. In this chapter, the authors focus more on the collaborative model of practice in acute care and the exciting roles that APNs are assuming in high-technology tertiary centers throughout the United States.

All of the chapters in Section II acknowledge the changing nature of healthcare delivery sites—the shift from hospital-based to community-based and home settings. Perhaps a sixth **P**, pecuniary factors, should be added to the change-producing factors cited by Venegoni in Chapter 6. *Pecuniary* is generally defined as pertaining to money. Consideration of healthcare costs and cost containment is the central and driving force in healthcare delivery and has therefore become the essential test that enduring changes must meet in healthcare delivery. This theme, carried through the clinical examples, institutional policies, and personal accounts included in the chapters, emphasizes the bases of many of the changes occurring in care environments. The chapter exemplars in Section IV provide additional clinical vignettes demonstrating how new environments are making advanced practice nursing more complex and how APNs are making unique contributions to the cost-effective provision of quality care that meets patients' needs.

The next section, Section III, addresses a variety of important issues related to advanced practice nursing, including accountability, professional licensure and credentialling, research utilization, empowerment, healthcare economics, and cost-containment initiatives. Exploring these chapters will assist the reader in understanding professional responsibility and accountability as they apply to the APN, and will further elaborate the economic culture imposed on advanced practice nursing and healthcare delivery by the predominance of the cost-containment imperative.

CHAPTER

6

Changing Environment of Healthcare

Sandra L. Venegoni

Whether a healthcare professional or healthcare consumer, one needs only to step back objectively for a few minutes from the present healthcare system to recognize the driving forces in our society that have an impact on the healthcare arena. This chapter discusses the major trends of a changing environment, a topic not addressed in the other chapters in this book.

Change. Depending on perception, individuals may interpret change differently. For some people, a change process is enriching, stimulating, and exciting. For many people, change is a troublesome process, causing undue stress and anxiety. Yet change is a phenomenon that most of us experience daily to one degree or another. A three-step process is necessary for effective change to occur: one must first *unfreeze* the old, then *remold* the new, and, finally, *refreeze* the new. Whether the change is a personal lifestyle change, a change in the manner of carrying out a task, or a change in the way an organization is structured or operates, the change process proceeds through a similar three-step transition: giving up something familiar, taking on something new, and then making the new a part of our nature and routine.

We have been forewarned by ancient and modern sages that change will happen and should be expected. In 5 B.C., the Greek philosopher Euripides predicted that the "only thing permanent in life is change." A modern sage, Stephen Covey (1991), in his literature of the 1980s and 1990s, likewise reminds us that there are only two constants: true principles and change. *Principles,* which are laws of nature and the universe, fall into two categories: the physical dimension (e.g., laws of gravity—the compass always points north) and the human dimension of relationships and organizations (e.g., people innately trust people who are trustworthy). Principles are constant and do not undergo change, but everything else is subject to change. Thus, change itself becomes a constant. These words of wisdom suggest that people should anticipate change as a routine, acceptable way of life.

The U.S. healthcare industry, like most other industries and organizations, has experienced major changes during the 20th century. Changes have occurred in the health or illness states of care recipients, characteristics of care recipients, sites of care delivery, and care reim-

Hickey JV: ADVANCED PRACTICE NURSING: Changing Roles and Clinical Applications © 1996 Lippincott–Raven Publishers

bursement. At the turn of the 20th century, healthcare was primarily delivered to individuals who experienced illness as a result of epidemics and unsanitary living conditions. Later, individual acute conditions predominated, followed by an increase in chronic conditions. Many chronic conditions are associated with an individual's lifestyle and behavior. Healthcare delivery sites have also changed; home care during the early part of the century was converted to institutional care, especially after World War II and the subsequent increase in the number and size of hospitals. Toward the end of the 20th century, we have witnessed a shift back to home and community care.

Most of these changes in healthcare delivery reflect major conditions and changes in society as a whole. It is society's economic and sociological phenomena that influence all aspects of healthcare delivery—the type of care to be delivered, the sites of delivery, and the systems of reimbursement for care. Before studying the major societal forces of change, a framework must be established for understanding the term *environment* and its relationship to healthcare organizations and the healthcare industry.

ORGANIZATIONAL ENVIRONMENT

Organizations have been the subject of study throughout the 20th century; however, they received major emphasis after 1950. In his review of the sociological study of organizational structure and behavior, Scott (1981) identified five essential components of all organizations: social structure, participants, goals, technology, and environment. Although analysts of organizations, perhaps, have focused on the study of only one component at a time, Scott reminds us that all components are interdependent.

In discussing the definition of organizations, Scott (1981) categorized all analysis of organizations into three perspectives: the rational system, the natural system, and the open system. The *rational system perspective* focuses on the specific goals and formalization of an organization's structure to distinguish it from other groups of individuals. The *natural system perspective* defines an organization not by its goals or structure but by its ability to survive. All participants in the organization carry out activities to this end: the survival of the organization. Both the rational and natural system perspectives tend to view the organization as a closed system with tight boundaries that separate the organization from the environment. The *open system perspective,* on the other hand, views the organization as a "coalition of shifting interest groups that develop goals by negotiation; the structure of the coalition, its activities, and its outcomes are strongly influenced by environmental forces" (Scott, 1981, p. 23). Open systems depend on exchange with other systems in their environment. They have permeable boundaries so that resources are imported from the environment and transformed into outputs that are then exported back into the environment. Open systems are influenced by, interact with, and are interdependent with elements in the environment.

Another method of describing environment is beneficial when considering the changing forces that influence healthcare. Two generally accepted, broad categories of environment are the societal (general) environment and the specific (task) environment (Hall, 1972; Jackson, Morgan & Paolillo, 1986). The *general environment* affects all organizations in a given society or culture. Every organization in a given geographic area, whatever its purpose or function, will feel the effects of forces in the general environment. Forces include local demographic and economic conditions and sociological, cultural, political, legal, and educational situations. For example, a large number of layoffs in a city will produce a ripple effect in many different types of organizations and groups in that area.

The *task environment,* on the other hand, is specific and affects each individual organization more directly. The task environment contains components that are most relevant to an organization and, yet, are different for each organization. For example, healthcare organizations in a city differ from other types of organizations such as industry, restaurants, and sales organizations. In his early work in which he coined the term *task environment,* Dill (1958) suggested that the task environment consists of customers, suppliers, competitors, and regulators. In applying these categories to healthcare organizations, the following examples come to mind. Customers are the consumers of healthcare—the patients. Some business organizations are both customers and distributors of healthcare services in their association with large hospitals. The hospitals provide their products—healthcare services—to the business organizations in a variety of community settings. For example, a hospital might provide physical examinations and blood and urine screenings for employees of a local organization at their place of business. Suppliers include those organizations that supply members of the labor market (e.g., schools of nursing), suppliers of equipment and materials (e.g., pharmaceutical firms or medical supply companies), and suppliers of capital (e.g., affiliated local religious groups or proprietary-owned organizations). Competitors in healthcare organizations include other local health organizations. Regulators of healthcare organizations differ from those of other organizations in a local area (e.g., local or state boards for certificate of need, licensure, and so forth).

For purposes of considering the changing environment and its effects on healthcare, this chapter uses the open system perspective and the categories of general environment and task environment. Healthcare reform at the national level will exert its influence on most healthcare facilities throughout the nation. Local factors will exert their effect on the local market organizations in states, cities, or rural areas. The factors described in the remainder of this chapter affect all healthcare organizations, wherever they are located.

MAJOR FACTORS IN THE CHANGING ENVIRONMENT

Although many forces in the environment are influencing healthcare systems and healthcare delivery in the United States, this chapter addresses the five most significant factors. They can easily be remembered as the five **P**s: **p**laces (the "where" of healthcare delivery); **p**eople (the "who" of healthcare delivery); **p**reventive model (the "type" of healthcare delivered); and the "how" of healthcare delivery, which includes the **p**aradigm shift and **p**rocess.

Change 1: Places (Sites) of Healthcare Delivery

In tracing the sites of healthcare delivery in the United States during the 20th century, a historian might be tempted to paraphrase the old adage, "What goes around, comes around." A contemporary explanation of this saying is provided by Peter Senge (1990) in his description of learning organizations. He states that "reality is made up of circles but we see straight lines. Herein lie the beginnings of our limitations as system thinkers" (p. 141). So that we are not limited in our understanding of healthcare systems, perhaps we need to think of their evolution as circular, changing over time but returning, in a somewhat different fashion, to its original point.

In the early period of the 20th century, most healthcare services were provided in the home setting, including those for the two most important events— birth and death. Early institutions for illness care were predominantly those involved with epidemics and infectious diseases, such as tuberculosis sanitariums. Following the world wars, but especially after World War II, the hospital increased in importance as the delivery site for acute healthcare. Several major factors led to this situation. The construction and renovation of hospitals, as well as the addition of equipment to hospitals, escalated in the mid-1940s when the government provided funding of these projects through the Hill-Burton Act of 1946. Along with the increased capacity for care, hospitals were assured a guaranteed source of payment with two new forms of reimbursement: the "Blues" and Medicare. Blue Cross and Blue Shield, a healthcare benefit offered to employees in rapidly increasing numbers, soon became a bargaining chip between labor and corporate management in our industrialized society. Acute care quickly began to be delivered in a hospital setting and employees abruptly forgot that, in essence, they were the bill payers for such healthcare. In a personal interview, one of the nation's foremost health economists, Uwe Reinhardt (cited in Rovner, 1994), stated that one of the biggest misconceptions Americans have about our healthcare systems is "that someone else, their employer, is paying their health bill" (p. 64). Employees, who forgot that the cost of healthcare benefits actually comes out of their paycheck, demanded more hospital care because it was covered through their benefits. True to the laws of supply and demand, the more and better hospitals that were available (supply), the greater the demand by employees. Along with increased supply and demand, came escalated hospitalization costs.

Use of hospitals for healthcare by older people also escalated with the passage of Medicare, the Title XVIII Amendment to the Social Security Act, in 1965. Medicare was the largest addition to the social security legislation since the 1930s. Of its two parts, Part A, which covers hospital insurance benefits for aged people, and Part B, which is the supplementary medical insurance benefits for aged people, Part A had the most effect on hospital care. In his 1965 State of the Union Address and Economic report to Congress, President Johnson defined Medicare as the "biggest single increase budgeted—a $2 billion annual rise in Social Security benefits for the aged" (*Facts on File Yearbook,* 1965, p. 277). In 1966, 18.9 million older people (almost all of those potentially entitled) were enrolled in hospital insurance and more than 6000 hospitals and 1200 home health agencies had been certified for participation in the program (Breslow, 1973, p. 17).

By the mid-1970s, spurious effects of the new policy were that hospitals and healthcare services "were able to receive compensation for services previously provided gratis, and at the same time to purchase new equipment and meet labor demands more readily. Costs . . . increased 10% annually between 1966 and 1973" (Smith & Hollander, 1973, p. 2). Physicians, likewise, increased their prices and reduced bad debts through Medicare. "Between 1966 and 1973, their fees increased 5–8% per year and their incomes increased nearly 11% per year" (Smith & Hollander, 1973, p. 1). Although extremely necessary, the passage of Medicare in 1965, with its later additional coverage of people with end-stage renal disease, has negatively affected the national budget throughout its approximately 30-year history.

As the United States rapidly approaches the beginning of a new century, healthcare delivery sites have begun to change dramatically. As healthcare reform continues to become included in state and national laws, it has escalated the switch of care delivery from inpatient hospital settings to outpatient ambulatory settings. Hospitals, recognizing their inability to stand alone as major care providers, have ceased being freestanding, independent players and have merged, entered joint ventures and alliances, and networked with other providers to establish "seamless" integrated delivery systems along a continuum of care and services. But what was the impetus for such change?

Historically, three major foci have driven most of healthcare reform during the post–World War II era: *access* to healthcare for all, *quality* of care, and *cost* of care. During the late 1970s and early 1980s, the escalating cost of healthcare, both in and out of hospitals, and cost containment became national issues. From 1965 to 1990, healthcare costs have increased from $42 billion to $647 billion, an increase from 5.9% of the gross national product spent on healthcare to 12.5% (Safriet, 1992). To curb the rising healthcare costs, three effective healthcare system changes were proposed. One dealt with how Medicare would pay for hospital care for senior citizens; the second dealt with the "gatekeeper" effect of managed care, competition, and capitation; and the third addressed the amazing advances in medical technology that have permitted an increasing number of procedures to be conducted in ambulatory outpatient settings. (Managed care is discussed in Chapter 9 and technological improvement is discussed later in this chapter).

A major revision to the Medicare method of paying for hospitalization for older people occurred with congressional passage of the Tax Equity and Fiscal Responsibility Act (TEFRA) of 1982. This act established a cost-per-case basis for hospital payment and placed a ceiling on the rate of increase in hospital revenues that Medicare would support. Congressional amendment to the Social Security Act in 1983 (P.L. 98-21) converted a retrospective form of inpatient care for Medicare patients to a prospective payment system. This new system, with its diagnosis-related groups, prospectively set the number of days an elderly person could be hospitalized, based on the individual's diagnosis. If the number of hospitalized days exceeded the preestablished number, the hospital suffered a financial loss and would have to absorb the cost. As a result of this new system, an increasing number of elderly people were being discharged from hospitals "quicker and sicker," consequently increasing the number of admissions to nursing homes and spurring a growth spurt of out-of-hospital delivery services, such as health maintenance organizations and home health services (Guterman, Eggers, Riley, Greene, & Terrell, 1988; Russell & Manning, 1988). Thus, the stage was set for more healthcare services to be delivered by community care delivery systems. This action has only escalated during the continued cost containment efforts and downsizing of hospitals and acute-care during the 1990s.

As the nation moves closer to the 21st century, the entire spectrum of healthcare delivery is undergoing modifications in an effort to reengineer and improve healthcare operations. The concept of "hospitals without walls" is readily understood. Newly created posthospital care programs, in addition to existing long-term care facilities such as nursing homes, accept and care for patients who are not yet ready for discharge to their homes. Two relatively new entities include the rapidly multiplying subacute units and assisted-living facilities. Subacute units, as a newly created step in the integrated delivery systems, are located in hospitals or nursing homes, or are freestanding units. They were created to provide a link between acute care and long-term care. As such, these facilities are especially able to care for individuals recovering from acute conditions; for a growing number of chronically ill elderly people (Griffin, 1994; McDowell & Brown, 1994); and for other people with special needs, such as ventilator-dependent residents (Griffin, 1994; McDowell & Brown, 1994). Assisted-living units, on the other hand, were created to fill the gap between nursing homes and home care. The number of assisted-living facilities, estimated between 30,000 and 40,000, "combines housing with a variety of personalized healthcare and supportive services, normally for frail elderly persons aged 82 and over" (Cerne, 1994, p. 72).

Ambulatory care programs, another category of posthospital care, provide a complete continuum of care. Some programs, such as the one at Stanford University Hospital in California, offer not only an adult day healthcare center but a home care program. Although home care has been a part of the healthcare industry for many years, this particular program, established in 1985, links together the home care provider and the case manager to provide skilled nursing needs in the home. The program has documented a decreased length of stay in the hospital and a yearly savings of between $10 million and $15 million (Day, McFarlin, & Friel, 1993). Other patients, who have special needs and still require some type of hospitalization can be managed through partial hospitalization programs. For example, the partial hospitalization program at Stanford University Hospital, an alternative for acute psychiatric patients, meets for 6½ hours every Monday through Friday, and includes different types of therapy sessions for participants based on individualized care plans. Members of an interdisciplinary team develop and review these care plans (Bronstein, 1993).

The preceding examples are only a few of the methods being created to contain costs of hospitalizations and healthcare delivery. More nontraditional delivery programs will likely be created based on consumer needs. This trend has already begun with the "customer focus" of quality care initiatives. In the future, more healthcare will be delivered at convenient sites such as schools, churches, and shopping malls—perhaps even at fast-food restaurants.

Change 2: People Receiving Care (Demographics)

One of the most significant trends in the changing healthcare environment is the demographic changes of the population, especially the increasing numbers of people aged 65 years and older. In a 1987 study conducted by the American College of Healthcare Executives (Wesbury, 1988), 1600 experts identified the aging of America as the "number one public policy issue and most critical issue affecting the future of our health care system" (p. 60).

Americans are experiencing an increased life expectancy due to improved healthcare and health status, a significant reduction in mortality rates for infants, children, and young adults, and a decreased number of maternal deaths. A child born in 1900 could expect to live to age 47 years, whereas a child born in 1990 can expect to live to approximately age 75.4 years, an additional 28.4 years since the turn of the century (U.S. Bureau of the Census, 1993).

Throughout the 20th century, the number of people aged 65 years and older has steadily increased from 4.1% of the population (3.1 million people) in 1900, to 12% (28 million) in 1987, to 12.6% (31.8 million) in 1991—a tenfold increase since the turn of the century. The number in 1991 represents about one in eight Americans (U.S. Bureau of the Census, 1993). In 1990, about 2.2 million people celebrated their 65th birthday (6000 per day), whereas only 1.6 million people older than age 65 years died during the same year. The total net increase for people older than age 65 years in 1990 was 645,000. The 1990 census demonstrated a daily net increase of approximately 1770 people who turn age 65 years. By the beginning of the next millennium, an estimated 35 million people (13% of the population) will be members of this group (U.S. Bureau of the Census, 1993).

During the Great Depression, relatively few babies were born. This small birth cohort will slow somewhat the number of people reaching age 65 years in the latter half of the 1990s and early years of the 21st century. However, when the post–World War II "baby boomers" who were born between the years 1946 and 1964 begin to enter the retirement age group, there will be a dramatic increase in people aged 65 years and older. This increase is projected to occur between 2010 and 2030. The estimated number of people who will reach age 65 years during 2010, 2020, and 2030 are 39 million, 52 million, and 66 million, respectively (U.S. Bureau of the Census, 1993).

The most rapid growth since 1985 has been in the age group of people aged 85 years and older—the oldest-old (National Institute on Aging, 1987). A comparison of age groups in 1990 to their counterparts in 1900 shows that, in 1990, the 65- to 74-year-old age group was eight times larger than in 1900; the 75- to 84-year-old age group was 13 times larger; and the 85-year-old-and-older age group was 25 times larger, representing 3.2 million people. Projections for the 85-year-old-and-older age group in the 21st century are also astounding. In 1987, 9.6% of the elderly population was aged 85 years and older. This percentage is expected to increase to 15.5% by 2010 (Shugars, O'Neil, & Bader, 1991, p. 32).

As the growth of the population of people older than age 65 years increases, this growing age group will greatly influence the U.S. healthcare system. For example, most older people have at least one chronic condition and many experience multiple conditions, which has led to a national shift from acute to chronic care. In 1990, the most frequently occurring chronic conditions in this age group were arthritis (47%), hypertension (37%), hearing impairments (32%), heart disease (29%), and orthopedic impairments (17%) (American Association of Retired Persons, 1992).

Although representing only 12% of the population in 1987, people aged 65 years or older accounted for 36% of total personal healthcare expenditures. Major health expenses for this age group included hospital expenses (42%), physician care (21%), and nursing home care (20%). In 1990, 34% of all hospital stays were by people aged 65 years or older. When hospitalized, their average length of stay (8.7 days) was longer than for people younger than age 65 years (5.3 days). Older people also experienced more physician visits (nine visits) than younger people (five visits). Healthcare expenditures for older people in 1990 cost $162 billion, or an average of $5360 per person annually. The average was four times higher than for younger people. One fourth of healthcare expenditures was paid out-of-pocket by older people. Two thirds of healthcare expenditures were covered by some type of third-party reimbursement: $72 billion from Medicare, $20 billion from Medicaid, and $10 billion from other sources (American Association of Retired Persons, 1992).

A moderate percentage of older people have assessed their health as fair or poor (28%), most likely because older people generally experience an increased number of days of restricted activities due to illness or injury. In contrast, only 7% of younger people have rated their health in the same categories. On average, each older person in 1990 experienced 31 annual days of restricted activity; on 14 of these days, they were confined to bedrest (American Association of Retired Persons, 1992).

It would behoove healthcare providers to heed the predictions of experts who have spent much time studying the aging population. These experts have stated that "health professionals who graduate between the years 1990 and 2000 will spend most of their practice lives caring for this generation . . . [and that] much of the nation's health care resources will be measured against the long-term care needs of this generation" (Shugars et al., 1991, p. 32).

Change 3: Preventive Model of Care (A Changing Focus)

Throughout most of the 20th century, Americans have experienced a model of care that had as its major orientation the treatment of disease and illness. This model is slowly being replaced by a model of "health" care that emphasizes health promotion and disease prevention. The national shift in attitude toward health has been reflected in major national health policy. In the 1979 landmark publication *Healthy People: The Surgeon General's Report on Health Promotion and Disease Prevention* (U.S. Department of Health, Education, and Welfare, 1979), the second public health revolution of the century was initiated by the Carter administration. This national report mirrored what was simultaneously occurring on the international front. In 1978, the World Health Organization (WHO) held an international conference on primary healthcare in Alma-Ata, USSR, and pronounced the desired goal of "attainment by all the citizens of the world by the year 2000 of a level of health that will permit them to lead a socially and economically productive life" (WHO, 1985, p.2). The new U.S. health policy emphasized prevention of disease and highlighted people's responsibility for their own health.

The *Healthy People* report launched a national shift from the previous focus on curative care and treatment of disease. Most of the common diseases of the late 1970s were those that could likely be prevented, hence, the recognized need for a change in attitude toward health. Throughout the 20th century, Americans have witnessed a change in patterns of morbidity and mortality (Orlandi, 1987; Taylor, Denham, & Ureda, 1982). During the early part of the century, infectious diseases such as smallpox, measles, mumps, rubella, diphtheria, and scarlet fever were the predominant conditions. Increased emphasis was placed on improving sanitation in housing, drinking water, and sewerage as well as enhancing immunization programs to eliminate these conditions. Since 1975, the major health conditions have been "contemporary epidemics of degenerative, neoplastic and stress-related disease. It appears that much of the morbidity and mortality of these new epidemics are self-inflicted" (Taylor et al., 1982, p. 1). Each of the three leading causes of death in the United States today—heart disease, cancer, and cerebrovascular disease—has a major component related to an individual's personal lifestyle behavior.

The *Healthy People* report outlined three broad prevention strategies to improve the health status of Americans: disease prevention, health promotion, and health protection. Each of these categories was then subdivided into areas of concern, each with its own specific objectives. A total of 226 objectives was written and an appropriate health and human services agency was assigned responsibility for each objective. The objectives were published in 1980 in *Promoting Health/Preventing Disease: Objectives for the Nation* (U.S. Department of Health and Human Services, Public Health Service, 1980), with the year 1990 established as the projected date to successfully meet these objectives. Although the objectives did not constitute a federal plan, they were intended as "national in scope and as a challenge to both the public and private sectors" (DHHS, 1980, p. 4). An emphasis on action to meet the 1990 objectives was established by creating an ongoing evaluative process and a midcourse review to report progress.

Since publication of the *Healthy People* report, there has been a surge of federal, state, and local government involvement with health promotion and disease prevention. The government assesses progress at the end of each decade and establishes goals for the next decade. For example, in 1990, DHHS reviewed the extent to which goals had been accomplished during the 1980s and established 300 measurable objectives for the following decade in *Healthy People 2000: National Health Promotion and Disease Prevention Objectives* (DHHS, 1990).

The emphasis on "healthcare" as opposed to "illness care" has permeated clinical practice in the health field, research arena, and professional journals. National guidelines for clinical prevention services in the practice and educational settings have been established and published in the *Guide to Clinical Preventive Services* (U.S. Preventive Services Task Force, 1989). These age- and gender-specific guidelines include suggested screening tests, targeted physical exams, immunizations, and counseling or health advice that are intended to become a part of periodic health visits. The guidelines are part of the national "Put Prevention Into Practice" program, which provides educational materials for patients and a clinician's handbook.

That America must focus on "health" care is evident from the 1993 data on overall cost of health (illness?) care in the country: $900 billion annually, 14% of the GNP, and $3000 per person annually, with 70% of the cost made up of preventable illness and its associated costs. The prevention of the following two common conditions, for example, can result in savings: preventing the treatment and rehabilitation of a hip fracture can save $40,000 per person and preventing bypass coronary surgery can save $30,000 per person (DHHS, 1990). James Fries, MD, professor of medicine at Stanford University School of Medicine and author of many books and articles on medical cost reduction and health improvement, has described positive results of the shift to a health focus. People reduce their use of services by 7% to 17% when they are provided medical information and guidelines for care to assist them in making health decisions. Quality health programs in the workplace have been effective in reducing the number of sick days and costs for outpatient and hospital care—a cost reduction ranging from 15% to 25% (Fries, 1993, p. 21). The emphasis of the prevention model is one of the most exciting changes occurring in the United States. It will not only continue, but probably escalate in the 21st century. Furthermore, it will produce a significant effect on the U.S. healthcare system.

Change 4: Paradigm Shift (Quality Improvement and Customer Satisfaction)

The emphasis on the quality of healthcare professionals and healthcare delivery systems has become a familiar concept in America. As early as 1910, Abraham Flexner, through funds from the Carnegie Foundation, studied the quality of medical schools in America. The Flexner Report found many medical schools to be inadequate in their education of "improperly and insufficiently trained" physicians (Wolinsky, 1980, p. 249). This study resulted primarily in the closure of medical schools that did not produce the quality physicians needed by society and the establishment of the American Medical Association Council on Medical Education to oversee medical education. Other means of assuring quality included the licensure of healthcare providers and certification of facilities and organizations.

Delivery of quality care in hospitals was boosted by voluntary participation in the Joint Commission on Accreditation of Hospitals review. This process provided one manner of documenting the provision of "quality care" to the public through its quality assurance program. Later renamed the Joint Commission on Accreditation of Healthcare Organizations, the organization continues to provide the same standards of quality for multiple healthcare organizations.

Another attempt to improve the quality of care has been the development of clinical practice guidelines for treating selected medical conditions. In 1990, both the General Accounting Office and the Institute of Medicine encouraged such guidelines (Shugars et al.,

1991). The Agency for Health Care Policy and Research (AHCPR), within DHHS, was established in 1989 under P.L. 101-239 (the Omnibus Budget Reconciliation Act of 1989) to "enhance the quality, appropriateness, and effectiveness of healthcare services and access to these services" (DHHS, 1992, p.1). The AHCPR has called together panels of experts to develop clinical guidelines to assist practitioners in clinical decision making as well as for consumers in making their health choices. Another function of the AHCPR, in its quality mission, is to conduct medical effectiveness/patient outcome research, develop a database, and research dissemination methods. Outcome research presents a unique challenge to the practitioner because it attempts to link the process of care (i.e., treatment or care) to outcome (e.g., improved functional status).

One of the monumental steps in the provision of quality care during the 20th century has been the paradigm shift begun in the industrial model of W.E. Deming (1986). A *paradigm* consists of rules, regulations, and attitudes involved in running an organization (Barker, 1989). Deming's model of Total Quality Management was adapted to healthcare organizations in the late 1980s. The National Demonstration Project on Quality Improvement in Health Care (Berwick, Godfrey, & Roessner, 1991) demonstrated that quality improvement principles and techniques could be modified and applied successfully to healthcare organizations. The continuous quality improvement movement, which is based on statistical control of variation, consists of three fundamental principles: customer satisfaction, participative management, and teamwork.

The critical element for any healthcare organization seems to be quality improvement, which has been demonstrated to lead directly to greater efficiency and cost reduction. Volumes have been written on the subject of quality healthcare improvement, yet, perhaps none speaks to the situation as well as *Restructuring Health Care: The Patient Focused Paradigm* (Lathrop, 1993) and *Total Quality in Healthcare: From Theory to Practice* (Gaucher & Coffey, 1993). *Restructuring Health Care* offers not only an analysis of the current healthcare model with its inefficient and ineffective delivery of care, but also presents a restructured model of patient-focused hospital care. As the 18th century author Voltaire once stated, "The world needs skeptics, not critics." The quality improvement movement will continue to have its share of both. *Total Quality in Healthcare,* classified by the authors as a how-to book, outlines a journey of implementing quality improvement in a large medical center. Futurist Joel Barker (1992) has stated that, for an organization to be successful in the future, the key elements of excellence, innovation, and anticipation must become an integral part of the culture (p. 12). Gaucher and Coffey (1993) demonstrated how these key elements can become a part of a health center's commitment to quality and the foundation for survival into the 21st century.

Change 5: Process Change (Modern Technology in Healthcare)

How does one describe the technological advances of the 20th century, especially as they relate to healthcare? Perhaps they can best be summed up by comparing the perspective of a centenarian to that of a 10-year-old at the beginning of the new millennium. For the child who has lived a brief 10 years of life, growing up in an automated, technologically sophisticated world, "modern inventions" are a part of life—not only the modern means of transportation and communication, but also the modern means of diagnosing and treating healthcare problems. The child, while eating a microwaved meal, can watch modern medicine performed nightly on television, where hospital scenes are common and accessible (search-and rescue programs are just one example).

The centenarian, on the other hand, can describe 100 years of a life filled with awestruck wonder. Imagine being able to relate first-hand the transitions that occurred in the world of automation; advances in transportation (from horse and buggy to automobile, airplane, and spaceship to the moon); the world of communication (telephone, television, answering machines, compact discs, and computers). The centenarian can also describe technological advances in the field of healthcare over his or her lifetime—the "wonder drugs" and costly devices we now take for granted. The centenarian can use familiar terms, so much a part of our world at the end of the 20th century, that were not a part of the healthcare system a mere 50 years ago—terms such as EKG (electrocardiogram), PET (positron emission tomography), CT (computerized tomography) and MRI (magnetic resonance imaging) that relate to sophisticated diagnostic equipment, or terms such as laparoscopy, angioplasty, and organ transplantation, related to remarkable advances in surgery. The list is infinite! Each of these technological advances represents an improvement in the way in which something was carried out in the past.

Consider, for example, the advances that computer technology, including both software and hardware, has brought to healthcare. Sophisticated information systems now exist that are an integral part of the data retrieval system used in the management of patients' medical records. It is now possible to maintain patients' records in a central database, to be tied together with all members of a healthcare system by way of voice systems and computerized telecommunications networks. A step beyond that includes the electronic information super-highways and community health information networks. These networks provide the potential to integrate multiple systems: hospitals, care providers in their offices and on clinical sites, payers, researchers, laboratories, and suppliers. Large central databases, such as FAMUS, the primary care project in Quebec, is collecting longitudinal data on 2000 patient visits per month. This information will be used to identify a risk register for cardiovascular disease and to determine the success of interventions based on clinical guidelines (Grant, Niyonsenga, & Bernier, 1994). It has been stated that the "rate of change in information systems technology is approaching exponential proportions" (DeLuca & Doyle, 1991, p. 1). This being so, it causes one to wonder what monumental changes will occur during the careers of today's graduating professionals.

Some of the advanced technology used in healthcare was initiated by the military in its ongoing preparation for the battlefield. Individual, handheld computers, with 6-inch, touchtype video screens, are expected to improve communications and information available to the soldier of the future. This equipment is being researched and tested by members of the U.S. Army, which plans to fully computerize at least part of an armored brigade by 1996 (Matthews, 1994). Such computers have unlimited potential for the advanced practice nurses (APNs) of the future as a means of communication linkage and storage of updated healthcare information.

The military is also investigating the use of telemedicine as part of battlefield medicine (LaNoue, 1994). *Telemedicine* is a form of remote clinical consultation system in which a clinical expert in the United States, for example, is linked with a care provider on the battlefield in a remote location. By way of computerized technology at both sites, the clinical consultant is able to provide direct guidance during treatment of casualties and surgical procedures. Identification of the casualties will be known instantly in the United States by way of a personal status monitor worn as part of each soldier's wristwatch. The monitor is then connected to a battlefield transmitter by medical corps personnel and the casualty information is instantly transmitted. If one has the creativity and vision to consider the potential of telemedicine for APNs, the ideas are unlimited. Visualize rural areas of care where an APN can connect with preceptors for clinical expertise in treatment of unusual cases. Perhaps the APN could link by way of telemedicine satellite to the National Library of Medicine in Bethesda, MD, or Library of Congress for article reprints. All, and more, is within the realm of possibility.

Yet, in the midst of all the technological advances in healthcare, some have spoken out regarding the appropriate use and inappropriate overuse of available technology. Although primarily referring to physicians, Cassell's (1993) comments apply to most healthcare practitioners. He questioned whether practitioners are running technology or if it is the other way around. Technologies frequently take on a life of their own and can be called on to fulfill the practitioner's need for certainty (in a professional world of frequent uncertainty); for control (in situations with patients in which conditions sometimes cannot be controlled); and for immediate answers. He has advised educators to teach practitioners "who are in themselves the primary instruments of diagnosis and treatment, to tolerate uncertainty, accept ambiguity, deal with the complete, and turn away from mere wonder" of modern technology (p. 39). Indeed, most of us can attest to the excitement generated by a new piece of technology when it first arrives in either a home setting or hospital. Along with the increased demand for what the technology can offer, it can also be the subject of abuse—too many unnecessary tests, too much time spent with the new piece of equipment and taken away from other activities, and so forth.

Summary of the Five Ps

Each of the five **P**s (**p**laces, **p**eople, **p**revention, **p**aradigm, and **p**rocess) exists as part of society's macroenvironment and will continue to affect open systems of healthcare. Furthermore, each of the five **P**s will continue to have a significant impact on the type of healthcare being delivered as well as the manner and place in which it is delivered. Most of the changing forces are beyond our ability to alter or control. So, then, the question arises: What difference does it make to the APN that these simultaneous forces are occurring in society? The most important point for us to remember is that we must change what is within our power to change: ourselves! We must change ourselves to adapt to the changing forces in the environment and the manner in which they affect our practice. Implications of change for APNs are critical and must be learned if we are to succeed, both personally and professionally. The remainder of this chapter provides suggestions for the way in which the APN can continue to work to adapt to the changing environment of healthcare.

IMPLICATIONS OF CHANGE FOR ADVANCED PRACTICE NURSES

Each individual must learn personal lessons if he or she is to survive healthcare reform and adapt to a changed environment. The intention of the discussion that follows is to serve as a stimulus for each APN to identify his or her own areas of needed change and to offer suggestions for the change.

Develop Survival Skills

First and foremost, it is essential to understand the changing environment and the effect it has on healthcare, in general, and specifically on the geographic area in which you practice. Keep an eye on the trends in the healthcare marketplace and stay ahead of the ever-changing horizon. If you have ever been on a ship headed toward the horizon, you realize you will never reach it—it always moves ahead of you. So, too, with the changing environment. Just when you think you have reached a point, you will find that something has changed. Individual strategies for succeeding in this type of environment must be mapped out and followed. This will include current and updated information from a variety of sources, such as readings, continuing education, and workshops.

A second survival skill is the ability to evaluate yourself and your individual reaction to change. What personal, emotional response to change do you notice (shock, denial, anger, bargaining?). All of these responses may, indeed, be normal, as long as they are time limited and you do not get "stuck" in a phase. "A tree that bends in the wind, doesn't break" is a Chinese proverb that expresses a timeless truth: to survive, you have to learn to be flexible, to bend in the wind, and to reset the sails in a storm. This can be accomplished by keeping a pulse on changes, anticipating them, and adapting to them. You may find that you have to let go of "sacred cows" in your effort to proactively plan for ways to change with the changing environment. It helps to be innovative and creative in reacting to the changes of society—to be able to do things differently from what was known before.

Practice What You Preach and What You Teach

Watch some of the health professionals you know, including yourself. We in healthcare spend many hours teaching people about ways to improve their health; but how much of the advice we give others do we actually follow ourselves? How well have you checked your lifestyle habits lately? What are your daily basic habits of eating, rest, sleeping, play time, stress management, and weight control? Do you have any addictive habits? It is especially necessary for health providers to be true exemplars and role models for others.

Become a Learner at Any Age

Never stop learning. There is an old proverb that states, "When you are through changing, you are through." Never be through! The times and technology will pass you by if you cease your ongoing learning. Be able to differentiate between memorizing facts and using critical thinking skills to exercise judgment and reason. To accomplish this, you must know what you need to learn by keeping abreast of general societal trends. Sometimes this may mean reading outside of your particular field to grasp the big picture. All too frequently, we find ourselves becoming narrow-minded and isolated in a small area of concern. It behooves us to keep our horizons broad. In addition to learning, you must use new knowledge, apply it to situations, and share it with others to make it stick in your mind. If at all possible, be a part of a learning organization (Senge, 1990), in which personnel are encouraged to keep their skills and knowledge updated. Be curious about what you do not know. Never stop asking why. Include areas such as healthcare financing and planning in your quest for new knowledge.

Keep Abreast of Technology

Selectively learn what you need to learn. Certainly, know the use of computers and how they will continue to be a part of our healthcare delivery system. It is essential that you keep your mind open to unlimited possibilities as you read about advancing technology. Frequently ask, How could I use that in my practice?

Be Politically Astute

So many changes in healthcare are part of an ongoing political process, yet many APNs are politically naive. You need to be extremely aware and informed of the political process and how it affects healthcare. Many people will choose to be politically active on a local, state, or national level. The more one knows about the political process, the more one tends to become involved; somewhat of a self-fulfilling prophecy. It becomes rewarding when APNs realize they not only can, but must, be politically involved to influence political changes in healthcare in the future.

Live Your Practice Standards

Know the practice standards for APNs and carry out the professional role accordingly. While doing so, there is the opportunity to demonstrate clinical outcomes with patients, to show that what you do makes a significant difference in the delivery of care and the functional outcome of the individual. Intuitively, many healthcare providers know they make a difference but fail to collect the data to portray their role to others in an objective, scientific manner. The demonstration of outcomes presents a wonderful opportunity for APNs to become increasingly involved in clinical research. A wealth of information has been generated over the years regarding the APN's role. But more research needs to be carried out in correlating the APN role with patient outcomes. How, by what we do in the process of healthcare (the provider–patient relationship of the APN and patient), can we demonstrate an improved patient outcome?

Avoid a "Victim" Identity

All too frequently one hears the "poor me" syndrome if something does not work out the way one wants it to work out. Take advantage of opportunities, get excited, move on physically and mentally, redesign your work, change your paradigm, and change your way of thinking if you are a negative thinker. If you get a lemon, seize the day and make lemonade!

Set Up an Individual Quality Improvement Program

Find something in yourself that needs to be changed and do it. Many times, this improvement may be in the realm of being a team player. Although many people belong to teams, they are not necessarily the most effective team members. How often do you recognize the good of others and show respect and appreciation? Or do you find yourself needing to criticize others? How often do you hold to your basic principles and standards when the easier route would be to go with the flow? We have within our power many ways to make life easier for ourselves and others with whom we work. It becomes a challenge to find the opportunities to improve. We have a choice; the choice to accept the challenge to improve is ours!

References

American Association of Retired Persons. (1992). *A profile of older Americans: 1992.* Washington, DC: Author.

Barker, J. A. (1989). *Discovering the future: The business of paradigms* (3rd ed.). St. Paul, MN: ILI Press.

Barker, J. A. (1992). *Future edge: Discovering the new paradigms of success.* New York: William Morrow.

Berwick, D. M., Godfrey, A. B., & Roessner, J. (1991). *Curing health care: New strategies for quality improvement.* San Francisco: Jossey-Bass.

Breslow, L. (1973). Quality and cost control: Medicare and beyond. In B.L.R. Smith & N. Hollander (Eds.), *The administration of Medicare: A shared responsibility* (pp. 17–44). Washington, DC: National Academy of Public Administration Foundation.

Bronstein, J. (1993). The partial hospitalization program: An alternative for acute psychiatric patients. *Stanford Nurse, 15*(2), 10–12.

Cassell, E. J. (1993). The sorcerer's broom: Medicine's rampant technology. *Hasting's Center Report, 23*(6), 32–39.

Cerne, F. (1994, June 5). Consumer choice could give big boost to assisted living. *Hospitals & Health Networks,* p. 72.

Covey, S. R. (1991). *Principle-centered leadership.* New York: Simon & Schuster.

Day, C., McFarlin, P., & Friel, S. (1993). Bridging the gap between hospital and home: Home care and case management. *Stanford Nurse, 15*(2), 3–5.

DeLuca, J. M., & Doyle, O. (1991). *Health care information systems: An executive's guide for successful management.* Chicago: American Hospital Publishing.

Deming, W.E. (1986). *Out of the crisis.* Cambridge, MA: Massachusetts Institute of Technology, Center for Advanced Engineering Study.

Dill, W.R. (1958). Environment as an influence on managerial autonomy. *Administrative Science Quarterly, 2,* 409–443.

Facts on File Yearbook, 1965 Index of World Events (1965). *Facts on File Yearbook, 25.* NY: Facts on File, Inc.

Fries, J. F. (1993). Reducing the need and demand. *Healthcare Forum Journal, 36*(6), 18–23.

Gaucher, E. J., & Coffey, R. J. (1993). *Total quality in healthcare: From theory to practice.* San Francisco: Jossey-Bass.

Grant, A., Niyonsenga, T., & Bernier, R. (1994). The role of medical informatics in health promotion and disease prevention. *Generations, 18*(1), 74–77.

Griffin, K. M. (1994). ISHA: Looking ahead. Working toward a seamless care continuum. *Transitions, 1*(1), 3.

Guterman, S., Eggers, P. W., Riley, G., Greene, T. F., & Terrell, S. A. (1988). The first 3 years of Medicare prospective payment: An overview (special report). *Health Care Financing Review, 9*(3), 67–77.

Hall, R. H. (1972). *Organizations: Structure and process.* Englewood Cliffs, NJ: Prentice-Hall.

Jackson, J. H., Morgan, C. P., & Paolillo, J.G.P. (1986). *Organization theory: A macro-perspective for management.* Englewood Cliffs, NJ: Prentice-Hall.

LaNoue, M. (1994, November). *Telemedicine as an agent of change.* Paper presented at the meeting of the Association of Military Surgeons of the U.S., Orlando, FL.

Lathrop, J. P. (1993). *Restructuring health care: The patient focused paradigm.* San Francisco: Jossey-Bass.

Matthews, W. (1994, August 29). Focus on technology: A grunt's "Grunt." *Army Times,* p. 32.

McDowell, T., & Brown, H. (1994). Integrated delivery systems: An introduction and case study. *Transitions, 1*(1), 9–15.

National Institute on Aging. (1987). *Personnel for health needs of the elderly through the year 2020* (NIH Publication No. 87-2950). Washington, DC: U.S. Government Printing Office.

Orlandi, M. O. (1987). Promoting health and preventing disease in health care settings: An analysis of barriers. *Preventive Medicine, 16,* 119–130.

Russell, L. B., & Manning, C. L. (1988). The effect of prospective payment on Medicare expenditures. *New England Journal of Medicine, 320*(7), 439–444.

Rovner, J. (1994). An interview with Uwe Reinhardt. *Modern Maturity, 37*(6), 64–72.

Safriet, B. J. (1992). Health care dollars and regulatory sense: The role of advanced practice nursing. *Yale Journal on Regulation, 9*(2), 417–485.

Scott, W. R. (1981). *Organizations: Rational, natural, and open systems.* Englewood Cliffs, NJ: Prentice-Hall.

Senge, P. M. (1990). *The fifth discipline: The art and practice of the learning organization.* New York: Doubleday.

Shugars, D. A., O'Neil, E. H., & Bader, J. D. (Eds.).(1991). *Healthy America: Practitioners for 2005: An agenda for U.S. health professional schools.* Durham, NC: Pew Health Professions Commission.

Smith, B.L.R., & Hollander, N. (Eds.). (1973). *The administration of Medicare: A shared responsibility.* Washington, DC: National Academy of Public Administration Foundation.

Taylor, R. B., Denham, J. W., & Ureda, J. R. (1982). Health promotion: A perspective. In R. B. Taylor, J. W. Denham, & J. R. Ureda (Eds.), *Health promotion: Principles and clinical applications* (pp. 1–18). Norwalk, CT: Appleton-Century-Crofts.

U.S. Bureau of the Census. (1993). *Statistical abstract of the United States, 1993* (113th ed.). Washington, DC: U.S. Government Printing Office.

U.S. Department of Health and Human Services, Public Health Service (1992). *Pressure ulcers in adults: Prediction and prevention.* (AHCPR Publication No. 92-0047). Washington, DC: Agency for Health Care Policy and Research.

U.S. Department of Health and Human Services, Public Health Service (1990). *Healthy people 2000: National health promotion and disease prevention objectives* (DHHS Publication No. PHS 91-50213). Washington, DC: U.S. Government Printing Office.

U.S. Department of Health and Human Services, Public Health Service (1980). *Promoting health/preventing disease: Objectives for the nation.* Washington, DC: U.S. Government Printing Office.

U.S. Department of Health, Education, and Welfare. (1979). *Healthy people: The surgeon general's report on health promotion and disease prevention.* Washington, DC: U.S. Government Printing Office.

U.S. Preventive Services Task Force. (1989). *Guide to clinical preventive services.* Baltimore, MD: Williams & Wilkins.

Wesbury, S. A. (1988). The future of health care: Changes and choices. *Nursing Economic$, 6*(2), 59–62.

Wolinsky, F. D. (1980). *The sociology of health: Principles, professions, and issues.* Boston: Little, Brown.

World Health Organization. (1985). *Handbook of resolutions and decisions of the World Health Assembly and the executive board.* Geneva: Author.

CHAPTER

7

Cultural and Ethnic Diversity: Cultural Competence

Angeline Bushy

COLORING OF AMERICA

Demographers have reported that the largest population increase in the United States is among people of all ages in minority groups of racial and ethnic origin. Some demographers have even forecast that white Anglo-Americans will be in the minority by the turn of the century. The changing complexion of American society has serious implications for healthcare providers in general and nurse practitioners in particular for planning, delivering, and evaluating services for target consumers: clients, patients, communities, and populations. People of color are an integral part of our national fabric, yet little is known about these and other underrepresented groups living in the United States (Coates, 1994; National Rural Health Association [NRHA], 1994; U.S. Bureau of the Census, 1991).

The literature is replete with citations describing diverse minority and vulnerable populations, as well as the concepts of multiculturalism, cultural awareness, cultural sensitivity, and cultural competency. Despite the national emphasis, the lifestyle and health beliefs of minorities within a community often remain foreign to caregivers who most often are of Anglo-American origins (Aamodt, 1976; Ailinger, 1985; Benedict, 1956; Bushy, 1992; Bushy & Rohr, 1990; Chance, 1966; Crowles, 1988, Dougherty, 1978, Dielu, 1982, Duffy, 1989; Fong, 1985; Leininger, 1984, 1985b; Mead, 1929; Princeton, 1988; Spradley, 1970, 1975; Tripp-Reimer, 1983; Turner, 1991; Wang, 1984; White, 1990).

The predominant racial minorities in the United States—African, Hispanic, Asian, Pacific Islander, Native, and Eskimo Americans—differ greatly in their social, political, and economic histories. Moreover, there are significant differences in their cultural beliefs, behavior norms, and the extent of their acculturation into mainstream American culture (i e , white, middle-class, and of Anglo-European descent). These differences also exist among other underrepresented subgroups who live, work, and seek healthcare from practi-

Hickey JV: ADVANCED PRACTICE NURSING: Changing Roles
and Clinical Applications © 1996 Lippincott–Raven Publisher

tioners in communities across the nation. Perhaps, for example, Anglo-American consumers have beliefs and lifestyles that appear quite unusual to practitioners of Anglo-American origin.

This chapter discusses the role of ethnocultural factors in an individual's perceptions of health, illness, and healthcare behaviors. The terms *multiculturalism, cultural awareness, cultural sensitivity,* and *cultural competency* are explored in relation to planning, delivering, and evaluating appropriate and acceptable healthcare to minority (i.e., underrepresented) groups. Included is historical content on self-care, folk remedies, and alternative healers. Strategies are presented that incorporate cultural factors to help nurse practitioners develop meaningful and appropriate treatment plans for culturally diverse patients.

PROFESSIONALLY UNDERSERVED COMMUNITIES

To provide care that is culturally appropriate and acceptable a subgroup requires that practitioners make an effort to define the community or population of interest. Some subgroups are easy to identify because they are isolated by a geographical boundary, biologic or racial features, lifestyle, attire, religion, political views, language, leisure activity, or occupation. For example, it is generally not difficult to identify an Amish or Mennonite county in a midwestern state or the Hispanic and Asian sections of a large city. However, other groups are not obviously bound in a given region or do not have a "distinct" lifestyle, such as Laotians, Vietnamese, Italians, Poles, Irish, Jehovah's Witnesses, Orthodox Jews, Latter-day Saints, Seventh-Day Adventists, smaller Native American Tribes, or Latinos of Cuban versus Filipino versus Mexican origin. Nonetheless, the perspectives of less noticeable groups are critical to providing appropriate and acceptable services for those consumers.

The problems associated with cultural insensitivity in the healthcare system are exacerbated because only a small percentage of individuals of minority origins enter the health professions, specifically as nurse practitioners. In addition to planning and delivering care, the cultural perspective also is not considered when measuring consumer satisfaction and acceptability of healthcare services for continuous quality improvement programs. This information deficit only serves to perpetuate a less than effective healthcare system because the services that are provided are neither appropriate nor acceptable to target consumers (Bushy, 1995).

APPROPRIATE AND ACCEPTABLE CARE

Available and accessible services do not equal appropriate and acceptable care. The terms *available* and *accessible* refer to services existing within a community, with an adequate number of professional healthcare providers to deliver those services at a reasonable cost to the consumer. The terms *acceptable* and *appropriate* infer that a particular service is offered in a manner that is congruent with the ethnocultural values of a target population. This means that the care is desirable and familiar to the person receiving it, and this preference often is based on ethnic and cultural factors.

Census data have revealed a number of health professional shortage areas in the United States that are most often found in the inner city and in rural counties (NRHA, 1994; U.S. Bureau of the Census, 1991; U.S. Department of Health and Human Services [DHHS], 1990). Underserved areas have been found to include a higher proportion of racial, ethnic, religious, and cultural minority populations. These vulnerable groups experience high levels of poverty, limited educational opportunities, poorer overall health status, and restricted access to professionals of similar cultural and racial backgrounds. It is laudable for nurse practitioners to establish a practice in an underserved area or with a minority population. However, that in and of itself may be not be sufficient to assure that underserved populations have access to healthcare.

Cultural preferences vis-à-vis cultural barriers is not a new concept to practitioners or a novel component of healthcare reform. Rather, the effects of cultural preferences have come into the forefront with recent epidemiologic reports that indicate the health status of minority groups is less than desirable. Inequities are especially evident when minorities are compared with middle-class Anglo-Americans. These epidemiologic findings are reinforced by the mandates put forth in *Healthy People 2000: National Health Promotion and Disease Prevention Objectives* (DHHS, 1990) that specifically target the special needs of vulnerable, minority populations across the United States.

The cultural factors that evoke consumer satisfaction go beyond appropriateness of dietary services, access to one's preferred pastoral care provider, or not offering an analgesic based on the belief that stoicism and suffering in silence are associated with the characteristic of machismo. Culture has been found to be a determinant in deciding the appropriate time to seek healthcare services and the manner in which to interact with a professional provider. Cultural values also influence a person's definition of health versus illness, choice of self-care behaviors, and perception of effective and ineffective caring behaviors (Bushy, 1992; Capra, 1983; Good & Good, 1986; Gums & Carson, 1987; Leininger 1969, 1978, 1985b; Reddick-Lynch, 1969; Simonson & Walker, 1988).

The following situations are other examples of cultural factors that may hamper acceptability of services:

- traditions of handling personal problems (e.g., self-care practices such as using over-the-counter medications, exercising, ingesting alcohol, resting, or praying)
- beliefs about the cause of a disorder and the appropriate healer for it (e.g, doctor, nurse practitioner, neighborhood nurse acquaintance, chiropractor, herbalist, community lay healer, medicine man, voodoo priestess, homeopathy, reikke [therapeutic touch], curandero, or shaman)
- lack of knowledge about a physical or emotional disorder and the place of formal services for preventing and treating the condition (e.g., being stoic and suffering in silence rather then seeking supportive care; paying for emergency care rather then spending money on health promotion or primary prevention; or expecting to receive a prescription, specifically an antibiotic or an analgesic, when paying to see the doctor or nurse practitioner)
- language barriers (e.g., English as a second language; functional illiteracy [reading below the 5th grade level—most healthcare literature is written at the 10th grade level or higher]; nonverbal [cultural] nuances associated with terminology that is used to educate about healthcare)
- difficulty in maintaining confidentiality and anonymity in a setting where many residents are acquainted
- cultural insensitivity by health professionals, particularly nurse practitioners; this insensitivity, coupled with the usual stress experienced by consumers when seeking care, especially publicly funded care, can further exacerbate mistrust of the healthcare system.

These situations reinforce the notion that even if a service is available and accessible, it may not be appropriate for individuals in a target population. Moreover, a consumer's evaluations of care-related services are usually rated as "satisfactory," "unsatisfactory," "acceptable," or "unacceptable." Subsequently, that rating often becomes a significant determinant in whether the person complies with prescribed treatment regimens or even uses a service that is readily available and accessible. Individual preferences ultimately can affect the overall health status of the consumer, his or her family, and the community as a whole. Ethnocultural data provide information about the target consumer's perceptions, attitudes, values, and expectations. The need for ethnocultural data is reinforced by the national agenda for healthcare reform that promotes more efficient use of existing resources, coupled with the increasing multicultural diversity in the U.S. population and consumers' mandate for care-givers who are culturally competent.

CULTURALLY COMPETENT CARE

Like other skills in the nurse practitioner's repertoire, cultural competency must be developed and refined. Before practitioners can become sensitive to and accommodate another's beliefs and values, however, they must first understand something about their own background. Practitioners must become aware of how their own cultural origins affect personal beliefs, behaviors, and ways of interacting with people on a professional and personal level. Of the many ways to reflect on one's circle of culture, making a personal assessment is probably the most popular. Questions in these self-appraisals tend to be similar, as follows (Yawn, Bushy, Dubbels, Pelage, & Hill, 1994).

How do you identify yourself in terms of race, ethnicity, religious or political beliefs, and socioeconomic class?

What has it meant to be part of that group?

Describe the customs or traditions in your family of origin that expressed your heritage.

What special foods, gifts, songs, and ceremonies were related to events such as birth, puberty, starting school, graduation, marriage, divorce, illness, hospitalization, and death?

How were feelings such as love and affection expressed in your family of origin?

How were feelings such as anger and sadness expressed?

What were the most valued and respected personal traits?

What has been the role of women and men in your family and culture?

How were decisions made? Who had the final say in those decisions?

What role was fate believed to play in a person's life?

How were time, work, leisure, health, and illness defined and valued?

What was your first experience with feeling different?

Reflecting and responding to these questions, first for oneself, and subsequently as they apply to a patient, is critical to a practitioner's developing awareness and sensitivity of the meaning of culture in everyday situations. Self-appraisal can help practitioners to understand people's personal expectations when they are ill and then compare those expectations with individual patients for whom they provide care. As with other problems practitioners encounter, an initial step in resolving cultural barriers to care is to recognize factors that prevent consumers from seeking care and following treatment plans (Leininger, 1978, 1984, 1985a, 1985b).

How can practitioners acquire ethnocultural knowledge about groups in a particular practice setting? It is difficult to learn about people who are not part of the community mainstream unless practitioners seek out subgroups. Consequently, one approach is for practitioners to become highly involved and subsumed in a community's social and political activities. Even with intense involvement, it is unlikely that an outsider will learn all the important cultural facts about a minority before making at least a few blunders. Rather, one learns gradually by working with patients in a community over time. Eventually, with a desire to learn, less obvious values and expectations become more obvious to the practitioner. For example, one becomes aware of and sensitive to consumers' manner of interacting with a health professional when seeking care and their self-care behaviors, folk remedies, and use of alternative healers (Agar, 1981; Boas, 1924; Filsted, 1970; Glasser & Strauss, 1967; Hartman, 1982; Johnson, 1990; Jorgenson, 1989; Kus, 1985; Langness, 1965; Langness & Frank, 1981; Pederson, 1988; Pelto & Pelto, 1979; Polit & Hungler, 1992; Rose, 1990; Spradley, 1979, 1980.)

Cultural awareness and sensitivity precede the development of cultural competence. This statement infers that practitioners have the ability to provide care that is appropriate and acceptable to a consumer, even though it is not part of their own belief system. The process of becoming culturally competent involves progressing from awareness and sensitivity to a more sophisticated understanding of the belief systems of minority individuals. This process requires a dedicated effort to learn about a minority's beliefs and lifestyle preferences by interacting with individuals in their environment and by consulting outside resources that provide additional information about their lifeways and belief systems (Bushy, Grassy, Kost, & Ramsdell, 1989; Capra, 1983; Fong, 1985; Simonson & Walker, 1988; Yawn et al., 1994).

ETHNOCULTURAL INFORMATION RESOURCES

The discipline of anthropology can be especially useful to practitioners desiring to glean information about a particular cultural or ethnic group. Not only is anthropologic information useful in the delivery of appropriate care but also for program planning and for measuring quality of and satisfaction with care. Practitioners can learn a great deal by studying the language, music, and customs of a defined group. With holistic group assessments, practitioners should also consider social structures, including religion, politics, economics, judicial system, kinship, education, and beliefs about the use or rejection of technology.

Of particular interest are a minority community's geographical setting, historical roots, natural resources, economic base, food preferences, art forms, folktales, myths, symbols, and rituals. For example, practitioners might read biographies and fiction or attend plays and movies presented from a specific group's point of view. These leisure activities can provide contextual information about a minority group to an interested outsider (Christy, 1975; Pederson, 1988; Reddick-Lynch, 1969; Shafer, 1974; Stanford, 1972; Thompson, 1989; Watson, 1979).

Individuals of a minority vary in the extent to which they exhibit or demonstrate political, religious, ethnic, racial, or cultural traits. For instance, with immigrants and refugees, the length of time they have been in the United States often makes a difference. Language barriers in both spoken and written communication can hinder an individual's assimilation into the major culture. Generational differences, too, influence the rate of assimilation in that younger generations generally assimilate more readily than do older community members. Economic status also is a factor, with poor people consistently displaying more ethnocentric behaviors.

It is important to keep in mind that the healthcare system, too, has a culture of its own. Culture, in this case, influences interactions between professionals as evidenced by the hierarchy of physicians, nurses, and technicians and the relationship between professionals and patient. Individuals at the top of the hierarchy function in a belief system defined by power and authority. Power, perceived or attributed, makes it difficult for individuals to ask questions unless specifically given permission to do so. Patients may choose not to ask for clarification on a pertinent issue related to the care they are receiving. This value is perpetuated by practitioners who inaccurately estimate what patients already know or understand as well as the clarity and appropriateness of their own explanations.

Nurse practitioners interested in reviewing or implementing research findings that focus on the culture of an underrepresented or vulnerable group are reminded that somewhat different approaches may be used for those kinds of studies. More familiar quantitative methodologies usually are associated with statistical analysis of surveys; experimental, quasi-experimental, or correlation studies; and epidemiologic reports. Studies using anthropologic methods, eliciting qualitative ethnocultural data, often obtain data by way of personal interviews using informants (i.e., subjects), community focus groups, ethnographies, oral histories, case studies, and information that is disseminated by the community's media sources (Polit & Hungler, 1992).

This is not to say that qualitative designs are better than quantitative, or vice versa. Rather, the two approaches yield complimentary information. Both are important to assess cultural beliefs accurately and measure the appropriateness of services from the consumer's perspective. For various reasons, qualitative methods are less likely to be in the nurse practitioner's repertoire. A comprehensive discussion on this issue is beyond the scope of this chapter. For more detailed information, the reader is encouraged to review citations included in the reference listing for this chapter.

As with any topic one wishes to learn more about, a literature review is an important step to determine what has or has not been written about a minority group. Not all information must be obtained from the professional literature. The popular media, including magazines such as *National Geographic* and *Newsweek,* plays, and television programs can be valuable resources for nurse practitioners regarding a particular group or an innovative program that has been implemented to meet the group's special needs. For example, a tertiary medical center plans to contract with the Indian Health Service to implement an alcohol treatment program for Native Americans, specifically the Chippewa Tribe. The innovative program will integrate traditional healing practices (e.g., participation of a tribal healer in the program, a sweat lodge, and other traditional rituals) with contemporary interventions (e.g., consumer-oriented education, psychotherapy, and group process). In this case, citations of probable interest to the practitioner include descriptions of similar programs for tribes in other geographical areas, histocultural reports on the Plains Indians, and general evaluation reports of other chemical dependency rehabilitation programs.

Popular literature in the past decade has featured articles describing innovative, cross-cultural programs that integrate traditional with contemporary healing practices. In brief, a review of the literature helps practitioners to build on the experiences of others and, it is hoped, to avoid some of the same pitfalls. A review of the literature also can provide background information on the ethnocultural perspective for measuring consumer satisfaction to determine if a program is appropriate and acceptable.

MULTICULTURAL PLANNING AND EVALUATION MODELS

Planning and evaluation models of healthcare that strictly lend themselves to the dominant (Anglo-European) culture no longer are acceptable. Such approaches do not work equally well for all groups and all individuals, at all times and in all situations. If consumers are expected to assume a greater role in their healthcare, planning and evaluation models must incorporate processes that consider consumers' ethnocultural bent.

To this end, anthropology, grounded theory, phenomenology, and other qualitative methodologies can be useful. Gradually the multidimensional data begin to tell an interested outsider, in this case the nurse practitioner, the minority group's story. Sometimes cultural competence may not be mandatory but may be helpful in planning and evaluating services that target consumers find appropriate and acceptable. At other times, the lack of cultural competence will doom a program to failure. For example, a group of primary care providers is deciding whether to add two outreach family planning clinics to their services; if implemented, how can services be appropriate and acceptable to each community? One of the proposed practice sites is located in a predominately Mexican-American community with a high percentage of migrant workers. The other proposed site is the student health center of a large university with more than 50,000 full-time students. The following questions should be asked in relation to both of the clinics.

What is the meaning of pregnancy to the group?

What are the community's predominant religious denominations and community members' theological positions regarding birth control, family planning, and pregnancy?

What are their beliefs, values, and perceptions about public support for family planning clinics?

What is the local fertility rate? Maternal–infant mortality rate? Adolescent pregnancy rate?

How is an unplanned pregnancy viewed by the "typical" family? A burden? A blessing? A fulfillment of assigned gender roles?

How are male and female gender roles defined?

What, if any, reproductive health concepts are included in the health curricula of local schools? Who is responsible for teaching the courses? What is the instructor's background?

What are the use patterns for accessing services, particularly obstetric providers?

What are their perceived barriers to accessing existing family planning services including the public health clinic; physicians (e.g., family practice physician versus obstetrician); and alternative care providers (e.g., midwife, nurse practitioner, physician assistant, or endogenous healer)?

Program planners may find the responses to these questions to be completely different because of demographic and cultural differences in the target community (Bushy, 1995; Yawn et al., 1994). The findings have definite implications in planning, delivering, and evaluating family planning services at each site. Once implemented, practitioners' increased cultural awareness and sensitivity will help to explain puzzling or annoying differences among individuals within the context of a particular health-related behavior. In turn, meaningful ethnocultural data will enable practitioners to plan, develop, and evaluate treatment plans that mesh with patient preferences.

CULTURE, SELF-CARE, FOLK REMEDIES, AND ALTERNATIVE HEALERS

In addition to seeking healthcare from professional practitioners, people who develop a problem can obtain relief in a number of ways, including using self-care with its folk remedies and ᴠice from alternative healers. The resources and the rationale for those behaviors ᴇpending on cultural, socioeconomic, environmental, geographical, and religious ᴄtors. Even so, self-care, folk medicine, and alternative healers have a strong his-ᴛhat is common across cultures. Knowledge about this phenomenon can provide ᴤ about modern self-care practices, and historical citations can offer a frame of ᴩractitioners about a minority person's health beliefs. Information of this nature is ᴉent of holistic and culturally competent care (Bricklin, 1982; Campbell, 1972; Copland, 1924; Evans, Magan, & Thompson, 1923; Fong, 1985; Gums & ; Hand, 1976; Heinerman, 1982; Kennett, 1976; Kidder, 1994; Levin, 1975; Robertson, 1987; Salmon, 1984; Thomas, 1988; Whealan, 1983; Whorton, ᴉs, 1994).

have always found life to be hard and filled with numerous stresses. Illness was a rrence for our ancestors but, unlike us, they did not have medical doctors to treat ᴀses of illness they relied on self-care practices that integrated ritualistic behaviors products. Remedies varied by geographical regions. Many of these practices had ᴏnes, which incorporated myth with the ritualistic use of objects from the environ-ᴀnimals or their body parts, plants, herbs, or personal belongings. Rituals, believed ᴇmedy's effectiveness, usually involved repetitious behaviors, such as dancing, ᴤaging with ointments, or ingesting the product in a carefully prescribed manner. ᴍore complicated and severe the disease, the more complex and ritualistic was ᴛeat it. This was especially true of treatments for communicable diseases for ᴠas no known effective cure, such as smallpox, venereal disease, tuberculosis, ᴦh, plague, cholera, cancer, and rabies. Over time, the name of a product may however, the products and rituals have remained the same for generations. ᴊlly, caring for the sick was usually a task assigned to women and some became with healing skills. Even the smallest tribes and communities had a well-and experienced midwives. The terms for *healer*—for example, *brauchfrua, curandara*—were based on the language and culture of a group. Before the advent of specialized social functions, care of the sick was an individual and family responsibility. In socially and geographically isolated communities, folk medicine and good neighbors were the traditional means of treating the ill. Today this is referred to as a "social support system"(Bushy, 1992; Bushy et al., 1989).

Religion and healing have long been interrelated. Likewise, good health and healing have often been associated with being in God's grace, ridding the body of bad spirits, or suffering in this world for one's wrongdoings. This belief system probably evolved from European priests well versed in demonology, who provided treatment for the sick. Over the centuries, religious leaders have played an important role in perpetuating the belief that headaches, mental illness, epilepsy, and birth defects are the result of God's wrath or demonic possession. Modern faith healers are just as readily accessible, through the television set. Moreover, many people contribute financially to those particular faith healers to maintain or restore good health for themselves or family members.

Common-folk have always had great respect for healers, often believing them to be God's representatives. Thus, when a family hired a healer to treat a family member, it was done to cast out evil spirits, make amends with God, and rid the patient of an illness. Based on repeated observations of sick people, healers gained knowledge about the patterns and symptoms of an illness as well as effective and ineffective interventions for that condition.

Traditionally, most families have had a healing authority; usually this was a grandmother, aunt, or uncle with acknowledged healing skills. With the increase in the size of communities, the task of healing was eventually assigned or relinquished to specialized resources, hence the evolution of witch doctors, healers, medicine men and women, priests, shamans, physicians, nurse practitioners, and hospitals. Community members never doubted that the community healer had the power to restore health to their sick. Like the contemporary practitioner, a healer's reputation was at stake when providing services to patients. If healing did not progress in an expected manner, the healer was likely to be declared a "witch" by the community at large. Likewise, contemporaries recognize that a satisfied customer's word-of-mouth reports are the most effective marketing strategy to recruit other patients.

For posterity, healers transmitted through the oral and written word remedies they believed were effective. Thus, the healer entrusted healing secrets to subsequent generations. With the advent of the printing press, books of popular and not so well known remedies were published and made available for public use. The *Doctor Book* was a comprehensive source of information for the prevention, treatment, and curing of ailments. A more expensive *Doctor Book* included two additional chapters, one focusing on reproductive health conditions in women and another on remedies for veterinary purposes.

Our ancestors were resourceful when it came to their healthcare. For instance, because the *Doctor Book* was expensive and money was scarce, several neighbors shared in the cost of purchasing the book. Then, when someone in the family became sick, a family member was dispatched to obtain the book from the neighbor who had most recently consulted it. Interestingly, the neighbors generally knew who had the book at any given time. To avoid traveling in an emergency, particularly in the winter, someone in the family who could read and write (often a female) would copy in the family's Bible or cookbook those suggestions believed to be most useful in an emergency.

In recent years, as part of local celebrations, groups typically comprising women (e.g., church circles, homemakers clubs, and women's clubs) have compiled community cookbooks. It is not unusual to find at the end of these books several pages of "time-tested" family remedies. Practitioners might want to find such books, which are another source of background information about a minority community.

Contemporaries are beginning to understand that emotions play an important role in healing and the body's ability to restore and maintain health. Now, as in historic times, the mind-over-body connection probably contributes to a healer's success. Yet, folk remedies and self-care originated and have remained popular because of
- a lack of available, accessible, affordable, and acceptable healthcare
- limited knowledge about body function and the disease process
- the reported effectiveness of a specific treatment by the highly regarded family healer.

Self-care is as old as humankind; therefore, it should be viewed as a healthcare resource. More than ever, especially with healthcare reform, society is relying on the individual and family to assume a significant role in their own care. Nurse practitioners must assume that most people, including health professionals, use self-care and folk medicine at some time in their lives. They may use more self-care remedies when they perceive themselves to be unhealthy or sick.

Furthermore, practitioners should be aware that it is not unusual for patients to use veterinary supplies for self-care, particularly antibiotics and ointments for skin and muscle conditions. Traditionally, for many families, domestic animals were of great financial value and a source of livelihood. Because a remedy was safe for humans, the treatment also was deemed appropriate for animals having similar conditions. However, modern science and the Food and Drug Administration (FDA) have reversed the priorities; that is, products are tested for safety first on animals before they are made available to consumers.

Even though self-care and folk medicine may seem inconsistent with scientific knowledge, without such practices any system of healthcare would be swamped. For many people, the major distinction between care provided by healthcare professionals and self-care is the remuneration factor. Practitioners may find self-care practices ridiculous, yet well-educated consumers continue to engage in those practices (Hamburg, 1994; Miller, 1994). According to national news reports, in 1990 alone, Americans spent more than $27 million on health-related products. In 1993, an estimated 38 million people tried one or more self-care products. The FDA speculated that 1 in 10 Americans suffers side effects from self-care treatments. The most profitable self-care products are arthritis remedies; spurious cancer clinics; cures for acquired immunodeficiency syndrome; weight-loss schemes; sex stimulants; baldness remedies; nutritional cure-alls; muscle stimulators (legitimate in many cases, but they do not get rid of wrinkles); treatment for "women's problems" such as premenstrual syndrome (PMS); remedies for hypoglycemia; remedies for generalized yeast infections; and feminine hygiene products. In essence, self-care, folk healing, and alternative providers must be considered by practitioners as integral to professional treatment plans, even if these self-care interventions are not formally acknowledged by the consumer.

Self-care continues to be used for health promotion, disease prevention, illness detection, and treatment of symptoms and encompasses a continuum of activities to retain and restore health. Health promotion focuses on wellness "approach" behaviors, primary prevention involves illness "avoidance" behaviors to prevent or ward off an ailment, and illness treatments usually focus on symptom management or curing the condition.

LEVELS AND CATEGORIES OF FOLK REMEDIES

Self-care should be viewed from two levels; personal health behavior skills and sociopolitical skills. Both levels contribute to individual and family well-being. Personal self-care skills are those used to maintain or restore an individual's health. Sociopolitical skills are inherent in the self-care used by a community or a family to treat unusual conditions that occur in its members, particularly physical and emotional consequences related to social and developmental transitions.

The literature has described three major categories of folk remedies that are used across all cultures: folk remedies that are used to prevent or treat short-term conditions, chronic incurable conditions, and psychosomatic conditions. "Well-informed" contemporaries continue to use variations of these remedies, as is evidenced by the continued popularity of literature available in supermarkets, bookstores, and convenience stores.

Remedies in the first category are used to prevent or treat undesired physical symptoms or short-term or self-limiting conditions. These remedies include vitamins; minerals; food supplements for body or muscle building; remedies for warts, cold sores, minor menstrual problems, muscle aches, constipation, diarrhea, indigestion, hay fever, "growing pains," sore throats, ingrown toenails, colds, influenza, nosebleeds, insect bites, impetigo, hiccups, bumps, bruises, pimples, rashes, colic, dandruff, enureses, ringworm, "jock itch," and athlete's foot; as well as childrearing advice and first aid for common emergencies. Many of these common conditions are the focus of advertisements for an ever-increasing number of over-the-counter medications used by the public.

Remedies in the second category are used to prevent or treat chronic and incurable conditions including arthritis, hypertension, allergies, weight gain, weight loss, baldness, asthma, ulcers, gallbladder problems, impotence, infertility, sinusitis, and chronic pain, especially of the back. These conditions vary in severity depending on weather, stress, diet, and physical activity. It is not unusual, however, for consumers to attribute improvement of the problem to a certain product they used during that particular interval.

Remedies in the third category are used to prevent or treat complex conditions that often are emotional, psychosomatic, or nervous in origin, including persistent skin conditions (e.g., psoriasis, eczema, or hives); stomach ulcers, severe persistent menstrual cramps, endometriosis, migraine headaches, seizures, insomnia, neurosis, and psychosis. "Nervous" conditions have been more difficult to treat and usually are long term. Interventions for those conditions historically have been directed "at" the victim and have included praying over the victim as well as physical abuse and torture through chaining, imprisonment, and shunning. Often the treatment is extended to members of the patient's family. The stigma associated with mental illness is an ongoing consequence of those interventions.

UNIVERSALITY OF FOLK HEALING RITUALS

Some remedies and rituals are common to a number of cultures including unusual occurrences in nature, select human behaviors, and touch (Capra, 1983; Fong, 1985; Gums & Carson, 1987; Hand, 1976; Kennett, 1976; Kidder, 1994; Levin, 1975; NRHA, 1994; Robertson, 1987; Stanford, 1972; Thompson, 1989).

Unusual Occurrences in Nature

Unusual occurrences in nature include eclipse, position of the moon with earth or other planets, prolonged weather patterns, severe storms, and circumstantial events in daily life, all of which have been given spiritual connotations. In some cultures, these occurrences are believed to affect health or healing. More significant events are viewed as a message from God or one's spiritual guides, or as omens.

Circumstantial events can also serve as a guide for childrearing and may play a role in life decisions such as the appropriate time to marry, procreate, bury a loved one, or plant a crop. For example, an old, partially intact family Bible included the following handwritten notation: "Proper weaning is done when the moon is in a zodiac sign that does not rule a vital organ—Aquarius, Pisces, Sagittarius, and Capricorn." Note the similarities between this remedy and the astrological advice given in a daily newspaper. The contemporary practitioner still encounters individuals with these beliefs, such as minorities who practice voodoo and witchcraft and underrepresented groups who have a particular religious bent.

Select Human Behaviors

Another universally held folk belief is the concept of the curse, or "evil eye." This occurs when a "spell maker" stares at another person who, in turn, believes that he or she has been cursed by the spell maker. It becomes a grave problem when the spell is cast on a child, because the family believes misfortune will follow this youngster.

The antidote to this imposed fate varies but often involves a ritual of anointing the cursed individual with the saliva (spit) of the spell maker. Other rituals that people believe will improve health or ward off misfortune and illness include wearing an amulet or stones or colored crystals, carrying a rabbit's foot or lucky charm, wearing a select piece of clothing, or wearing an item that has religious significance (e.g., crucifixes, medals of religious figures, or scapulars and other garments).

Touch as a Therapy

Touch is another universal component of self-care and healing rituals. Touching rituals can involve various body parts of the healer as well as the person being healed. Touch also has symbolic or metaphorical connotations, hence the rationale for an old practice that involves touching the possession of an ill person or a blessed person.

A common theme in folk healing is that certain people have a magical, God-given healing touch. For example, people of royal birth, those exhibiting unusual (bizarre) behaviors, and those having a distinguishing physical characteristic such as a birthmark or physical anomaly often are believed to have a magical or healing touch. Consequently, individuals having the "blessed touch" are sought by a community or family to treat sick members.

A popular ritual used by these blessed individuals is to suck on an afflicted body part to draw out evil. Bloodletting is a variation of this theme, as are several popular remedies for the common cold, such as placing an onion pack on the feet to draw out a cold or putting a mustard plaster on the chest to draw out germs and irritants that cause a person to cough. These remedies may seem antiquated but some patients still espouse the curative powers of liniment, goose grease, onion packs, mustard plasters, or petroleum jelly. Some people also believe the practice of rubbing a mentholated ointment on the chest and feet of a person with a cold is more effective when the sick person also ingests a small dab of the ointment. Also, they believe putting a little of the salve into a hot steamer helps to clean the air and helps the sick person's breathing.

Touch continues to be an important part of healing by contemporary health professionals. There has been a resurgence in research on the relationship between touch and caring and curing. A proposed explanation is that touch promotes the generation of chemicals in the body's immune system, thereby promoting healing. Examples of therapeutic touch in which nurse practitioners engage are the "rituals" of a routine physical examination: taking vital signs, checking the height of a fundus, providing comfort measures in the form of a back rub administered to an elderly person, therapeutic massage, hugging a child after giving the child an intramuscular injection, touching the hand of a grieving person to demonstrate empathy or support, or initiating pet therapy for a lonely patient.

The list in Box 7-1 includes other commonly used folk remedies popular in many cultures. Most practitioners will at some time encounter one or more of these remedies in their practice. However, researchers frequently cannot explain how and why folk remedies work. In recent years, scientists have found several long-standing remedies to be effective. Practitioners of modern medicine continue to use a few of these remedies to treat diseases. Even so, the treatments were used centuries before people could explain how the body responded to an intervention. For example, the remedy of placing a spider web on a wound to enhance the clotting process and help stop bleeding was used centuries before physiologists identified the clotting mechanisms of the blood. People ate rose hips for generations to help them stay healthy long before biochemists recognized the importance of vitamin C in the diet.

Many popular and universal remedies still do not have physiologic explanations, including wearing copper bracelets to help reduce arthritic pain, ingesting garlic to reduce high blood pressure and prevent upper respiratory infections, or drinking aloe vera or applying it to affected body parts for a medicinal effect. Still, people who use these treatments typically are convinced of their effectiveness. For this reason, practitioners need to be aware that disapproval of those practices will do little to deter the patient from continuing to engage in them.

CONTEMPORARY SELF-CARE PRACTICES

Despite the increased availability of healthcare services and professionals in the 20th century, self-care continues to be popular, partly because of the high cost of healthcare and the inherent skills of human survival and partly because consumers lack faith in the effectiveness of the healthcare system. The consumer movement has created a receptive audience for the distribution of a wide range of self-care literature, at-home diagnostic devices, and the ever-increasing number of over-the-counter medications.

BOX 7.1   COMMONLY USED FOLK REMEDIES

For Burns
Scald milk and moisten a piece of bread in it. Squeeze out the excess moisture and place
　　bread on the burned area.
Place sliced raw potato on the burned area.

For Boils
Cover a boil with axle grease three or four times a day.
Cover the boil with a piece of adhesive tape for 24 hours, then remove the tape—the core
　　will stick to the tape.
Make a poultice with camomile tea and apply three to four times a day to the lesion until it
　　comes to a head and drains.

For Digestive/Alimentary Problems
For an upset stomach and nausea, drink fresh ginger tea.
For treating and preventing ulcers, eat fresh cabbage.
For hemorrhoids, apply witch hazel packs.

For Babies With Colic
Administer fennel tea.

To Stimulate a Baby's Appetite for Breast Milk
Eat fresh garlic 1 hour before breastfeeding.

For Feminine Itching
Bathe with vinegar, ginger, salt, or baking soda.

For Smallpox
Carry an onion in your pocket.

For the Prevention of Childhood Colds
With breakfast, give your children two cherry flavored vitamin C tablets every day. Take an
　　extra tablet in winter.

For the Treatment of Menstrual Problems (PMS)
Take at least one tablet of each of the following daily: dolomite, multiple vitamins with iron,
　　vitamin B_6, vitamin E, magnesium, and evening primrose oil.

For the Regulation of Blood Pressure
Take two or three garlic tablets every day and reduce salt intake.

Several contemporary self-care publications were first printed around the turn of the 20th
century; they probably evolved from the practice of updating early *Doctor Books*. These popular magazines still are available at many newsstands, and based on their widespread distribution, one can assume that modern consumers still are interested in the content. The content in
these self-care publications includes nutrition, over-the-counter medications, illness diagnosis,
treatment for health problems, and symptom management. The publications prescribe the
most advantageous ways to use a variety of naturally occurring resources, such as teas, herbs,
fruits, and vegetables. In each issue, one may find numerous advertisements informing readers
how to purchase a particular remedy discussed within. Some of the products are proven "fad-
scams." Most, however, have never been validated as either effective or ineffective, despite
the prolonged popularity of the product.

In light of the widespread use of self-care and folk remedies, practitioners must be sensitive to patients' alternative conceptions of causation and remediation of illness.

IMPLICATIONS FOR NURSE PRACTITIONERS

Health professionals in general and practitioners in particular must accept that self-care, in many instances, may be an effective therapy. Because of ethnic diversity, many Americans use a wide range of therapeutic systems as alternatives to conventional medicine. In addition to those described in this chapter, some of the more popular remedies are psychic healing, Rolfing, chiropractic care, faith healing, therapeutic massage, osteopathy, meditation, and visualization. Perhaps a user's belief in nontraditional modalities contributes to their effectiveness.

Even though practitioners of conventional western medicine may not formally acknowledge self-care and, in many instances, may deny its effectiveness, they must recognize self-care as a significant aspect of primary healthcare. Self-care interventions, however, may interfere with or actually be detrimental to the individual. For this reason, practitioners must become informed of the fine line between folk medicine and scientifically based healthcare; but differentiating the two can become problematic in some cases.

To elicit information about a patient's use of self-care and folk remedies, practitioners must learn to tactfully ask pertinent questions during assessment. Practitioners then summarize this information in the patient's database and integrate the information into the patient's care plan for effective, appropriate, and acceptable education (Leininger 1985a, 1985b; Pelto & Pelto, 1979; Spradley, 1979; Sudman & Bradburn, 1983). Questioning by caregivers must always be nonjudgmental, and include the following:

Does the patient rely on self-care or traditional folk practices? If so, what are they?

Which remedies does the patient use for health promotion? Disease prevention? Illness intervention?

Is the patient currently being treated by a cultural healer? If so, is he or she willing to share information about the nontraditional interventions?

Does the patient prefer having a cultural healer as a part of the traditional healthcare plan? If so, who is this healer and how can this individual be contacted?

Are there certain individuals or relatives the patient wishes to have present during treatment? What role are they to take during the healing process?

Should a patient's belief system include folk remedies such as drinking herb tea, eating certain foods, using natural products, or using over-the-counter drugs, practitioners should respect these beliefs. Respect, however, does not require negating the use of scientifically based treatments. Instead, it means assessing the benefits and risks of a remedy. Then, if appropriate, incorporate the self-care as an adjunct to prescribed scientific interventions.

Nurse practitioners must be sensitive to the fact that when they present scientific knowledge that appears incompatible with a patient's traditional beliefs, the patient probably will accept the traditional way and reject the best health information. Nurse practitioners likely can anticipate noncompliance behaviors on the part of these patients. Taking time to have the patient explain, in his or her own words, the treatment plan and how to take any prescribed medicines can go a long way toward improving practitioner–patient communication. Such explanation can also alert the practitioner to cultural beliefs and values that could promote or hinder patient compliance with prescribed regimens. Practitioners demonstrate an even greater measure of cultural competency by asking a patient for his or her point of view. This approach supports collaborating with the person rather than imposing a treatment plan, although it is initially time consuming. A collaborative approach can prevent many follow-up phone calls or office visits due to misunderstood treatment protocols.

Practitioners can learn a great deal about effective patient teaching from consumer-oriented, self-care publications. Congruency between traditional beliefs and an emphasis on measures to promote health and prevent illness partially accounts for the success of self-care magazines. The information in such publications is typically presented in a clear, concise manner, making sense to the readers. Even though the logic may lack scientific accuracy, the content has an element of truth to it. Essentially, the "new" information expands on what most consumers already know about a particular topic. This marketing approach is highly effective for promoting a particular product or remedy. Collaborative efforts on the part of practitioners to integrate self-care with scientifically based intervention encourage compliance behaviors, especially if the remedy is not detrimental and will not compromise the patient's therapeutic regimen. Instead of negating culturally based folk remedies and implementing a totally unfamiliar regimen, practitioners should consider the highly effective strategy used by popular self-care magazines. Allow the patient something that is culturally familiar, such as folk remedies and self-care behaviors. As a result, the consumer is apt to adhere more closely to the scientifically based therapeutic regimen and perceive the care that he or she is receiving as appropriate and acceptable.

Overall, cultural competency is one of the most important elements of providing holistic nursing care to patients in this culturally diverse country. With that in mind, nurse practitioners must always be aware of, and sensitive to, the role of ethnocultural factors in an individual's perceptions of health, illness, and healthcare behaviors. Cultural competency is reflected by the coordination of a meaningful and appropriate treatment plan. Cultural competency is also an important factor in planning, delivering, and evaluating appropriate and acceptable healthcare for patients, especially those of minority origins.

References

Aamodt, A. (1976). Observations of a health and healing system in a Papago community. In M. Leininger (Ed.), *Transcultural health issues and conditions for health care dimensions*. Philadelphia: F.A. Davis.

Agar, M. (1981). *The professional stranger: An informal ethnography*. New York: Academic Press.

Ailinger, R. (1985). Beliefs about treatment of hypertension among Hispanic older persons. *Topics in Clinical Nursing, 7*(3), 26–31.

Benedict, R. (1956). *The chrysanthemum and the sword*. Boston: Boston Press.

Boas, F. (1924). The methods of ethnology. *American Anthropologist, 22,* 311–321.

Bricklin, M. (1982). *Rodale's encyclopedia of natural home remedies*. Emmaus, PA: Rodale Press.

Bushy, A. (1992). Cultural considerations in health promotion: Where does self-care and folk medicine fit? *Holistic Nursing Practice, 6*(3), 10–18.

Bushy, A. (1995). Ethno-cultural sensitivity and measurement of consumer satisfaction. *Journal of Nursing Care Quality, 9*(2), 16-–25.

Bushy, A., Grassy, B., Kost, S., & Ramsdell, K. (1989). *Folk medicine on the prairie*. Bismarck, ND: Medcenter One.

Bushy, A., & Rohr, K. (1990). The Plains Indians: Cultural considerations in the use of fetal monitors. *NeoNatal Network, 8*(4), 1–6.

Campbell, J. (1972). *Myths to live by*. New York: Bantam Books.

Capra, F. (1983). *The turning point*. New York: Bantom Books.

Chance, N. (1966). *The Eskimo of North Alaska*. New York: Holt, Rinehart & Winston.

Christy, T. (1975). The methodology of historical research. *Nursing Research, 24*(3), 189–192.

Coates, J. (1994). The highly probable future: 83 assumptions by the year 2025. *The Futurist, 28*(4), 29–38.

Copland, R. (1924). *The health book*. Cleveland, OH: Press of the Commercial Bookbinding.

Cowles, K. (1988). Personal world expansion for survivors of murder victims. *Western Journal of Nursing Research, 10*(2), 163–180.

Dougherty, M. (1978). Becoming a woman in rural black culture. New York: Holt, Rinehart & Winston.

Drehr, W. (1982). *Working men of Ganja*. Philadelphia: Institute of Human Issues.

Duffy, M. (1989). The primary support received by recently divorced mothers. *Western Journal of Nursing Research, 11*(6), 676–693.

Evans, N., Magan, P., & Thompson, G. (1923). *The home physician: A guide to health*. Omaha, NE: Pacific Press Publishing Association.

Filsted, W. (Ed.). (1970). *Qualitative methodology*. Chicago: Markam.

Fong, C. (1985). Ethnicity and nursing practice. *Topics in Clinical Nursing, 7*(3), 1–11.

Glasser, B., & Strauss, A. (1967). *The discovery of grounded theory: Strategies for qualitative research*. Chicago: Aldine.

Good, B., & Good, M.D. (Eds.). (1986). *Mental health research and practice: Development of culturally sensi-*

tive training programs. Rockville, MD: National Institute of Mental Health/U.S. Department of Health and Human Services.

Gums, J., & Carson, D. (1987). Influence of folk medicine on the family practitioner. *Southern Medical Journal, 80*(2), 209–212.

Hamburg, J. (1994, July 31). Can home remedies work? *Parade Magazine,* pp. 4–5.

Hand, W. (1976). *American folk medicine.* Berkeley: University of California Press.

Hartman, D. (Ed.). (1982). *New directions for methodology of social and behavioral sciences: Using observers to study behavior.* San Francisco: Jossey-Bass.

Heinerman, J. (1982). *Aloe vera, jojoba, and yucca.* New Canaan, PA: Keats Publishing.

Johnson, J. (1990). *Selecting ethnographic informants.* Newbury Park CA: Sage Publications.

Jorgensen, D. (1989). *Participant observation: A methodology for human studies.* Newbury Park, CA: Sage Publications.

Kennett, F. (1976). *Folk medicine: Fact and fiction.* New York: Crown Publishers.

Kidder, R. (1994). Universal human values: Finding an ethical common ground. *The Futurist, 28*(4), 8–14.

Kus, R. (1985). Stages of coming out: An ethnographic approach. *Western Journal of Nursing Research, 7*(2), 177–194.

Langness, L. (1965). *The life history in anthropologic science: Series of studies in anthropologic method.* New York: Holt, Rinehart & Winston.

Langness, L., & Frank, G. (1981). *Lives: An anthropologic approach to biography.* Novato, CA: Chandler and Sharp Publisher.

Leininger, M. (1969). Ethnoscience: A new and promising research approach for the health sciences. *Image, 3*(1), 2–8.

Leininger, M. (1978). *Transcultural nursing: Concepts, theories, and practices.* New York: John Wiley & Sons.

Leininger, M. (1984). *Ethnohealth, ethnocareing and eth-nonursing of six cultures.* Detroit, MI: Wayne State University Press.

Leininger, M. (Ed.). (1985a). *Qualitative research methods in nursing.* New York: Grune & Stratton.

Leininger, M. (1985b). *Transcultural care diversity and universality: A theory of nursing.* Thorofare, NJ: Charles B. Slack.

Levin, L. (1975). The lay person as the primary health care practitioner. *Public Health Reports, 91*(3), 206–210.

Mead, M. (1929). *Coming of age in Samoa.* New York: New American Library.

Meyer, C. (1973). *American folk medicine.* New York: The American Library.

Miller, L. (1994, August 1). Non-traditional medical options: U.S. spends $13 million on studies. *USA Today,* p. D1.

National Rural Health Association. (1994). *Proceedings of the National Rural Health Association Conference on Minority Health: A shared vision, building bridges for rural health access.* Kansas City, MO: Author.

Pederson, P. (1988). *A handbook for developing multicultural awareness.* Chicago, IL: American Association of Counseling and Development.

Pelto, P., & Pelto, G. (1979). *Anthropologic research.* New York: Harper & Row.

Polit, D., & Hungler, B. (1992). *Nursing research: Principles and methods.* Philadelphia: J.B. Lippincott.

Princeton, J. (1988). A diphtheria epidemic in a religious sect: An anthropologic assessment. *Medical Anthropology Quarterly, 2*(1), 76–92.

Reddick-Lynch, L. (1969). *The cross cultural approach to health behavior.* Rutherford, NJ: Fairleigh Dickinson University Press.

Robertson, M. (1987). Home remedies: A cultural study. *Home Health Care, 5*(1), 35–40.

Rose, D. (1990). *Living the ethnographic life.* Newbury Park, CA: Sage Publications.

Salmon, W. (1984). *Alternative medicines.* New York: Tavistock Publishers.

Shafer, R. (1974). *A guide to historical method.* Homewood, IL: Dorsey.

Simonson, R., & Walker, S. (1988). *Multicultural literacy: Opening the American mind.* Ellensburg, WA: Greywolf Press.

Spradley, J. (1970). *You owe yourself a drunk.* Boston: Little, Brown.

Spradley, J. (1975). *The cocktail waitress: Women's work in a man's land.* New York: John Wiley & Sons.

Spradley, J. (1979). *The ethnographic interview.* New York: Holt, Rinehart & Winston.

Spradley, J. (1980). *Participant observation.* New York: Holt, Rinehart & Winston.

Stanford, B. (1972). *Myths and modern man.* New York: Washington Square Press.

Sudman, S., & Bradburn, M. (1983). *Asking questions: A practical guide to questions design.* San Francisco: Jossey-Bass.

Thomas, J. (1988). Kill or cure. *Nursing Times, 84*(7), 38–40.

Thompson, C. (1989). *Magic and healing.* New York: Bell Publisher.

Tripp-Reimer, T. (1983). Retention of folk healing practices (Matiasma) among four generations of urban Greek immigrants. *Nursing Research, 32,* 97–101.

Turner, T. (1991). Black rural elderly. In A. Bushy (Ed.), *Rural nursing* (Vol. 1, pp. 347–372). Newbury Park, CA: Sage Publications.

U.S. Bureau of the Census. (1991). *Characteristics of the U.S. population.* Washington, DC: U.S. Government Printing Office.

U.S. Department of Health and Human Services, U. S. Public Health Service (1990). *Healthy people 2000: National health promotion and disease prevention objectives* (DHHS Publication No. PHS 91-50213). Washington, DC: U.S. Government Printing Office.

Wang, J. (1984). Caretaker–child interactions observed in two Appalachian clinics. In M. Leininger (Ed.), *Care:*

Essence of nursing and health (pp. 370–385). Thorofare, NJ: Charles B. Slack.

Watson, J. (1979). *Nursing: The philosophy and science of caring.* Boston: Little, Brown.

Whealan, E. (1983). *The nutritional, purely organic, cholesterol free, megavitamin, low carbohydrate, nutrition hoax.* New York: Atheneum.

White, E. (1990). Black women's health care book: Speaking for ourselves. Seattle, WA: Seal Press.

Whorton, J. (1987). Traditions of folk medicine in America. *JAMA, 257*(12), 1632–1635.

Williams, G. (1994). The healing power of prayer. *American Legion, 137*(2), 19–22.

Yawn, B., Bushy, A., Dubbels, K., Pelage, M., & Hill, C. (1994). Making your practice palatable for your patients: Cultural competency. In B. Yawn, A. Bushy, & R. Yawn (Eds.), *Exploring rural medicine* pp. 253–271). Newbury Park, CA: Sage Publications.

8

Case Management and the Advanced Practice Nurse

Catherine Borkowski Benoit

The 1990s will undoubtedly be remembered as the era of healthcare reform. As changes in healthcare delivery evolve, the nursing profession will continue to face critical issues in providing care. Increased acuity, reduction in length of hospital stay, escalating healthcare costs, and constant advancement in technology all challenge the ability of advanced practice nurses (APNs) to deliver quality patient care. In addition, we will be asked to uphold standards of quality in an environment of ever-increasing financial constraints.

Nursing case management is one model of care that addresses the issue of meeting complex patient needs in an environment of increasingly limited healthcare and economic resources. *Case management* is a systematic process of mobilizing, monitoring, and controlling the resources that a patient uses over the course of an illness. In doing so, a controlled balance between quality and cost is achieved (Giuliano & Poirier, 1991).

This chapter provides an overview of the key concepts to understanding case management. Although abundant examples of variations of the model exist in the literature, all of the models share a common focus of enhancing continuity of care and timely and effective management of resources. The critical role played by APNs is discussed in detail because it is clear that they make a unique contribution in a resource-driven model of healthcare. The author's personal experience in the role of a nurse practitioner with a case management focus also is presented.

TRENDS IN PRACTICE: EVOLUTION OF THE CASE MANAGEMENT MODEL

The advancement of nursing practice since the 1960s illustrates remarkable strides toward preparation for the challenges of the 1990s. In the 1960s, the healthcare system in general showed little regard for cost-containment. Patient length of stay was rarely scrutinized, and nurses, who demonstrated little autonomy in their practice, viewed themselves as having almost no effect on the patient's overall course of hospitalization.

Hickey JV: ADVANCED PRACTICE NURSING: Changing Roles and Clinical Applications © 1996 Lippincott–Raven Publishers

The evolution of primary nursing as a philosophy and model of care mandated a new focus on the nurse's professional responsibility and accountability for providing quality patient care. Enhanced patient satisfaction with nursing care, continuity of patient care, and improved professional satisfaction for nurses were other documented benefits (McClelland, Kolesar, & Bailey, 1987).

Other models of care delivery developed in the 1970s and 1980s. However, none clearly spoke to the management of cost and the issues of quality that are paramount in the 1990s. Although we have made notable strides in the delivery of quality care, our energies have had little impact on the bottom line: significantly decreasing the cost of healthcare. Clearly, the successful healthcare organizations of the future will be consumer driven rather than product driven (O'Malley, Cummings, & Loveridge, 1989). Changes in patient care delivery, therefore, need to reflect this trend. The case management model has evolved in response to this need.

The literature contains references to case management as early as the 1950s. Emerging from the concept of managed care, the model came into use after World War II in the context of assembling the extended community services necessary to care for veterans who were psychiatric patients (Grau, 1984). By the 1960s, the federal government was using the term *case management* to describe programs designed to overcome the barriers of fragmented, duplicated, and uncoordinated services. In 1962, the President's Commission on Mental Retardation recommended that a "program coordinator" help patients gain access to services and expedite their delivery. This role is similar that of the contemporary case manager. By the early 1970s, the case management idea was apparent throughout public health and social welfare literature and social work practice.

The 1981 Omnibus Budget Reconciliation Act and the Medicare prospective payment system of reimbursement (diagnosis-related groups [DRGs]) broadened the focus of case management from that of making more services available to a wider range of patients to making the existing services more economically efficient for specific patient populations. Today, case management is most clearly illustrated by health maintenance organizations and preferred provider organizations, in which the goal is to strive for more efficient use of services by comprehensively coordinating care. For example, a particular primary care physician manages a designated group of patients. The primary care physician must provide or authorize all care for those patients, except in extreme emergencies, or insurance companies will not reimburse the cost.

NURSING CASE MANAGEMENT: DEFINING A MODEL

The onset of prospective payment moved case management into the acute-care setting. Case management has been described by numerous authors. Four key features commonly associated with most models of case management are

1. standardizing appropriate use of resources within an appropriate length of stay and aimed at identified patient care, care-giver, and system outcomes
2. promoting collaborative team practice among disciplines
3. promoting coordinated continuity of care over the course of an illness
4. promoting job satisfaction, job enrichment for caregivers, patient and physician satisfaction with care delivery, and minimization of cost to the institution.

The model described by Olivas and colleagues (Olivas, Del Togno, Armanasco, Erickson, & Harter, 1989) includes these features and describes case management as a multidisciplinary care delivery process aimed, by case type, at achieving a purposeful and controlled connection between the quality and cost of care.

Zander, from the New England Medical Center Hospitals in Boston, pioneered efforts to incorporate the concept of case management into hospital-based nursing in the 1980s. She defined case management as a technology for structuring care for all patients. It is a system that uses the nurse's clinical and management skills to organize the patient's healthcare needs (Zander, 1988a). Ultimate accountability for the clinical and financial outcomes for each patient rests with the nurse case manager and the attending physician. In a more global sense, the American Nurses' Association (ANA, 1988) has defined case management as a healthcare delivery process with the goals of providing quality healthcare, decreasing fragmentation, enhancing the patient's quality of life, and containing cost.

Clearly, the definitions of case management are broad and conceptual. Therefore, it is appropriate that models of practice have been operationally defined in many ways, depending on the setting and the unique needs of the population. The many definitions, however, share a common base within the nursing process that consists of assessment, planning, coordination, implementation, and evaluation of nursing care (Bower, 1992).

ROLE OF COLLABORATION IN THE SUCCESS OF A CASE MANAGEMENT MODEL

Although each version of case management is operationalized somewhat differently, the importance of coordination and open communication among disciplines is stressed. Clearly, collaboration among providers is essential to high-quality, cost-effective patient care. Senge (1990) used the term *aligned* to describe a group of individuals functioning as a whole:

> The fundamental characteristics of the relatively unaligned team is wasted energy. Individuals may work extraordinarily hard, but their efforts do not translate to team effort. By contrast, when a team becomes more aligned, a commonality of direction emerges. There is less wasted energy. A synergy develops. Individuals do not sacrifice their personal interest to the larger team vision; rather, the shared vision becomes an extension of their personal visions.

The energy generated by this synergy allows the team to appreciate a patient's entire trajectory of illness and anticipate integrated care needs accordingly.

The development of collaborative practice is based on the existence of three essential components: diverse professional skills and contributions, effective communication processes, and a common purpose (Spross, 1989). A common purpose is essential, because fragmentation and ambiguity occur when a common purpose is not understood. In case management, the common purpose of providing quality patient care is guided by practice standards from each discipline and communicated effectively among disciplines.

Each member of a multidisciplinary team brings unique abilities and ideas to the approach to patient care. Physicians and nurses often view patients from different vantage points: physicians may have a relationship with patients that spans over time, whereas acute-care nurses typically know patients intimately from a single episode of illness. When their talents need to work in a complementary fashion to contribute to the overall goal of quality patient care, there is then no one member who holds authority over other team members. The approach is a cooperative venture between the patient, family, and clinicians. This effect gives care providers an understanding of patient situations that is far more comprehensive than any individual practitioner could achieve alone (Pike, 1991).

ROLE OF THE ADVANCED PRACTICE NURSE AS CASE MANAGER

The ability to work in a collaborative practice as an effective case manager requires superb communication skills and clinical expertise. However, the selection criteria for nursing case managers is as varied as the practice settings in which they work. The ANA (1988) publication *Nursing Case Management* recommends a bachelor of science in nursing (BSN) degree as the minimum level of educational preparation for a nurse case manager. Other authors have stated that the BSN is the logical choice for case manager because the nurse coordinates patient care 24 hours a day (Lynn-McHale, Fitzpatrick, & Shaffer, 1993). The BSN–prepared case manager, as a primary caregiver, plans nursing care for the patient's entire length of stay and delegates care to other nurses (who are members of a group practice) acting as associates on other shifts.

Cronin and Maklebust (1989) identified both positive and negative aspects of having nurses prepared at the baccalaureate level as case managers. They reported improvement in overall quality of patient care as well as increased job satisfaction on the units where these case managers were practicing. However, these nurses expressed frustration and an inability to manage cases effectively while they were involved in the delivery of direct patient care. In addition, they reportedly felt ill prepared by their curricula or needed advanced education or experience to institute change at the system level and to delegate and collaborate effectively.

With the proliferation of subspecialties in healthcare, the scope of nursing knowledge has vastly expanded. Nurses prepared at the advanced practice level (Master's degree) not only possess the necessary expertise to meet the demands of the clinical setting, but have also developed confidence in their practice abilities as well as skills in collaboration and critical thinking.

In addition to being an expert practitioner, the APN is also a manager, teacher, researcher, consultant, and change agent. He or she is a role model of effective collaboration between nursing and other members of a multidisciplinary team. In this way, nursing practice as a whole is moved from a reactive to a proactive, effective, and efficient model of care delivery. It is this expertise in clinical decision making and an understanding of the overall functioning of the healthcare delivery system that separates the APN from other nurses who might act as case managers (Nugent, 1992).

ROLE OF THE ADVANCED PRACTICE NURSE AS CASE MANAGER IN A PRIMARY NURSING SYSTEM

The role of the APN case manager in a primary nursing system presents particular challenges if role confusion is to be avoided. Zander (1988b) reported that APNs can succeed as case managers, but care must be taken to ensure that the professionalism and accountability of the staff nurse are not adversely affected. Although certain authors have expressed the belief that if primary nursing is functioning effectively, many case management responsibilities can be assumed by the nursing staff, others have supported and valued the role of the APN case manager as one that is separate but complementary to the role of the primary nurse.

As a case manager, the APN can be called on to provide consultation, support, and backup when a primary nurse is unavailable or when patient needs move out of the realm of the primary nurse's expertise. The APN can assist the primary nurse with goal setting and work with new staff members as they develop their own skills in the areas of clinical expertise and decision making. The APN may handle problematic interactions with patients and physicians at the request of the primary nurse for the purposes of providing support and a role model (Trella, 1993).

Above all, it is imperative that the APN remain sensitive to the unique relationship between the primary nurse and the patient. This mutual respect and recognition of each other's clinical expertise and contribution will move the team toward their goal of a truly integrated approach to patient care. Clifford and Wandel (1993) stated that "primary nursing and case management have helped to develop a greater understanding of the nurse's role in providing continuity in the care of patients" (p. 268). Working in collaboration with an APN case manager, the primary nurse is able to more effectively organize and deliver care throughout the spectrum of an illness.

IMPLEMENTATION OF CASE MANAGEMENT: SELECTING A TARGET POPULATION

Most authors have agreed that it is important to determine which patients would benefit most from case management (Table 8-1). Groups of patients thought to be most appropriate are

TABLE 8-1 **Selecting a Target Population for Case Management**

Target population should include patients for whom the course of treatment

· is costly

· is unpredictable

· involves frequent or chronic readmissions

· involves significant variances in length of stay

· involves multiple physicians or multiple disciplines.

Examples of target populations

· frail, chronically disabled clients (e.g., physically or mentally challenged)

· clients with long-term, complex medical problems (e.g., human immunodeficiency virus or transplants)

· individuals severely compromised by an acute episode of illness.

those whose illnesses consume a great deal of healthcare resources, who have a long length of stay, and who are part of a high-volume population for a particular institution. Examples of these groups of patients have been articulated by the ANA (1988) and are listed in Table 8-1. In addition, case management can be effectively used with a surgical population whose length of stay and hospital course is predictable but can be prolonged by potential for complication or fragmentation when many disciplines are involved (e.g., the surgical population that has epilepsy).

Once a target population is chosen, the next logical step is to identify and establish the collaborative team that will provide care for the patients. In the acute-care setting, the team might consist of physicians, nurses, therapists from the rehabilitation team (e.g., physical therapists, occupational therapists, and speech pathologists), dietitians, and utilization review nurses. This team will establish outcomes for patients, including expected length of stay, common problems encountered, and expected outcomes for each of the identified problems. Medical and nursing activities are expected to achieve these outcomes within a predetermined length of time.

Establishing a Case Management Plan

In some settings, this expected course is outlined informally, and the emphasis is on the flexibility of nurses to network services across the system for their patients (Ethridge & Lamb, 1991). In other areas, more formal case management plans and critical pathways are developed and used to structure care (Zander, 1988a). A *case management plan* is a design tool, used to standardize care delivery, that identifies interventions and goals for all disciplines involved. The *critical pathway* is an abbreviated, more user-friendly version of the case management plan. It is an outline or protocol of how the hospital stay is to proceed for a patient with a particular diagnosis. It serves as a day-to-day guide for patient care, and tells the nurse what care needs to be given and when so that the patient can move through hospitalization during the time frame allotted by the particular DRG (Dunston, 1990). Tables 8-2 and 8-3 contain an excerpt from a sample case management plan for a patient with an anterior cervical diskectomy and fusion and show the critical pathway appropriate for this patient.

Patients with complex problems create a special challenge. With these individuals, many confounding factors make it difficult to predict their course accurately. In such cases, it may be necessary to incorporate aspects of several plans or to develop the pathway on a day-to-day basis, always being certain that care is goal oriented and resource conscious.

TABLE 8-2 **Case Management Plan: Anterior Cervical Diskectomy and Fusion (Expected Length of Stay: 3 days)**

Problem	Outcome	Process
Knowledge deficit regarding discharge instructions and home care	Patient will demonstrate an understanding of the following discharge instructions regarding care at home: States purpose of medications; demonstrates understanding of wound care; demonstrates an understanding of signs and symptoms that should be reported to the physician; demonstrates an understanding of the importance of wearing cervical collar; demonstrates an understanding of activity restrictions; states knowledge of follow-up appointment	Instruct patient regarding the: use of medications (narcotics, muscle relaxants, avoidence of NSAIDS) Instruct patient regarding care of an incision: Keep wound covered with waterproof dressing; report any drainage to physician Instruct patient regarding activity restrictions: No exercise except walking; no lifting > 5lb for 6 weeks Arrange follow-up appointment with nurse practitioner for suture removal Inform patient that neurosurgery office will call patient to arrange follow-up appointment with neurosurgeon

Performing a Variance Analysis

The benefit of using a well-documented plan or care pathway is the ease of identifying both positive and negative patient variances to meeting expected outcomes. Variance tracking is a means of quality assurance and the stepping stone to quality improvement with a case-managed population.

Identification of variances is generally not difficult. The patient either is or is not meeting the predetermined goals in the care plan. A positive variance is achieved when a patient

TABLE 8-3 **Critical Pathway: Anterior Cervical Diskectomy and Fusion**

	Operating Room Day	Postoperative Day 1	Postoperative Day 2	Postoperative Day 3
Activity	Out of bed	Physical therapy/ occupational therapy involved p.r.n	Discontinue pneumatic boots if ambulating t.i.d.	
Comfort	Morphine/Demerol Patient-controlled analgesia/Intramuscular	Evaluate for change to p.o. Add Flexeril/Valium for spasms	Discontinue patient-controlled analgesia	
Nutrition	Intravenous fluids Ice chips Advance diet if tolerated	Advance diet		
Labs/Tests			Anterior posterior/ lateral cervical spines	
ʰher medications		Colace		
ʰd care	Phili collar on at all times	Obtain second collar for discharge		Change dressing
ʰ	Monitor urinary output and bowel sounds	Discontinue Foley	MOM p.r.n.	Dulcolax

progresses more quickly than expected. For example, a postoperative patient is able to tolerate the switch from intravenous to oral pain medication on postoperative day (POD) 1 rather than on the expected POD 2. The patient, therefore, is able to be discharged from the hospital 1 day early. Conversely, negative variances occur when specific outcomes are not met.

Variances from the care map have a wide variety of origins. Selker, Beshansky, Pauker, and Kassirer (1989) have identified nine specific areas associated with variance and subsequent delays in discharge. These include delays related to:

1. test scheduling (e.g., the patient is unable to have a test performed on a weekend)
2. availability of test results (e.g., the results of a test are unavailable within a standard turnaround time)
3. surgery (e.g., there is difficulty getting a patient on a busy operating room schedule)
4. consultation (e.g., the consultation is not done within a standard time)
5. the patient (e.g., the patient or family is undecided about a therapy or referral facility)
6. physician responsibility (e.g., medical management decision making is delayed by an inability to discuss the case with the entire team)
7. education, training, or research (e.g., an interesting patient is kept in the hospital for teaching purposes)
8. discharge planning or scheduling for outside support and care (e.g., the patient remains in the hospital because of a late request for home services)
9. availability of appropriate level of outside care and resources (e.g., the patient is waiting for a bed in a rehabilitation or nursing facility).

The first step in reducing hospital costs is to engage in research to identify variables that influence cost in a particular patient population. It is the case manager's responsibility to identify and document variances and communicate them to other members of the collaborative team for their review. In this way, specific actions can be taken to prevent continued deviation from the case management plan. For long-range planning, variance data will be useful in guiding practice changes and alterations in the work system and environment.

Evaluating the Model: Measuring Effectiveness

Evaluating a case management model involves consideration of the effect case management has on cost of care, as well as quality of care, nursing satisfaction, physician satisfaction and patient satisfaction with both nursing care and the overall care received. Several studies have described the effect of case management on decreasing cost of care. VanTassel (1990) described more than $3 million in cost savings realized as a result of interventions by case managers who used resources efficiently. Other data have revealed reductions in length of stay, decreases in cost per patient day, and increases in reimbursement indices (Trella, 1993). In these populations, specific factors related to cost savings included

- enhanced communication with patients and families, enabling them to make fully informed decisions and to better plan for care
- identification of patient problems in a timely way, allowing them to be addressed proactively or concurrently rather than retrospectively
- more effective communication among disciplines
- reduction or elimination of duplicate or overlapping care, tests, and treatments through improved sequencing and coordination of care activities
- minimized or eliminated delays in required tests, treatments, or care
- enhanced knowledge among clinicians regarding the financial aspects of care
- attention to patient needs and the issues and problems encountered in providing efficient, effective care at both the individual and aggregate patient levels.

Addressing these issues provides the case manager with useful data that can facilitate system changes that improve the cost and quality of care (ANA, 1988). It is important to look simultaneously at quality and cost savings so that cost containment is not achieved at the expense of quality. If, for example, an increased rate of readmission is noted while working toward the goal of decreasing overall length of stay, it is critical to look at quality issues that might account for the readmissions.

Role satisfaction leads to the retention of qualified and experienced nursing staff and positively influences patient care at the bedside. Nurses working in collaboration with an APN case manager generally believe (Cronin & Maklebust, 1989) that case management not only improves the quality of care on the unit, but positively affects their own nursing practice as well. Additional benefits include decreased job stress, increased job satisfaction, and decreased turnover rate. These benefits translate to a decrease in expenditures for recruitment and orientation. Ownership, recognition, and increased involvement with a patient's complete episode of illness allow nurses greater control over the most important aspect of their job: caring for patients.

A unique study by Newman, Lamb, and Michaels (1991) looked at the process of case management as practiced by a group of nurses at Carondelet St. Mary's Hospital and Health Center in Tucson, AZ. In this setting, high-risk adults were followed from the acute-care area into the community by nurse case managers. The case managers were interviewed regarding their practice and relationships with the patients. Several of the nurses interviewed believed that patients were implementing positive changes in their health behaviors to an extent that had not been seen previously in their practices. Nurses believed they were working differently with patients as a result of the case management model. Their practices were having a greater effect on the overall health of their patients as they assisted them to make choices that lessened the risk of illness and maximized wellness.

With pressure on physicians to maintain quality care while cutting costs and reducing length of stay, it is understandable that physicians would support a case management model of practice. Trella (1993) reported that, with case managed populations, physicians believed the staff were better able to communicate patient needs and progress. Tests were completed and results were reported in a more timely manner, nursing documentation contained more pertinent information, and overall care was more highly rated.

The patient's perspective of working with a nurse case manager is clearly of paramount importance in evaluating the effectiveness of the model. The nurse case manager, through his or her actions, strives to optimize patient outcomes by coordinating care through an entire illness. It is expected that these actions will ensure that patient outcomes are met and will enhance patient and family satisfaction.

Lamb and Stempel (1994) interviewed 16 individuals who had worked with or were in the process of working with a nurse case manager. Participants were asked to describe their experience working with the nurse case manager within the context of their own illness. The basic theme that emerged from the data was the process of the patients' becoming their own "insider–experts." That is, the patients made cognitive and behavioral changes as they worked with nurse case managers.

In the Lamb and Stempel study, patients initially viewed the nurse case manager as an expert—someone who was knowledgeable about his or her physical status and could teach the patients ways to take care of themselves. As an aspect of routine practice, the APN monitored physical status and collaborated with the physician regarding salient physical findings. As patients' physical status stabilized, the focus of the relationship often shifted to emotional and spiritual concerns, and patients began sharing intimate concerns with the nurse. Bonding occurred between patient and nurse, allowing the patient to feel known and cared for as an individual. In the context of this bonding, the patients began to think differently about their situations, gain confidence in their ability to care for themselves, and accept greater responsibility for performing the role of insider–expert. The patients came to believe that the nurse case manager knew his or her "stuff" and that working together could positively affect what was occurring in their lives.

Respondents reported other valuable activities performed by the nurse case manager including listening, validating, counseling, supporting, confronting, offering choices, and praising. A frequently mentioned behavior described that of "going beyond." That is, the nurse case manager's actions were more than or over and above patients' expectations or what they had experienced with a nurse in prior interactions (Lamb & Stempel, 1994).

Patients described their relationship with the nurse case manager as clearly different from the relationship they had with their physician. Interactions with the two healthcare professionals seems to be governed by different sets of rules. One woman believed that her doctor might be willing to listen to her concerns, but she was reluctant to begin the discussion, because she was conscious of the busy waiting room and felt uncomfortable "taking up his time." With the nurse, however, she felt a sense of ease and was able to form a more intimate relationship. She was better able to sit and talk and discuss her concerns. She sensed that the nurse wanted to make sure she was "on the right track" (Lamb & Stempel, 1994).

Overall, patients of nurse case managers demonstrated improved self-care skills, were hospitalized less often, and enjoyed an enhanced quality of life. The perspectives of the individuals involved in the study offer important information as we look to justify the role of the nurse case manager in the delivery of quality care (Lamb & Stempel, 1994).

Future Directions

The APN's role will continue to change and be challenged as the current healthcare delivery system continues to evolve. The APN possesses the educational and clinical expertise that is so necessary for meeting the economic and clinical demands in the resource-driven healthcare climate of the 1990s. Using the model of case management empowers the practitioner to function as facilitator toward bridging the gap between cost and quality of care.

ROLE OF THE NURSE PRACTITIONER WITH A CASE MANAGEMENT FOCUS: A PERSONAL PERSPECTIVE

In the late 1980s, the changing face of healthcare prompted administrators at Boston's Beth Israel Hospital to look carefully at issues of length of stay, efficiency, and quality improvement. On the neurosurgery service in particular, it was clear that measures needed to be taken to decrease length of stay and improve the continuity of care between the outpatient and the inpatient areas. Historically, this population is one that presents complex medical and nursing care challenges and frequently exceeds its DRG–allotted length of stay. A group of nurses and physicians worked together to examine the options. This section describes the events that led to a needed change in practice, a new approach to care, and ultimately an improvement in the collaborative relationships of the healthcare professionals involved in the care of this patient population.

Overview of the Neurosurgery Service

The Division of Neurosurgery at Beth Israel Hospital is staffed by three attending neurosurgeons and one general surgery intern. The population of patients is consistent with any university-based teaching hospital with a strong emphasis on spine and epilepsy surgery. The neurosurgeons perform an average of 425 operations per year; the average daily inpatient census is 12. Patients are primarily located on one patient care unit, whereas those patients needing more intensive monitoring are cared for in the surgical intensive care unit or the postanesthesia care unit.

The patient care unit is a 30-bed unit dedicated to the care of neuroscience patients. The primary nursing model of practice is used there, and all nursing staff are prepared at a baccalaureate level. A unit-based clinical nurse specialist is available to consult with staff on difficult patient care issues, to facilitate staff education, to integrate research into practice, and to provide direct patient care.

Inception of the Role

A careful look at the current model of patient care revealed three primary areas of concern. First and foremost, the length of stay for patients on the service needed to be carefully evaluated in a concurrent and ongoing way. It was clear from data compiled in the 12 months before the project onset that closed-head trauma patients and spinal surgery patients were two groups that dramatically exceeded their DRG length of stay. These two subsets of the population would need to be examined closely and strategies would need to be developed to decrease their time in the hospital while still ensuring that quality care was being provided.

A second concern was the continuity and quality of care for patients as they moved from the inpatient to the outpatient area. Typically, patients were evaluated by their neurosurgeon during an outpatient office visit. If they were deemed to be surgical candidates, they would be scheduled for a subsequent office visit, during which they would meet with their neurosurgeon to sign their surgical consent and undergo preoperative testing. They would be admitted to the hospital on the morning of their procedure and would be cared for by a team that consisted of their attending neurosurgeon, a general surgery intern who was rotating through the service, a primary nurse, and associate nurses. On discharge from the hospital, they would return periodically for office visits with their neurosurgeon.

This model of care, which is traditionally used with the surgical population, seemed cumbersome and ineffective with this group. Patients expressed a lack of communication with their attending physician during the preoperative period and believed that many of their questions regarding upcoming hospitalization were left unanswered. The neurosurgeons spent long hours in the operating room each day and were often unavailable to answer patient questions in a timely manner. In the hospital, patients enjoyed the relationship with their primary and associate nurses and generally expressed a feeling of being well cared for. Unfortunately, this nursing relationship was not extended into the outpatient area, and patients once again expressed feelings of isolation and frustration when they were unable to consistently communicate with their attending physician. Clearly, these issues needed to be addressed.

The third area of concern focused on collaborative relationships. Lack of communication among team members was a common complaint of all healthcare professionals involved in the care of the neurosurgery patients. The team, consisting of an intern acting under the supervision of the attending physician, rotated onto the service at monthly intervals. By the time the intern became familiar with the latest innovations and the common patient responses in the postoperative period, it was time for the intern to move on to the next rotation. The intern often expressed feelings of frustration regarding the lack of attending physician guidance. In turn, the intern was unable to effectively communicate the patient care plan to the nurses.

Other professionals involved in the care of this population expressed similar concerns. For example, the physical and occupational therapists who play such a strong role in the rehabilitation process for these patients expressed feelings of working in isolation and of a perceived lack of value by other team members. It is obviously unacceptable for one discipline to provide patient care working in isolation. It was decided that there needed to be a single, integrated care plan for each patient that was developed jointly and proactively by physicians, nurses, and other involved healthcare professionals.

Redesigning: Implementation of a New Role

Early thoughts regarding the problem looked at the addition of a utilization review nurse to the neurosurgery team. Although this change would certainly place an expert on the "front lines" to concentrate on the problems of length of stay and delays in discharge, the issues of continuity of care and collaboration would continue to go unaddressed.

Those involved in planning the redesign believed that a strong clinical base was an essential component of the new role. If inroads were to be made in this already well-established system, it would be necessary to use clinical expertise as a basis for change. Other pre-requisites included superb communication skills, a willingness and ability to form and maintain interdisciplinary relationships, and the ability to practice "across the system," or to move freely between the inpatient and the outpatient areas.

An APN with a case management focus was the ideal choice for the position. It was believed that either a nurse practitioner or a clinical nurse specialist would bring the necessary skills to the role. Working between the inpatient and the outpatient areas, this nurse would work collaboratively with the neurosurgeons and the nurses to facilitate efficient, quality care that would begin on initial contact with the neurosurgeon and continue throughout hospitalization and into the posthospital period. Early goals for the position included:

- improvement in the continuity and quality of care for both inpatients and outpatients on the neurosurgery service
- improvement in collaboration among all disciplines involved in the care of the neurosurgery population
- identification of delays in discharge and implementation of interventions to decrease the overall length of stay for inpatients hospitalized on the neurosurgery service.

Role Responsibilities

Although not a case manager by title, the concepts of case management are strong components of this role. As a member of the inpatient team, one of the nurse practitioner's primary responsibilities involves monitoring the delivery of care to ensure quality and cost-effectiveness. This goal is facilitated by establishing and maintaining collaborative relationships with all healthcare professionals involved in the care of the patients on the service. The physicians, primary and associate nurses, physical and occupational therapists, social workers, utilization review nurses, and nutritionists are all members of one team who are working toward the common goal of improving patient care. No one member is more important than the other. Each brings unique abilities and ideas in the approach to patient care.

In this system in which the practice of primary nursing is so strong, the nurse practitioner's role in no way replaces or interferes with the relationship between the primary nurse and the patient. Instead, the nurse practitioner acts as a consultant to the primary nurse in situations that warrant advanced practice nursing intervention. As a facilitator, the nurse practitioner's role supports that of the primary nurse in the delivery of more effectively organized, quality care.

In the outpatient area, the role responsibilities are not as clearly defined. At the onset of the position, the components of the case management role as they applied to the inpatient area were easily operationalized. The application of these concepts in the outpatient area were not as straightforward. Bridging the gap between the inpatient and outpatient areas, a primary area of focus, involved establishing relationships with providers in the ambulatory area and in the community in much the same way as was done in the inpatient arena. Meetings occurred with outpatient rehabilitation therapists who cared for patients of Beth Israel Hospital. Site visits were arranged to tour local inpatient rehabilitation hospitals where Beth Israel Hospital patients were frequently referred. Contact was made with the visiting nurse and hospice services to which most patients commonly were referred. Relationships were developed that would later serve to improve the ease and effectiveness of communication and enhance the overall continuity and quality of care.

Initially, role responsibilities were broad and the means in which to operationalize them was flexible. A copy of the original job description is contained in the Special Display 8-1.

Further Development of the Role

Implementation and evolution of the role made the needs of this patient population even clearer, and interventions were put into place to meet these needs. As a result, the process of expert

JOB DESCRIPTION

Title: Nurse Practitioner/Neurosurgery

General Summary

Exemplifies and promotes excellence in neuroscience nursing practice with an emphasis on the neurosurgical population. Works in a collegial relationship with the nursing staff and the neurosurgical team to ensure continuity of patient care with special attention given to those hours when the neurosurgeons are in the operating room. Uses the consultation process with nurses and surgeons to facilitate continuity of patient care, conformance with standards, and achievement of identifiable outcomes. Participates in interdisciplinary rounds and patient care programs for patients on the neurosurgery service. Contributes to the ongoing care and management of inpatients on the neurosurgery service and to a designated group of outpatients determined by the department of nursing and neurosurgery.

Role Responsibilities

1. Is an integral member of the neurosurgical team and assumes selected responsibilities to ensure continuity of patient care.
2. Serves as a consultant to the nursing staff.
   - Responds to pages when the neurosurgical team is in the operating room or as the need arises.
   - Assists the primary nurse/associate nurse with assessment and clinical decision making regarding changes in patient status.
   - Collaborates with the primary nurse/associate nurse to determine when physician input or intervention is necessary to ensure safe standards of patient care.
   - Provides liaison consultation between the primary nurse/associate nurse and the neurosurgeon and house officer when they are in the operating room or otherwise not immediately available.
   - May perform tasks mutually agreed on by the departments of nursing and neurosurgery, following completion of appropriate inservicing.
3. Promotes individualized care planning consistent with efficient and thorough assessment of patients.
   - Contributes to a common database through active sharing of relevant information.
   - Assists physicians and nursing staff in setting priorities and maximizing resources to develop an optimal care plan for patients.
   - Reviews routine orders for appropriateness and frequency.
   - Actively participates as a representative of the neurosurgical team in social services rounds, patient care conferences, and interdisciplinary team meetings.
   - Facilitates with the primary nurse and neurosurgeons early discharge planning and timely completion of appropriate discharge referral forms.
   - Participates in all activities of the neurosurgery team, including morning rounds and conferences.
4. May assume an ongoing caseload of selected patients as determined by the departments of nursing and neurosurgery.
5. May assume responsibility for following a selected group of outpatients in collaboration with the neurosurgeons (i.e., preoperative patients for the purpose of teaching or postoperative patients for wound assessment and functional assessment).

6. Participates in the orientation and teaching programs for new house staff and clinical nurses.

7. Monitors patient care outcomes in accordance with defined patient care standards.

    • Identifies pertinent nursing care problems appropriate for further investigation.

    • Evaluates the effectiveness of nursing care and recommends approaches to practice based on research findings.

    • Assists physician and nurse colleagues in their research efforts.

8. Collaborates with other health care disciplines within the hospital and community to develop effective patient care programs.

Accountability

The neurosurgical nurse practitioner is accountable to the director of surgical nursing for the totality of work performance. Any participation in medically related decisions will be monitored by a designated attending physician on the neurosurgical team.

1. Current nursing registration in the Commonwealth of Massachusetts.

2. Master's degree in neuroscience nursing.

3. In-depth, current knowledge and demonstrated experience in neuroscience nursing practice, and the ability to translate professional and institutional goals into effective programs.

4. Experience in teaching or program planning. Knowledge of adult learning principles.

5. Knowledge of, or experience with, primary nursing.

6. Knowledge of the research process and application to practice.

7. Ability to organize resources appropriately; ability to work independently with other services and departments in the hospital.

8. Strong interpersonal skills, especially a commitment to interdisciplinary and collaborative practice.

The preceding statements are intended to describe the general nature and level of work being performed by people assigned to the classification. They are not intended to be construed as an exhaustive list of all responsibilities, duties, and skills required of personnel so classified. (Beth Israel, 1990)

---

care now begins in the outpatient setting. As a direct care provider, the nurse practitioner meets with each patient before his or her scheduled surgery to perform a patient history and physical exam and to provide patient and family teaching. This visit offers the opportunity to screen for potential problems that might occur during hospitalization or during the posthospital phase of care. The nurse practitioner makes a tentative plan for discharge and provides information regarding rehabilitation hospitals and home services to the patient and family as needed. Perhaps most important, a relationship begins to form between the patient and a consistent care provider who will follow the patient across the spectrum of illness.

The nurse practitioner directs information obtained during this preoperative visit to other members of the team involved in the patient's care. He or she reviews background health and social history with the primary nurse so that he or she can better meet the patient's needs. The nurse practitioner also reviews pertinent physical exam findings with the attending physician and the intern. He or she alerts the social worker regarding all patients who will potentially need a rehabilitation hospital admission before returning home. The nurse practitioner also consults physical and occupational therapists about patients with baseline functional deficits. In this way, the team can plan proactively for early interventions, ultimately improving the quality and cost-effectiveness of care.

In the inpatient area, the nurse practitioner is responsible for routine postoperative management as well as monitoring and treating common patient problems in collaboration with the intern and the attending physician. He or she gives particular attention to facilitating communication among team members and between the team and the patient. Each morning following rounds, the nurse practitioner allots time to meet briefly with the primary and associate nurses to discuss patient care goals for the day. On a weekly basis, the nurse practitioner formally discusses rehabilitation goals with the team in "rehab rounds." However, pertinent information of this nature is shared daily among team members. The utilization review nurse is available each morning to address issues of justification and length of inpatient stay, and the nurse practitioner discusses discharge planning with the social worker.

The nurse practitioner openly communicates goals of care and other pertinent information to patients and families. On a daily basis, he or she discusses progress and planning. A conversation with a patient might be as follows:

> Our goals for you today would be to have you walk in the halls at least three times and to begin taking clear liquids, if you can. Tomorrow we will stop your PCA [patient-controlled analgesia] pump and switch you to pain medication by mouth. If your pain is well controlled, if you don't have a fever, and if your incision is clean and dry, you will be able to go home the day after tomorrow. How does this plan sound? Is someone available to pick you up from the hospital that day and help you get settled at home?

This interactive approach to care and discharge planning ensures that the team's goals for the patient as well as the patient's own goals are met. If a patient fails to progress at the expected rate, the variance can be identified early and the appropriate interventions put into place. If there are issues with organizing support services at home, these issues can be addressed immediately so that a delay in discharge does not result.

Before discharge, the nurse practitioner spends time with each patient and the primary and associate nurses to discuss discharge instructions and follow-up care. For problems that occur at home, the patient is given the option of calling the nurse practitioner during regular office hours or contacting the primary or associate nurses who are always available to answer questions and triage problems. A follow-up appointment for suture removal and a functional evaluation is organized with the nurse practitioner. The patient returns to the patient care unit for this appointment to facilitate the involvement of the primary nurse.

The nurse practitioner is involved in long-term, postoperative follow-up in collaboration with the attending neurosurgeon. Patients may be referred for independent consultation with the nurse practitioner regarding the management of common problems, including pain management, activity intolerance, impaired wound healing, mobilization problems, and monitoring of anticonvulsant levels.

CASE VIGNETTE

The following case vignette illustrates the role of the nurse practitioner as a facilitator of quality, cost-effective care across the system.

As a nurse practitioner, my initial contact with J began when she was admitted to the neurology service following a generalized seizure. She was a previously healthy 56-year-old woman who had experienced a seizure while at work that morning. A CT [computerized tomography] scan done in the emergency unit revealed a large, bifrontal, infiltrative mass. The neurosurgery service was consulted and plans were made for biopsy. I became involved in her care postoperatively.

The first of several postoperative days involved a flurry of activity. The biopsy results indicated that the tumor was a glioblastoma multiforme, a highly malignant, primary brain tumor. J's neurological exam revealed a moderate amount of left-sided weakness, which impaired her ability to ambulate safely. She was scheduled to begin radiation therapy the next day. Her postoperative progress following the biopsy was typical. She worked with physical and occupational therapists on her ambulation and functional deficits.

Her primary nurse approached me with concerns regarding the discharge plan. On POD 1, we had met with J, J's husband, and their adult daughter to discuss the diagnosis and the care plan. At that time, the neurosurgeon felt that her hemiparesis would improve before discharge and that she would be able to safely return home. Forty-eight hours later, we were still seeing significant functional deficits. The primary nurse and the therapists agreed that the patient would benefit from an inpatient rehabilitation stay. Concurring with their assessment and realizing that our initial plan was no longer feasible, I scheduled a second meeting to give the team an opportunity to discuss their suggestions with J and her family.

When the suggestion was presented, J and her family expressed agreement and relief. They, too, felt that J was not ready to be at home. The social worker was contacted by the nurse practitioner and the complex needs of the patient were presented. J would need to enter a short-term rehabilitation program that would enable a patient with a brain tumor to address issues related to that condition. J would also need to be transported back to the hospital on a daily basis for radiation therapy treatments. Above all, J was anxious to begin a program immediately, because she wanted very much to be back at home as soon as possible.

Our efforts to expedite the referral process were successful and J was transferred to an appropriate facility the following day. She remained there as an inpatient for 2 weeks, during which she was transported back to the hospital for daily radiation treatments. I maintained contact with her husband during this time and was able to provide emotional support and answer questions as they arose. As an outpatient, J was managed by the visiting nurse and hospice services in her town.

She did well for approximately 6 months, when her family began to notice further functional decline and mental status changes. At this point, my relationship with her husband and the hospice nurse proved to be of key importance in the management of the terminal phase of J's illness. She had expressed the wish to be pain free and to die at home. These wishes guided our care over the next 3 months. J died at home with her husband and daughter 9 months following the diagnosis.

The case management skills used by the nurse practitioner were key to a positive outcome with this patient's care. Her medical and nursing care needs were complex and the goals of that aspect of her care required careful integration with her social situation and overall philosophy of death and dying. Most important, the continuity of care was maintained despite the involvement of multiple caregivers across a variety of settings.

Special Projects

The changes in practice on the neurosurgery service prompted an intensive look at the problems of prolonged length of stay and delays in discharge. One of the primary goals of the nurse practitioner's role involved the identification of factors that delayed discharge and prolonged length of stay for this population. Based on this goal, a task force was organized to examine the problem. Task force members included the nurse practitioner, two primary nurses representing the general patient care unit, the three attending neurosurgeons, the neurosurgery social worker, and the physical and occupational therapists.

The task force was initially charged with generating a list of potential causes for delays in discharge that resulted in lengthened hospital stays. Early ideas included:
- delays in transfer of patients to rehabilitation hospitals and nursing homes
- a time lag between generation of a physical therapy order and the actual evaluation of the patient
- lack of communication with families regarding discharge plans

Although task force members all had intuitive ideas about areas of delay, little quantitative data had been collected to validate these ideas.

The *Delay Tool* (Selker et al., 1989), developed at the New England Medical Center in Boston, is a reliable and easy-to-use tool that identifies medically unnecessary delays and the epidemiology of these delays. We chose to use this tool as a means of gathering and quantifying data regarding delays in discharge.

The tool classifies all medically unjustified delays into one of nine categories previously discussed in the section Performing a Variance Analysis (see p. 112). Subclassifications into one of 166 subcategories allow further specification of the etiology of each delay. A patient is considered to have experienced a delay when one or more hospital days are unnecessary or inappropriate, that is, no medical reason exists for the patient to be in the hospital that day. *Delay days* are the actual number of calendar days of delay. A delay day occurs whenever a patient has to spend an additional night in the hospital.

Using this tool, we looked retrospectively at the medical records of all patients admitted to the neurosurgery service during a 4-month period. All charts were reviewed by the nurse practitioner, who had extensive experience with the Delay Tool as well as with the patient population and the practices of the neurosurgery service. Every delay observed was assigned to a single Delay Tool category. The minimum delay counted was 1 calendar hospital day.

During the 4-month period, 99 adult patients were admitted to the neurosurgery service, using 746 hospital days. The average length of stay was 7.54 days. Of the study participants, 40 patients (40.4%) experienced delays during their hospitalization. Of those 40 patients, 37 experienced one delay each and three patients experienced two delays each, for a total of 43 delays. There were 129 delay days, representing 17.29%. The average length of delay was 4.74 days, with a range from 1 day to 33 days.

Figure 8-1 illustrates the percentage of total delays by category as described in the Delay Tool. Physician responsibility (category 6) and discharge planning or scheduling outside support or care (category 8) were the most frequently identified causes of delays, accounting for 28% and 37% of delays, respectively. In cases in which physician responsibility was the basis for the delay, we commonly found that the medical management of the patient was conservative beyond the standard of practice. For example, at POD 5 following a lumbar diskectomy, a 28-year-old woman was afebrile, her pain was well controlled with Tylenol With Codeine No. 3 (acetaminophen with codeine phosphate), and she was independently ambulating. All other monitoring parameters were within normal limits. Her attending neurosurgeon chose to keep her in the hospital for 1 additional day "just to see how the day went." Delays of this type usually resulted in just 1 extra day in the hospital; however, these single days multiplied by a large number of patients result in a significant financial burden on the system.

In cases in which discharge planning or scheduling of outside support or care was identified as the area of delay, problems were found to be related less to the organization of outside services and more to organizing patients and families to enable the discharge to happen. For example, at POD 4 following an anterior cervical diskectomy and fusion, a 37-year-old man was doing well and was ready for discharge, but requested to stay 1 additional day because he lived 3 hours from Boston and did not feel well enough to withstand a long car ride.

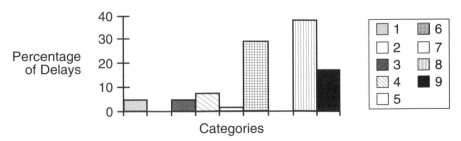

FIGURE 8–1. Percentage of total delays.

BOX 8.1 COST OF A 1-DAY DELAY ON A GENERAL PATIENT CARE UNIT	
Room rate (semiprivate)	$730.00
Physical therapy	75.00
Occupational therapy	75.00
Pharmacy charges	75.00
Lab testing	50.00
	$1005.00*

Estimated in October 1993.

As initially suspected, a significant number of delays (16%) occurred with patients waiting for available outside care in nursing homes, chronic care facilities, and rehabilitation hospitals (category 9). Box 8-1 illustrates the estimated cost per day of a delay.

Most important, the Delay Tool helped us to identify areas in which change in individual or hospital operations might ultimately reduce length of stay. Based on the results, we targeted our energies toward the areas of physician responsibility and discharge planning, putting into place the following interventions:

- establishing critical pathways for common diagnoses; these mutually agreed on care plans would guide our decision making with patients
- addressing the issue of length of stay during the preoperative interview and providing patients with written instructions regarding discharge planning and organization of supports at home
- addressing clearly the progress and discharge planning with the patient and family on a daily basis during morning rounds
- organizing preadmission and preoperative social services and rehabilitation referrals to decrease delays in the involvement of these services.

Above all, our work with the Delay Tool proved to be a consciousness raising effort for all team members. Length of stay and discharge planning have now become an integral part of preliminary goal setting for each patient.

Outcomes

Evaluation of the effect of the nurse practitioner working within a case management model of practice has proven to be more difficult than originally thought. Subjectively, responses have been positive. Primary nurses have cited a feeling of empowerment in their own role as a direct result of working with the nurse practitioner. Because communication has been enhanced, they feel more a part of the team and are more often able to articulate the overall care plan for their patients. Some of the more experienced primary nurses have begun to take on aspects of the nurse practitioner's role with respect to case management. They are more proactive in their approach to patient care and have been able to mentor less experienced staff in this regard.

Physician satisfaction with the role has been evident from the start. The house staff have reported a sense of increased support regarding the presence of a consistent team member on the service. Often consumed by the medical management of the patient, they have little time to devote toward discharge planning and patient education. The nurse practitioner is able to address these issues and ensure their integration into the overall care plan. Management of common problems is mastered more quickly, and less time is spent "reinventing the wheel." The attending physicians, too, appreciate the positive effect of improved communication on patient outcomes. There is now more consistency in patient care and significantly fewer situations are overlooked.

Patients and their families have reported an improvement in the continuity of care while moving across the system. They have described a feeling of being "known" by the nurse practitioner and have appreciated the ability to access the nurse practitioner easily if problems arise. Before the implementation of the role, they were frustrated by unavailability of the neurosurgeons. The nurse practitioner is available on page for emergencies during regular office hours and has consistent telephone office hours each afternoon for routine questions. Patients have found it reassuring to "just touch base" regarding their progress during this time.

Objective data regarding the effectiveness of the role have been more difficult to collect. Certainly the impact of the role on delays in discharge and length of stay has been addressed most successfully. The data obtained with the use of the Delay Tool have guided a number of interventions that have positively affected length of stay. Great strides were seen initially with the spinal surgery population. Average length of stay for lumbar diskectomy patients, which was 6 days at project onset, was decreased to 5 days 1 year after onset of the project. Four years after project onset, the population stayed an average of 4 days, with some patients being discharged after only 2 days. These advances can be attributed to vigilant attention to variances in the usual postoperative trajectory, as well as a willingness to make changes in what was once considered "routine" practice. For example, this patient population was routinely medicated for pain until POD 2 using a PCA pump. However, selected patients have recently been encouraged to change to oral analgesics on POD 1. If pain is well controlled, they are often able to be discharged the following day, 1 day earlier than if they had remained on PCA.

With the outpatient population, emergency room visits have notably decreased as a result of the nurse practitioner's availability. Because the nurse practitioner is easily accessible and can address patient concerns and answer questions in a timely way, some situations can be prevented from escalating to emergencies. The issue of pain management is a good example of a problem that, if left unattended, frequently results in an emergency room visit. The nurse practitioner's intervention by telephone, and, if necessary, during a scheduled office visit, encourages patients to attend to their pain management needs during regular office hours rather than resorting to the use of the emergency room during the night or on weekends.

It is clear to all members of the team that patient care is enhanced with the involvement of a clinical expert who is designated to ensure the delivery of quality, cost-effective care. Future goals of the group include more concise measurement of the effect of these interventions.

CONCLUSIONS

The APN's role will evolve and be challenged as the healthcare system continues to demand more cost-effective approaches to care. As a profession, nursing must maintain the accountability for the resources required to provide quality care.

The functions of direct care provider, educator, change agent, manager, and researcher are inherent components of the APN's role. These components, operationalized with a case management focus, create a clearly defined and differentiated role for the APN. In today's resource-driven healthcare environment, the marriage of these two concepts offers a solution toward bridging the gap between quality and cost of care.

References

American Nurses' Association. (1988). *Nursing case management.* Kansas City, MO: Author.

Bower, K. (1992). *Case management by nurses.* Washington, DC: American Nurses Publishing.

Clifford J., & Wandel, J. (1993). Creating a supportive work environment. In D. Mason, S. Talbot, & J. Levant (Eds.), *Policy and politics for nurses: Action and change in the workplace, government, organizations and communities* (pp. 268–279). Philadelphia: W.B. Saunders.

Cronin, C., & Maklebust, J. (1989). Case managed care: Capitalizing on the CNS. *Nursing Management, 20*(3), 38–47.

Dunston, J. (1990). How managed care can work for you. *Nursing, 90*(20), 56–59.

Ethridge, P., & Lamb, G. (1991). A Nursing HMO: Carondelet St. Mary's experience. *Nursing Management, 22*(7), 22–29.

Giuliano, K., & Poirier, C. (1991). Nursing case management: Critical pathways to desirable outcomes. *Nursing Management, 22*(3), 52–55.

Grau, L. (1984). Case management and the nurse. *Geriatric Nursing, 13*(6), 372–375.

Lamb, G., & Stempel, J. (1994). Nurse case management from the client's view: Growing as insider-expert. *Nursing Outlook, 42*(1), 7–13.

Lynn-McHale, D., Fitzpatrick, E., & Shaffer, R. (1993). Case management: Development of a model. *Clinical Nurse Specialist, 7*(6), 299–307.

McClelland, M., Kolcsar, M., & Bailey, M. (1987). From team to primary nursing. *Nursing Management, 18*(10), 69–71.

Newman, M., Lamb, G., & Michaels, C. (1991). Nursing case management: The coming together of theory and practice. *Nursing Health Care, 12,* 404–408.

Nugent, K. (1992). The clinical nurse specialist as case manager in a collaborative practice model: Bridging the gap between quality and cost of care. *Clinical Nurse Specialist, 6*(2), 106–111.

Olivas, G., Del Togno Armanasco, V., Erickson, J., & Harter, S. (1989). Case management: A bottom-line care delivery model. Part II: Adaptation of the model. *Journal of Nursing Administration, 19*(12), 12–17.

O'Malley, J., Cummings, S., & Loveriage, C. (1989). The new nursing organization. *Nursing Management, 20*(12), 29–32.

Pike, A. (1991). Moral outrage and moral discourse in nurse–physician collaboration. *Journal of Professional Nursing, 7*(6), 351–363.

Selker, J., Beshansky, J., Pauker, S., & Kassirer, J. (1989). The epidemiology of delays in a teaching hospital. *Medical Care, 27*(2), 112–129.

Senge, P. M. (1990). *The fifth discipline: The art and practice of the learning organization.* New York: Doubleday.

Spross, J. (1989). The CNS as collaborator. In A. B. Hamric & J. A. Spross (Eds.), *The clinical nurse specialist in theory and practice* (2nd ed., pp. 205–226). Philadelphia: W.B. Saunders.

Trella, R. (1993). A multidisciplinary approach to case management of frail, hospitalized older adults. *Journal of Nursing Administration, 23*(2), 20–26.

VanTassel, M. (1990). Effective applications of critical pathways. *Michigan Nurse, 63*(5), 5–6.

Zander, K. (1988a). Nursing case management: Resolving the DRG paradox. *Nursing Clinics of North America, 23*(3), 503–520.

Zander, K. (1988b). Nursing case management: Strategic management of cost and quality outcomes. *Journal of Nursing Administration, 18*(5), 23–30.

9

Advanced Practice Nurse in a Managed Care Environment

Marjorie A. Satinsky

The financing and delivery of healthcare have changed dramatically within the past decade, bringing communities in most parts of the United States into a managed care environment. Although state, regional, and local variations exist, almost everybody will be affected somewhat by managed care. As advanced practice nurses (APNs) determine their place in this new environment, it is important that they understand the concepts and assumptions that are the essence of managed care.

This chapter provides background information on managed care. It explains why managed care exists, defines related terms, and describes the characteristics of a mature managed care market. The chapter also addresses the effect of managed care on consumers and providers and describes the implications of managed care for APNs.

WHY MANAGED CARE?

Managed care has existed in the United States for many years, although the term is relatively new. For example, California visionaries created the Kaiser Health Plan and many of the foundations for medical care long before the 1970s, when the term *health maintenance organization (HMO)* was coined and federal legislation enacted. Managed care in the 1990s is related to, but not the same as, many earlier efforts. Why the current popularity?

Traditionally, the provision of healthcare and reimbursement for services have been unrelated. Physicians and hospitals provided as much care as they chose, and payers reimbursed providers on a fee-for-service basis. Payers devoted minimal attention to the level and appropriateness of service, let alone to cost, quality, and efficiency.

Technological advances in medicine have been a mixed blessing. As new techniques have become available, providers have been eager to use them, regardless of the cost to the system. So long as the payers footed the bill, consumers were eager to take advantage of new treatment modalities, and they welcomed state-of-the-art care.

Hickey JV: ADVANCED PRACTICE NURSING: Changing Roles
and Clinical Applications © 1996 Lippincott–Raven Publishers

For people fortunate enough to be covered by commercial health insurance or by public entitlement programs, such as Medicare and Medicaid, expectations grew. Oregon was a pioneer in limiting the availability and accessibility of care, but most states have not confronted the rationing issue.

The healthcare industry flourished under this scenario, growing to represent a significantly large share of the gross national product (GNP). By 1993, 13.9% of the GNP was devoted to healthcare. Not only did healthcare represent a disproportionately large share of the national economy, but the growth rate for healthcare exceeded that for other sectors of the economy. For example, between 1982 and 1991, the medical care price index rose by an annual average of 7.9%, whereas the annual average for the general economy rose by 4.1% (Nighswander, 1994).

The cost and growth rate of healthcare affected both the private and public sectors. Traditionally, American healthcare has been employer based, and so the private sector was negatively affected. Healthcare costs for some companies were so prohibitive that they began to lose their competitive advantage over companies based in other countries. To make matters worse, the concept of *cost shifting,* in which not all payers pay the same price for healthcare, had an increasingly negative effect on the private sector, because the government sought to limit federal healthcare spending in entitlement programs.

At some point, the market began to push for limits on healthcare costs that would not compromise the excellence in quality that technological advancement had brought. The market also did something else. When the Clinton healthcare reform proposal captured national attention, fear of national healthcare reform mobilized many states, many insurers, and many providers to make their own changes. That is why managed care exists.

To understand the implications of managed care for healthcare professionals, it is important to gain knowledge about management structure (eg, who manages), examples of managed care plans, public sector managed care, special niche plans, centers of excellence, integrated financing and delivery systems, transitional strategies, and the characteristics of a mature managed care market. The following sections address each of these areas.

OVERVIEW OF MANAGED CARE

When experts predict that the country is moving toward a scenario in which most population groups, including those covered by commercial insurance, Medicare, and Medicaid, will be covered primarily by managed care health insurance, they are not all speaking the same language. In a narrow sense, *managed care* means a type of health insurance plan. In a broader sense, *managed care* means a "wide range of health care delivery and payment strategies designed to hold down costs while assuring quality of care" (Lewin-VHI, Inc., 1993). Managed care applies to both plan types and to global strategies. A point that is often overlooked is the obligation to manage. Whose obligation is it? The obligation to manage is shared among providers, consumers, and payers (Satinsky, 1995):

> *Providers*—physicians, facilities, and others—have historically played the most important role in determining when, if, and how patients will receive care. As the relationships between insurers, providers, and plan enrollees change, however, providers have taken on a new role. They no longer dictate what care will be rendered at a particular price. Rather, they negotiate to provide care within a limited budget. As providers assume financial risk for a specific population of enrollees assigned to them, they develop internally driven, but externally sensitive standards for delivering high-quality, cost-effective care.

> *Consumers* also have a responsibility to manage care. Many individuals covered by commercial health insurance already have fewer choices of health plan coverage and more financial responsibility (e.g., copayments and deductibles). In many states, both Medicare and Medicaid populations are required or have the option to select managed

care insurance, and so these groups, too, must seek care according to the rules and regulations of particular health plans. For consumers, then, accessing the healthcare system is no longer the free-for-all it once was when indemnity plans dominated the market. They need to manage their health and the way that they seek care when they need it.

Payers—health plans, employers, and third-party administrators—are another group that manages care. The payers no longer pay for whatever care is ordered by providers. They are smart shoppers, and they have learned to manage their healthcare dollars through benefit design, selective contracting, and the shifting of financial risk to providers.

EXAMPLES OF MANAGED CARE PLANS

Health plans that fall under the generic heading *managed care plans* can be distinguished by organizational structure, freedom of access to providers, risk-sharing, and cost-containment techniques. The most common types of managed care plans are health maintenance organizations (HMOs); preferred provider organizations (PPOs); point-of-service (POS) plans; and managed fee-for-service plans.

Within each type of managed care plan is significant variation. Insurers confuse distinctions even more by packaging two or more products together for marketing purposes. Purchasers can then take advantage of buying from a single source.

Unfortunately, there is no "standard" managed care plan. Some but not all plans have chosen to meet federal or National Committee for Quality Assurance (NCQA) qualifications standards. Requirements for state licensure vary. The North Carolina Department of Insurance, for example, has promulgated HMO licensure requirements. In late 1994, however, the department determined that a number of plans were operating as "stealth HMOs" and did not comply with the law. Although these plans were jeopardizing their continued licensure to the general public and to their enrollees, they were HMOs.

Health Maintenance Organizations

HMOs are the most common type of managed care plan. By mid-1994, national HMO enrollment had reached 52 million, representing 20.3% of the population (Marion Merrell Dow, Inc., 1994). HMOs offer a set package of benefits, identified in advance. The HMO premium level is driven by the market; what payers can afford to pay determines price. The HMO benefit package includes preventive care as well as inpatient and outpatient care after the onset of symptoms or illness. HMOs contract with providers (e.g., community and tertiary hospitals, physicians, and other health providers) to provide care to enrolled subscribers. The providers are at financial risk for the care provided and therefore have an incentive to provide cost-effective, high-quality care. Each HMO enrollee selects a primary care physician (PCP), who manages that person's total care by authorizing specialist visits, hospitalization, and other services. Many plans call these PCP managers "gatekeepers," and compensate them for managing their patients' care.

Models of HMO plans include the staff model, group model, and open panel (independent practice association [IPA]) plans. In *staff model plans*, physicians who are salaried by the plan provide care, and income generated belongs to the plan. Some services may be provided on a fee-for-service basis. The plan physicians provide outpatient care at plan-owned ambulatory sites, often called "health centers." Some staff model plans own their own hospitals and other facilities; others contract for these services. The term *closed panel* is often used to describe staff model plans to acknowledge that physician care is only available from salaried physicians.

Because staff model plans own both physicians and, in some cases, hospital facilities, their opportunity to control unnecessary costs is great. During early HMO development, they were best able to sell their plans at the lowest premium. More recently, other model plans have improved their ability to deliver care and lower their premiums as well. Staff model physicians are salaried, but they do have a financial stake in overall plan success.

In *group model plans,* care is provided by a group of primary (and often specialty) physicians who see enrollees in their own offices. The group has a contractual relationship with the health plan. There are at least three variations in the group practice model. Sometimes, the physician group is organized as a separate legal entity but provides care only to members of the HMO with which it is affiliated. The Kaiser-Permanente groups are an example. Or, the physician group may have existed before its decision to affiliate with the HMO and it may provide care not only to that HMOs enrollees, but to enrollees in other plans and fee-for-service patients as well. In another kind of group arrangement that is not mutually exclusive with the first two, two or more groups may be part of a network that contracts with the health plan. Under the group model, the HMO generally contracts selectively with hospitals and other non-physician providers. Opportunities for controlling costs and managing quality are not as great as in the staff model, but they are good.

Open panel plans offer enrollees more provider choice than staff or group model plans. Providers provide outpatient care in their own offices and they are financially at risk for the care they provide. In some open panel plans, the physicians are legally organized into an IPA; the IPA as well as individual physicians are then at financial risk for the care provided. Hospital and other institutional care is provided by selected providers with whom the health plan contracts.

Both open and closed panel plans use different methods to reimburse physicians and hospital providers, depending on the degree of risk that is shifted or shared. For example, hospital reimbursement methods include discount from charges, per diem, per case, global case rate (including physician component), or capitation. Physician reimbursement ranges from discounted fee-for-service to capitation. In some open panel plans, the plan may also withhold a percentage of the physician's fee, keeping it in a separate pool until the end of the fiscal year. If the physician delivers care within his or her budget, the withheld money (or a portion of it) is returned. For both hospitals and physicians, the capitation method of reimbursement shifts the most risk to providers. Most HMOs move gradually toward full capitation and are likely to reimburse providers using a variety of methods, some of which may have conflicting financial incentives.

Theoretically, all types of HMOs spend less on healthcare services than indemnity plans, PPOs, or other managed care plans. Control mechanisms such as coordination of care by PCPs, provision of preventive care, utilization review, and quality assurance programs enable HMO plans to save dollars and to pass them on to plan members in premiums. Enrollees save on out-of-pocket costs as well, because most HMOs have relatively small copayments for office visits and other services. Still another advantage to HMO enrollees is the lack of paperwork; the HMO premium, paid in advance, pays for covered services, and enrollees do not submit bills for payment.

Preferred Provider Organizations

PPOs are a compromise managed care option that came into existence as an alternative somewhere between indemnity and HMO insurance. In general, PPO plans use financial incentives, not controls, to influence consumer and provider behavior. There is no standard PPO plan; the term refers to a variety of arrangements between insurers, providers, and third-party administrators.

PPOs, like HMOs, have the option of meeting qualification standards set by professional organizations. The American Accreditation Program, Inc., established in 1989, is the leading PPO accreditation organization (Kongstvedt, 1993). There are no federal PPO requirements, and state licensing requirements vary.

Many PPOs are owned by large insurance companies. For example, Travelers, Prudential, Metropolitan Life, Provident, Aetna, and John Hancock have developed PPO products. In general, these companies develop provider networks, compensate providers on a discounted fee-for-service basis, and perform administrative tasks such as marketing and claims administration. In other PPO arrangements, a corporate entity may develop a network of insurers, develop a provider network, and provide or arrange for the provision of administrative services. Private Healthcare Systems in Lexington, MA, is an example. The varieties of preferred provider arrangements are numerous.

PPOs are available primarily to the employed commercial population. Employees are encouraged to use participating hospitals and physicians, but they have the option to use "out-of-network" providers for an additional out-of-pocket cost. As in open panel HMOs, physicians provide care in their offices. The PPO contracts with hospitals and other providers. Most PPOs use some methods to control utilization; preauthorization for inpatient admission and for certain outpatient procedures is common.

The premium for PPO insurance usually falls between that of indemnity and HMO plans. Out-of-pocket costs vary, depending on whether the patient chooses to use in-network or out-of-network providers and pay a copayment or deductible. Unlike HMOs, PPOs do require paperwork, and eligible subscribers do submit bills, particularly when they use out-of-network services.

Point of Service Plans

In response to both employer and employee demands, some plans have modified either their HMO or PPO products, adding a feature that enables consumers to decide at the "point of service "whether to use the provider network or seek care outside of the network. If the POS plan is a variation of an HMO plan, enrollees use PCPs to coordinate all care but, if they wish, can seek care outside the HMO network. If the POS plan is a variation of a PPO plan, enrollees have the option to opt into the provider network at a lower cost to themselves.

Given their flexibility, it is no surprise that POS plans are growing more rapidly than other types of managed care. For example, during the first half of 1994, enrollment in *hybrid HMOs,* that is, licensed HMOs with an out-of-network option and open-ended panel (ie, POS) HMO plans with a separate license, grew by 18.7%. By mid-1994, enrollment in these types of plans accounted for 16.7% of all national HMO enrollment (Marion Merrell Dow, Inc., 1994).

Managed Fee-for-Service Plans

Managed fee-for-service plans are the least managed of the managed care options. These plans generally do not shift financial risk to providers and limit member access to care by selectively building networks of providers. Use controls are minimal; common ones are preauthorization for hospitalization or specific procedures.

PUBLIC SECTOR MANAGED CARE

Like the private sector, the public sector has been faced with dramatic increases in healthcare costs. The Federal Employees Health Benefits Program, Medicare and Medicaid programs, and the Department of Defense have all looked to managed care as a way to not only control costs, but to improve the coordination and quality of care.

In 1994, the Federal Employees Health Benefits Program offered HMO coverage to 2.1 million workers (Marion Merrell Dow, Inc., 1994). Most of the government enrollees in HMOs were in group model and IPA type plans.

Over the years, Medicare beneficiaries have had the opportunity to select a variety of managed care options. By mid-1994, 2.9 million Medicare enrollees had HMO coverage

(Marion Merrell Dow, Inc., 1994). For example, Medicare risk contracts offer HMO coverage as a total Medicare replacement. Controversy over the adequacy of federal reimbursement for elderly patients with complex medical problems has deterred some plans from taking the full-risk approach. An alternative managed care plan strategy for the Medicare population is to offer a Medicare wraparound or supplement (Kongstvedt, 1993). Medicare Select supplemental programs already exist in 15 states under a federal pilot program.

Medicaid recipients have also had the opportunity to participate in HMOs. By early 1995, eight states had obtained the necessary Health Care Financing Administration waiver (Section 1115) to develop programs (Somerville, 1995). Some states mandate managed care participation for particular categories of Medicaid recipients, and other states offer recipients the option of selecting HMO or traditional coverage. Another state-specific variation is the development of Medicaid–specific managed care plans instead of a Medicaid component within a commercial plan. Although the concept of managed Medicaid programs has resulted in significant cost savings and improved quality of care, in some states, such as Tennessee, others have experienced significant difficulties. One explanation for variation in success of Medicaid managed care is timing. In states which introduce Medicaid managed care before providers have experience managing commercial enrollees, operational problems often arise.

Healthcare programs for members of the armed forces, dependents, and others entitled to Department of Defense (DOD) medical care have also moved toward managed care (Kongstvedt, 1993). The medical benefits provided under the Civilian Health and Medical Program of the Uniformed Services (CHAMPUS) traditionally have been generous and costly, and the DOD has tested a variety of managed care mechanisms through demonstration programs. Unlike Medicare, though, the DOD did not attempt to make sweeping national changes. Examples of the Department's demonstrations are as follows:

The CHAMPUS Reform Initiative (CRI) requested competitive bids by at-risk contractors who would underwrite CHAMPUS services. Foundation Health Corporation was awarded the initial contract to conduct the program in California and Hawaii. CHAMPUS PRIME and CHAMPUS EXTRA were added to the standard CHAMPUS program. The PRIME product was similar to an HMO, and EXTRA was similar to a PPO.

New Orleans Managed Care Demonstration tested managed care techniques in an area without an inpatient medical treatment facility.

Catchment Area Management Demonstration projects were developed to contain costs at the local level. Local military hospital commanders assumed responsibility for managing the financing and delivery of healthcare for the entire beneficiary population in each catchment area.

The demonstrations achieved good results; consequently, the DOD introduced TRICARE on a national level (Bartling, 1995). The system created 12 health services regions and designated major military centers as lead agents. The triple option benefit includes TRICARE Prime (HMO with POS option), TRICARE Extra (PPO), and TRICARE Standard (indemnity insurance). Medical treatment facility commanders have the tools, authority, and flexibility to focus on the delivery of care, organization of the delivery of care, accountability, and to control or measure costs. The program, which began in fiscal year 1992, had a 3-year phase-in period.

SPECIAL NICHE PLANS

As purchasers have become more sophisticated about the design of their benefit plans, they have "carved out" specific problem areas and purchased service-specific coverage and management from companies with a particular expertise. For example, provision of mental health and substance abuse care has been a costly item for many employers, and they have turned to companies that specialize in the insurance and management of this benefit. A prescription drug plan, too, is a benefit often managed separately from the traditional benefit package.

In the early 1990s, the Massachusetts Division of Insurance coined an appropriate term for the many varieties of managed care that it regulated—or tried to regulate. That term is *OWAs*, which stands for "other weird arrangements!"

CENTERS OF EXCELLENCE

Particularly for high-cost tertiary care, some payers have developed special arrangements with networks of providers covering a large geographic area. The providers have agreed to accept a particular level of reimbursement, with the understanding that the payer will direct patients to them in a preferred relationship. Among the services for which centers of excellence are commonly developed are cardiovascular care and transplantation (e.g., bone marrow and solid organ).

An example of centers of excellence is the Medicare network for coronary artery bypass graft surgery. In 1991, the government selected seven U.S. hospitals to participate in the demonstration program (American College of Cardiology, 1993).

INTEGRATED FINANCING AND DELIVERY SYSTEMS

In a managed care environment, the financing and delivery of healthcare are likely to come together in integrated systems. Although the process of integration differs by market, all such systems will have at least four common characteristics: vertical integration of services, payment by capitation, emphasis on low-cost/high-quality services, and a rationing of resources. A 1993 report issued by The Advisory Board (1993b) describes these features:

Vertical integration of services means different levels of care (e.g., primary and specialty, acute, subacute, long-term, ambulatory, home care, and rehabilitation) are combined into a seamless *continuum of care*. Patients who access care at any point will be able to move smoothly among the different components.

Payment by capitation means financial risk is shifted from payers to providers and the unit of value is cost per member per month. In capitated systems, providers are responsible for a specific target population for which they receive an age- and gender-adjusted budget. To manage care within that budget, providers will strive to keep the target population healthy.

Low-cost/high-quality services, a goal of integrated systems, add value to what buyers purchase.

Rationing of resources emphasizes providing appropriate, but not unlimited, care. Rationing will occur in several ways. PCPs with a gatekeeper role will assume responsibility for the provision and management of care, and will direct their patients to specialty and institutional care, if and when necessary. Rich benefit packages may be redefined.

Integrated financing and delivery systems, like managed care, have already developed in some parts of the country. For example, California, Minnesota, and more recently, Massachusetts, are well on their way. KPMG-Peat Marwick, Center for Health Services and Policy Research, and J.L. Kellogg School of Management at Northwestern University in Evanston, IL, have jointly spearheaded a comprehensive study of nine hospital-driven systems, documenting their similarities and differences in structure, operations, and four-stage development (Shortell, 1993).

Systems develop for different reasons. The literature suggests that those systems that develop for market-related reasons, rather than in response to the needs of specific immigrant or religious groups or to the need for capital formation, are well-positioned to meet the needs of the future (Jones & Mayerhofer, 1994).

As integrated systems evolve, a critical issue in their success will be their ability to capture, share, and manage information from all parts of the system. If, for example, a system includes preventive services, physician's office, outpatient clinics, urgent-care centers, hospitals, home health, rehabilitation, and long-term care, the goal would be for all of these entities to exchange and use information about patients who receive care at one or more points. In an even more advanced concept for information sharing—Community Health Information Networks (CHINS)—multiple integrated financing and delivery systems share data electronically, not only among systems but with the community. CHINS have the capability to eliminate costly duplication and greatly enhance quality of care (Work & Mackevicius, 1995).

TRANSITIONAL STRATEGIES

Integrated financing and delivery systems have not yet come to most parts of the country. Indeed, they may never come at all to some rural areas. Most places are in a transitional stage and are experimenting with a variety of transitional strategies, including, but not limited to, the following:

management service bureau: generally a wholly-owned hospital subsidiary created to provide practice management services to physicians; examples of these services are physician recruitment, office staff training, group purchasing, and computerized billing

group practice without walls: individual physicians continue to practice in their separate offices, but form a grouplike practice to recognize economies of scale in marketing, centralizing services, and negotiating with managed care plans

open or closed physician–hospital organization: this organization may be open to all medical staff members or more selective in membership; having a physician–hospital organization is considered an advantage when negotiating with managed care plans that prefer one-stop contracting

comprehensive management service organization: going one step beyond the management service bureau, the comprehensive version not only provides practice management services, but also purchases the hard assets of practices, manages the practices, and negotiates managed care contracts

foundation: the health system buys the tangible and intangible assets of physician practices; the foundation is a not-for-profit wholly-owned system subsidiary that signs professional services agreements with physicians remaining in a separate professional corporation

staff model: the health system employs physicians, generally under a physician-managed clinic; it has more control over physicians than the foundation model

equity model: a for-profit group practice owns the facilities of an integrated system; physicians are employed, generally on a salaried basis, and have the opportunity to share in the system's equity (The Advisory Board, 1993b).

Regardless of where providers and payers are in the development of integrated financing and delivery systems, a key to future success will be the ability to coordinate the clinical delivery of care (Conrad, 1993).

CHARACTERISTICS OF A MATURE MANAGED CARE ENVIRONMENT

In a mature managed care environment, market forces, reimbursement, and service delivery contrast sharply with those same forces in a nonmanaged care environment. Their effect is felt by consumers and providers. Most parts of the country fall somewhere between these extremes and so have components of both, often with conflicting financial incentives.

In examining the differences between managed care and nonmanaged care environments, it is important to understand that successful systems respond to market forces. Attention to payers' wants and budgets helps systems and their components shift gears and provide evidence of value.

Market

The market in a mature managed care environment contrasts with that in a nonmanaged care market in at least two important ways: (1) competition is among integrated financing and delivery systems, not individual components, and (2) health plans and employers use many strategies to contain healthcare cost while ensuring quality of care.

Systems Competition

In a mature managed care environment, integrated financing and delivery systems compete for business, and competition is fierce. In nonmanaged care environments, competition is among such system components as hospitals, physicians, and health plans. In the Boston area, for example, there has been a rapid shift toward competition among three emerging systems: (1) Lahey Clinic/Harvard Community Health Plan/Pilgrim Health Care/Mary Hitchcock Clinic and a number of community or teaching hospitals; (2) Partners (Massachusetts General and Brigham and Women's Hospitals, Blue Cross and Blue Shield, and selected community hospitals); and (3) New England Medical Center/Deaconness Hospital/Baptist Hospital/Tufts Associated Health Plan and a number of community hospitals. On the surface, these competing systems will have similar features such as vertical integration of services, equity partnerships between insurers and providers, and community providers who are competing for regional business. California and Minnesota have an even more intense competition among integrated systems.

Health Plan and Employer Strategies for Balancing Cost Containment and Quality of Care

Purchasers, both health plans and employers, wield considerable influence in a mature managed care environment. Each has developed a number of strategies (Satinsky, 1995) to balance cost containment and assurance of quality care.

Health Plan Strategies

Health plans, for example, use strategies such as product diversification, plan consolidation, selective contracting, risk-shifting and demonstration of value. These are added to keep costs under control and make sure that providers deliver high quality care.

Product Diversification

Many managed care plans seek to convince employers to replace existing multiple health insurance offerings with a single product. To encourage the total replacement decision, these plans adopt a multiple option strategy, offering closed panel, group practice, open panel, and PPO options under a single umbrella. An example of this approach exists in the New England market. Harvard Community Health Plan began as a staff model plan. Mergers with Multi-Group and Rhode Island Group Health Association and a linkage with the Lahey Clinic and Mary-Hitchcock Clinic organizations added a group model to its portfolio. An agreement with John Hancock added a PPO option. The recent merger of Harvard Community Health Plan and Pilgrim Health Care added other options to the offering package.

Linking workers' compensation coverage to health insurance benefits is another diversification strategy. The Tufts Associated Health Plan in Massachusetts created the Managed Comp product to fill this niche.

Health Plan Consolidation

The number of managed care health plans has decreased over time. Some plans have indeed gone out of business, but others have merged, creating megaplans that can compete for business on a regional level. A recent example is Healthsource's strategic alliance with Provident. Similarly, Metropolitan Life and Travelers have combined their managed care efforts. In Minneapolis–St. Paul, a hotbed of managed care activity, 80% of the HMO enrollment in

1993 was covered by three large health plans, HealthPartners, Allina, and Blue Cross/Blue Shield/Blue Plus (Nighswander, 1994).

Selective Contracting

Many health plans have taken the selective approach to contracting with healthcare providers, working to establish partnerships in lieu of contractual relationships. The partnership approach facilitates a joint focus on problem areas. An obstacle to the selective approach has been the emergence in some states of *any willing provider laws* that require plans to contract with all qualified providers who are willing to accept their payments.

Risk-Shifting

Financial risk-shifting is another strategy that health plans use to control costs. Plans move from discounted fee-for-service arrangements to alternative methods of reimbursement that hold providers more accountable for the cost and utilization of care. Examples of risk-shifting are: per case payment, global rate payment covering both technical and professional components, and capitation.

Demonstration of Value

Managed care plans have always had financial targets and worked toward achieving budgets by managing use. In response to employer demands, they are now looking seriously at showing value for the dollar. Many are using a report card format to demonstrate their achievements in quality and outcomes.

For example, in 1993, Kaiser's northern California region developed a model "quality report card" (Kenkel, 1994). Kaiser measured quality, defined as service delivery, not clinical outcomes, for seven areas: childhood health, maternal care, cardiovascular disease, cancer, common surgical procedures, other adult health, and mental health and substance abuse. It also looked at member satisfaction with medical care, experience of care, access, and service. United HealthCare in Minnesota and U.S. Healthcare, Inc., in Blue Bell, PA, are two other managed care plans that have devoted significant effort to the report card approach.

Report cards vary, depending on the sponsoring organization. The Health Care Advisory Board (Health Care Advisory Board, 1994) summarizes the following indicators that plans might use to monitor themselves.

Access measures show enrollee ease in accessing the system.

Appropriateness measures compare actual care rendered with expectations.

Service quality measures show enrollee perceptions of the care they have received.

Encounter outcomes measures show the results of specific clinical encounters.

Disease management measures show the effectiveness of treating a disease in its entirety across the continuum of care.

Prevention measures indicate the frequency and effectiveness of preventive care.

Enrollee health status measures show the ability of the plan to maintain the health of its population.

In addition to producing report cards on their performance, many plans are now seeking recognition from two accrediting organizations, the Joint Commission for Accreditation of Healthcare Organizations and the NCQA. The NCQA, along with representatives of employers and health plans, has developed the Health Plan Employer Data and Information Set (HEDIS) criteria so that purchasers and eventually consumers can select health plans on the basis of quality of care and value. The plans themselves are expected to use the data to measure and improve their own performance. Criteria for quality under HEDIS 2.0 include access to care, appropriateness, efficacy, technical outcome, and member satisfaction (NCQA, 1993).

Employer Strategies

Employer strategies for cost containment and maintenance of quality include, but are not limited to, limiting choice of options, methodologically evaluating health insurance options, forming purchasing coalitions, increasing employee cost-sharing, creating carve-out products, using direct contracting, and, more recently, developing their own healthcare systems (Satinsky, 1995).

Limiting Choice of Health Insurance Options

As their healthcare costs have soared, many employers have taken draconian steps to bring them under control. A common strategy is to reduce the health insurance options available for employees and primarily to offer types of plans that incorporate cost controls into their structure and organization. Many employers, especially large national ones, have cast their lots with specific plans and have entered multiyear relationships. Examples are the innovative Allied Signal–CIGNA partnership and the General Electric Corporation preferred provider arrangement strategy.

Methodologically Evaluating Health Insurance Options

Many employers who once delegated decisions on health insurance up to a mid-level staffperson are more often turning to people with a new area of expertise: healthcare cost containment. Many have hired individuals and even staffs to manage the evaluation of health insurance options and, once a decision has been made, the management of care.

Forming Purchasing Coalitions

Employers in many communities have recognized the value of banding together to analyze healthcare costs, obtain and organize data, and negotiate with providers. For example, in Minneapolis–St. Paul, 13 of the largest employers formed the Business Health Care Action Group. The group ultimately contracted with HealthPartners, a large HMO, and its decision forced the plan to demonstrate commitment to cost and quality management by developing a joint effort with several important providers (i.e., Park Nicollet Medical Center, Mayo Clinic, and Methodist Hospital).

The Greater Cleveland Health Quality Choice Coalition is one example of the effect an employer purchasing group can have on care providers. When it released its fourth report on hospital performance in 1994, the coalition believed its data were sufficiently reliable to assess the quality and value of care provided by 29 participating institutions ("Employers Go To Bed With Cleveland's Latest Performance Report," 1995).

Employers can influence not only provider performance, but health plan performance and pricing as well. For example, an 11-member employer coalition in San Francisco, part of the larger Bay Area Business Group on Health, was able to obtain rate concessions from more than a dozen HMOs (Kenkel, 1994). The group also linked premium payment to health plan ability to meet criteria for customer service, quality of care, and data reporting.

Introducing Employee Cost-Sharing

It is no surprise that the person who pays has more of an interest in cost than the person who gets a free ride. Once somewhat reluctant to shift a portion of healthcare costs to employees, many companies are now willing to increase employees at financial risk by introducing copayments and deductibles, and, on a more positive note, by offering financial incentives for "good behavior" (e.g., participation in exercise and health education programs).

Creating "Carve-Outs"

The carve-out approach described earlier in the section Special Niche Plans (see p. 131) is another popular employer strategy for cost containment.

Using Direct Contracting

Self-insured companies in particular have bypassed insurance intermediaries to contract directly with providers. They use third-party administrators to handle administrative, marketing, and claims payment functions.

Developing Healthcare Services

Some large employers have decided that they prefer to produce rather than purchase healthcare services (Solovy, 1994). Delta Airlines, for example, has built a primary care center near Hartsfield International Airport in Atlanta. The John Deere Family Healthplan in Des Moines now has three primary care centers that provide services not only to company employees, but to local employers as well.

Reimbursement

In an aggressive managed care environment, providers (i.e., both physicians and hospitals) agree to accept financial risk for the care they provide to a specific population of enrollees. They are paid on a capitated basis. They receive capitation payments in advance, and the payment level reflects the expected utilization by the enrolled population for which they are responsible. To manage risk and live within the capitation budget, providers must control both volume and cost. They are usually rewarded for efficiency. For example, bonus payments may be related to operating within budget and to achieving specific goals for quality and efficiency. PCPs are key players when providers are at financial risk. They generally act as gatekeepers who steer enrollees to other providers, if and when necessary.

In contrast, in a nonmanaged care environment, providers are reimbursed when they actually provide care. Compensation for care offers incentives for performing high volumes of service. Physicians, for example, receive fee-for-service payments and have no financial incentive to monitor the amount and intensity of care they provide. Likewise, hospitals may be paid on a discount from charge basis and may be rewarded for every day that patients remain in the hospital. Specialty care is highly compensated, and PCPs do not become involved in determining which patients will need specialty care or other services.

In most of the country, provider reimbursement has elements of both managed care and nonmanaged care systems. In a 1993 report on capitation, The Advisory Board (1993a) suggested that "very few Americans are capitated for the whole course of their care" (p. 37). In Massachusetts, for example, where more than 40% of the population was covered by managed care insurance by 1995, provider reimbursement still contains conflicting financial incentives. The one health plan that made an early commitment to capitate PCPs continues to pay specialist physicians according to a plan-specific fee schedule. Hospital reimbursement is not completely aligned with physician reimbursement, creating a system of complex financial incentives. Hoping to avoid a similar situation, Duke University Medical Center in Durham, NC, chose to capitate both primary care and specialist physicians and Duke Hospital when it revised the health insurance program for university employees in 1995.

Service Delivery

Service delivery in a managed care environment differs from that in a nonmanaged care environment in at least three areas: emphasis on continuity of care, focus on nonhospital alternatives for care, and collaborative practice. In a managed care environment, providers have a financial incentive to provide less, rather than more, care and to ensure that care is provided at the appropriate level. Benefits include preventive care, such as well-child or well-adult visits, under the assumption that preventive health contributes to enrollee health and well-being.

Providers and payers use many techniques to facilitate the integrated provision of care across the continuum and to monitor resource utilization. Both health plans and healthcare providers may use case management to ensure that enrollees receive the care they need in the appropriate setting. Useful tools are practice guidelines, clinical protocols, and care-mapping (Zender, 1995).

In contrast, in a nonmanaged care environment, patients generally have more freedom to access providers without much input from and coordination by PCPs or payers. Fragmented care is the norm. Providers have a great deal of autonomy in ordering. In addition, provider participation is inclusive, not selective, making the payers' job of monitoring cost and quality more difficult.

Market forces affect use of resources as well. Payers do not tolerate overuse of ancillary services, unlimited prescriptions, or provision of care in a costly setting that could have been rendered more appropriately. The scope of covered benefits and plan rules encourage providers to provide outpatient, not inpatient, care, provided the healthcare can be rendered in a medically safe way. As a result, there is a significant shift from inpatient to outpatient care.

Service delivery in a managed care environment is collaborative. The collaboration occurs both among providers and between provider and health plan staff. On the provider side, for example, enrollees are expected to move through a continuum of care, and there is need for healthcare professionals at different points along the continuum to work together. When providers develop close working relationships with insurers, there is a necessity for the two to work together—again, with the patient and family as the focus.

EFFECT OF MANAGED CARE ON CONSUMERS

In mature managed care markets and in places that fall somewhere between nonmanaged care and managed care, consumers behave differently than they do in nonmanaged care environments. Consumers who are covered by managed care health insurance have the advantage of access to comprehensive care. When managed care works properly, consumers thus trade up. Their healthcare dollar now buys coordinated care, possibly with a PCP to coordinate use of the system. Health plan or provider staff may offer case management services to guide enrollees through the different components of care. Prevention and wellness are included in the benefits. Depending on the cost of their previous health insurance plan, many enrollees see their health insurance premiums or out-of-pocket costs decrease.

The transition from nonmanaged to managed care does not happen easily, however. Enrollees who are new participants in managed care plans are often confused by the rules of their health plans, and they look not only to plan member relations departments but also to providers themselves to clarify the requirements for access and reimbursement.

EFFECT OF MANAGED CARE ON PROVIDERS

The provider role in a managed care environment also changes (Satinsky, 1995). Hospitals are no longer the hub of all healthcare activity. Rather, they become revenue centers of a total system that also includes nonhospital providers such as home care agencies, long-term care facilities, and so forth.

As health plans exert pressure for more efficient care, there are significant changes in the balance of inpatient versus ambulatory care. Predictions have indicated that by 2000, 30% to 40% of traditional admissions will shift to outpatient encounters as a result of changing demographics, technological advances, and payer pressure.

Internally, many hospitals have looked at *reengineering,* defined by Hammer (cited in Bergman, 1994) as "the radical redesign of the critical systems and processes used to produce, deliver, and support patient care in order to achieve dramatic improvements in organizational performance within a short period of time" (p. 28).

In a managed care environment, providers concentrate on *patient-focused care,* in which the enrollees, not providers, are the target for changes in service delivery. Some hospitals use physical redesign. For example, previously centralized ancillary services such as laboratory and radiology may be decentralized into satellites so that the diagnostic testing can occur within inpatient units.

Another critical component of patient-focused care is the ability to develop and link patient-specific information. The idea of a computerized patient-focused information system is the glue that can hold together service provision at multiple delivery points.

As their roles in the healthcare scenario change, both hospitals and physicians are linking closely together. Transitional strategies (e.g., physician hospital organizations, management service organizations, and so forth) have brought these two groups together.

Another change on the provider side has been the recognition of provider responsibility to manage the health and wellness of a specific population. The American Hospital Association's vision for reform set forth in 1993 focuses on the community care network (American Hospital Association, 1993). The essence of the concept is that collaboration will improve a community's health status through the provision of a seamless continuum of services by healthcare providers operating within a fixed budget. The provider's accountability is to the community (Satinsky, 1995).

To compete and survive in a managed care environment, providers and their staffs must learn to behave in new ways. The opportunity for APNs is a good one.

EFFECT OF MANAGED CARE ON ADVANCED PRACTICE NURSES

The managed care environment gives APNs significant opportunity for professional growth and effect on the healthcare system. Advanced practice nurses have the training and experience that, combined with new skills, places them in an ideal position to assume a variety of important roles.

Skills for the Future

Advanced practice nurses in a managed care environment need proficiency in organizational, professional, and interpersonal skills. Managed care involves a major shift in organizational relationships, within each provider organization, among provider organizations, and between providers, payers, and consumers. Some organizations will change and thrive; others will not. Similarly, some health professionals will fit well and contribute to the change; others will seek opportunities elsewhere.

In his book *The Fifth Discipline,* Senge (1990) described the important characteristics of the leaders, that is, the "learning organizations": personal mastery, mental models, shared vision, team learning, and systems thinking. These characteristics, described as follows, are most appropriate for healthcare organizations and their employees in the 1990s.

Personal mastery: "the discipline of continually clarifying and deepening our personal vision, of focusing our energies, of developing patience, and of seeing reality objectively" (p. 7). Personal mastery in an organization contributes to that organization's strength.

Mental models: "deeply ingrained assumptions, generalizations, or even pictures or images that influence how we understand the world and how we take action." In a learning organization, the staff is aware of these pictures and willing to challenge them" (p. 8).

Ability to build a shared vision: perceiving a vision of the future that thrives on "commitment," not "compliance."

Team learning: thinking together on an ongoing basis.

Systems thinking: understanding the interconnectedness of the component parts.

In addition to skills that will enable them to contribute to the success of learning organizations, APNs need to master new professional and interpersonal skills, including, but not limited, to understanding the managed care environment, combining clinical and financial information, functioning comfortably when roles remain ambiguous and negotiable, interacting with multiple professionals both within and outside the organization, and finding new solutions. Each of these skills is described in the sections that follow.

Understanding the Managed Care Environment

Managed care, that is, the health plans themselves and the techniques for managing, are continuously evolving. Advanced practice nurses need to understand not only what managed care is today, but what it is likely to be tomorrow, as they work toward framing their own roles in the new environment.

To learn about managed care in its current stage, APNs can develop working relationships both inside and outside of the settings in which they work. Internally, most organizations have a managed care "guru" whose primary responsibility is managed care contracting and operations. That individual is a good resource for both managers and staff. Educational programs sponsored by external organizations are also important. Some of the most useful are not directed specifically toward the nursing profession, but are geared toward other professionals who also need to learn about managed care.

Another way for APNs to learn about managed care is to talk and visit with colleagues in parts of the country that are already characterized as mature managed care markets. California, Minnesota, and the Boston metropolitan area are good examples.

Combining Clinical and Financial Information

Advanced practice nurses in a managed care environment need clinical and financial skills and the savvy to combine them. For most, clinical skills are a given. There may be less proficiency in other skills such as healthcare finance, accounting, and computer applications.

Effective ways to learn some of these newer skills are to attend courses and conferences. Another approach is to talk with ANPs who are already using some of these techniques; they can provide concrete examples of new skills they learned and provide guidance on how to acquire and apply them. Some organizations have developed comprehensive managed care continuing education programs by using in-house experts on finance, "care mapping," case management, and so forth to educate each other.

Functioning Comfortably When Roles Remain Ambiguous and Negotiable

Of all the characteristics of the managed care environment, the most difficult to comprehend is the ongoing change and evolution. With this change comes a never-ending ambiguity about the role of ANPs and of other professionals as well. An example from the case management literature illustrates the point (Satinsky, 1995). At the Malden Hospital in Malden, MA, a new case management program was developed to integrate the previously separate functions of utilization review, discharge planning, and social services. Although case management was initially envisioned as focusing on the inpatient population, it quickly became clear that the case managers could go well beyond the walls of the hospital. The director of case management, an APN with experience in both provider and payer organizations, perceived an opportunity to expand the case manager role, not stopping at the official job description. Other institutions with case management programs have similarly encouraged the function to evolve.

Similarly, case managers who are employed by managed healthcare plans, usually HMOs, have also experienced an evolution of roles. In many plans, case managers exercise a high degree of autonomy for managing both clinical and financial aspects of care. Their roles expand and shrink as needed.

Interacting With Multiple Professionals Inside and Outside the Organization

Mature managed care markets are very competitive. Each healthcare professional plays a major role in ensuring that relationships with health plans, with employers, and with patients and families are good.

Advanced practice nurses are in a particularly good position to perform this function. By virtue of their knowledge, experience, and formal place within an organization, they are well suited to facilitate both internal and external linkages. The more skilled they are at identifying and resolving problems of coordination, the more they can contribute to their organization's functioning as a cooperative partner. For example, many academic medical centers and community hospitals have initiated comprehensive efforts to measure quality of care and to implement cost-containment programs, and APNs frequently hold key jobs. They interpret external demands for information, collect and interpret data, and collaborate with other professionals to make improvements.

Within many health plans, APNs perform similar roles to those in medical centers. Some are responsible for maintaining good relations with the plan enrollees. Others act as the liaison with the providers with which the plan contracts.

Finding New Solutions

Although the evolution from a nonmanaged care to a mature managed care market will occur in many parts of the country, it will not occur in exactly the same way in multiple places. The challenge to APNs is to look at the experience of others, to take risks, and to find solutions that are appropriate in a particular setting.

Again, the example of APNs in a case management role is a good one (Satinsky, 1995). Stanford University Hospital in California and New England Medical Center in Massachusetts are both academic medical centers that developed creative case management programs. Their case management programs differ, however, according to institutional cultures and local market conditions. Similarly, in a systems context, Friendly Hills HealthCare Network and Sharp HealthCare in California, and Lutheran General HealthSystem in Illinois took different case management strategies. Each is a success in its own unique way.

Potential Roles for Advanced Practice Nurses

There are many roles for APNs in a managed care environment (Hicks, Stallmeyer, & Coleman, 1993). If care is indeed provided along a continuum, the provision and management of care at different levels is the shared responsibility of providers and insurers. Advanced practice nurses have the opportunity to function at any one or multiple points in the continuum. Combining clinical, financial, and administrative skills makes the field wide open.

Opportunities for APNs in a managed care environment include, but are not limited, to primary care, case management, utilization management, patient advocacy, member services, education, triage, quality assurance, and resource management. Each role is described in the following sections, and examples are provided.

Primary Care

Conceptually, the idea of primary care has multiple meanings. As Goeppinger explains in Chapter 5, it may mean health promotion and disease prevention at the individual, family, and community levels. It may also mean secondary prevention, that is, the resolution of health problems in their early stages, such as screening for cervical cancer and vision and hearing testing. Primary care might also mean building capability and enhanced problem solving in health promotion at the community level.

Within a managed care context, primary care has even broader implications. PCPs, often called gatekeepers, not only provide care, but also coordinate appropriate referrals and ensure that enrollees for whom they are responsible have access to a variety of wellness and preventive services. As care shifts away from the institutional setting, the ability of the PCPs to manage enrollees' total care requires familiarity with a vast array of services, settings, and intervention techniques. Plans often pay a management fee to PCPs in recognition of their dual role as providers/coordinators.

Because primary care in a managed care environment is so comprehensive, many health plans and private practices employ APNs to work with physicians in the provision and collaboration of care. As explained in Chapter 10 on Collaboration and Advanced Practice Nursing, the collaborative role of APNs in a primary care setting can vary. In some instances, both the nurse and physician maintain independent practices of patients, collaborating when necessary. In other instances, the provision of all care is collaborative.

Case Management

As the financing and delivery of healthcare evolve, the popularity of the case management concept has grown. Although the term has many different meanings and applications, a good working definition includes the following three concepts (Satinsky, 1995):

1. comprehensive and applicable to a patient's entire episode of illness, regardless of the pay class or location in which the service is provided
2. organized around a system of interdisciplinary services and resources needed to provide high-quality care in the most cost-effective way
3. coordinated by clinical and financial management of care by coordinators, not direct caregivers, who have a financial incentive to manage risk and maximize the quality of care.

All case managers perform at least the following tasks: assessment, planning, intervention, monitoring, and evaluation. They perform their roles in a variety of settings. For example, managed healthcare plans use case managers to manage high-risk, high-cost, or other segments of the total enrollee population. Acute-care hospitals use case managers to manage the use of resources by patients. Large hospitals, particularly academic medical centers, often focus case management activities on patients with particular diseases such as cardiovascular disease, cancer, or renal disease. Employers, too, may use case managers to work with particular segments of the employed population. The list of possibilities is long.

In all settings in which case management has been implemented, APNs have proven to have the knowledge and skills to do the job. Examples of innovative program development exist in single hospitals (e.g., Winchester Medical Center in Virginia); in integrated systems (e.g., Friendly Hills HealthCare Network and Sharp HealthCare in California); and in separate ambulatory settings (e.g., Carondelet St. Mary's Hospital and Health Center in Arizona). Although each case management program is different, all offer unique opportunities for nurses to creatively coordinate the clinical and financial management of care.

Utilization Management

The concept of utilization management is a broad one, including prospective, concurrent, and retrospective review of care being rendered and resources being used. Many organizations have incorporated utilization review, discharge planning, social services, and sometimes quality assurance under a utilization management umbrella. In more advanced situations, case management may replace utilization management. In all of these situations, APNs can play an important role.

Patient Advocacy

The change from nonmanaged to managed care insurance can be difficult for enrollees who may have been previously accustomed to relatively free access to the healthcare system. Although managed care benefits may be clearly explained in subscriber information packages, most people welcome assistance in interpreting the fine print. Many institutions, particularly hospitals, have expanded the roles of their existing patient advocates or ombudsmen to include health insurance–related questions. For example, at North Shore Medical Center in Salem, MA, the patient ombudsman is responsible for responding to patient complaints. When managed care began to grow in popularity, she found that many patients' questions dealt with insurance coverage and plan rules and regulations. Patients tended to blame the hospital if the health plan limited acute-care coverage and worked to move the patient to a less intense and more appropriate setting. The patient ombudsman worked closely with the hospital's director of managed care and with the different health plans to resolve all problems.

Member Services

All managed healthcare plans have member services departments, and they often use APNs in key staff roles. Member services staff answer enrollee questions about covered benefits. They can also go one step beyond the explanation of benefits and actively assist enrollees to use the plan in the right way. For example, many managed care plans have altered their maternity benefit to cover 1-day admissions for normal vaginal deliveries and short stays for cesarean section births. Plan member services and other staff may provide information not only on benefit coverage but on home care and other alternative services.

Education

Advanced practice nurses have many opportunities as educators in a managed care environment. Their targets may be patients, physicians, or institutions, and other staff. Enrollees, for example, may benefit from several different kinds of education. On enrollment in a plan, they may need special instruction about the plan rules and regulations and benefit coverage. Or, they may need details on plan programs for health education and prevention. Plan member services departments can provide this information.

Physicians, as well, benefit from managed care education. Although all managed care plans have similarities, each plan has its own set of rules. Many plans use APNs to recruit, educate, and maintain ongoing relationships with network physicians.

Institutions, like physicians, need education on health plan operations. Some have many contracts, each with a different set of rules. Health plans often use APNs in a provider relations role to explain the rules and act as an ongoing problem solver.

In addition, there is an opportunity for education among professionals. In a managed care environment, care is collaborative, and it is important for all team members to share information with each other as well as with patients and their families.

Triage

Nurses have several opportunities to participate in the triage function that is intrinsic to managed care. Most health plans use telephone triage systems to answer enrollee inquiries after regular business hours and direct people to the appropriate level of care.

Triage opportunities exist in provider settings as well. For example, managed care enrollees are discouraged from inappropriately using costly emergency room services in lieu of accessing their PCPs. Many hospital emergency departments have made staffing changes and designated triage nurses to assess and steer patients appropriately.

Quality Assurance

Quality of care in a managed care environment is of concern to both health plans and providers. Plans take pains to protect themselves against unjust accusations of poor quality because their structure emphasizes cost containment. Furthermore, payers have become adamant that plans be held accountable for the quality of the services they provide. For both of these reasons, health plans take careful steps to ensure that quality standards are set, measured, and communicated to participating enrollees, providers, and purchasers. The use of report cards as a tool has already been described. Providers, like the health plans, need to ensure that the quality of care meets certain standards—their own, those of regulatory agencies, and those of the health plans with which they have relationships. In both health plan and provider settings, ANPs can play key roles in identifying problems, developing solutions, and communicating results.

Resource Management

Managed care emphasizes the provision of high-quality, cost-effective care. Both health plans and providers have learned that care may be costly because of inappropriate resource use, and each has taken steps to address the problems.

Health plans have the advantage of access to provider-specific information generated from claims data. Plan staff can use this information to work with individual providers. At the provider level, too, there is growing sophistication in physician profiling. Advanced practice nurses play an important role in both cases. An example is Duke University Medical Center, which employs an APN as the associate chief operating officer of medicine. A part of her function is to focus on clinical cost containment. That is, she identifies diagnosis-related groups that are high cost for the medical center and works with physicians to find more appropriate and less costly ways to deliver care (see Chapter 16).

References

The Advisory Board. (1993a). *Capitation I: The new American medicine.* : Washington, DC: The Advisory Board Company.

The Advisory Board. (1993b). *The grand alliance: Vertical integration strategies for physicians and health systems.* : Washington, DC: The Advisory Board Company.

American College of Cardiology. (1993). *Managed care primer.* Bethesda, MD: Author.

American Hospital Association. (1993). *Transforming health care delivery: Toward community care networks.* Chicago: Author.

Bartling, A. (1995). Trends in managed care. *Healthcare Executive, 10*(2), 6–11.

Bergman, R. (1994). Reengineering health care. *Hospitals and Health Networks, 68*(3), 28–36.

Conrad, D. A. (1993). Coordinating patient care services in regional health systems: The challenge of clinical integration. *Journal of the Foundation of the American College of Healthcare Executives, 38*(4), 491–507.

Employers go to bed with Cleveland's latest performance report. (1995, January 12). *Report on Medical Guidelines and Outcomes Research, 6*(1), 5–7, January 12, 1995.

Health Care Advisory Board. (1994). *Volume II. Quality measures: Next generation of outcomes tracking, implications for health plans and systems.* : Washington, DC: The Advisory Board Company.

Hicks, L., Stallmeyer, J. M., & Coleman, J. R. (1993). *The role of the nurse in managed care.* Washington, DC: American Nurses Publishing.

Jones, W. J., & Mayerhofer, J. J. (1994). Regional health care systems: Implications for health care reform. *Managed Care Quarterly, 2*(1), 31–44.

Kenkel, P. (1994). *Straight As: How to use quality report cards to win market share.* New York: Thompson Publishing Group.

Kongstvedt, P. R. (1993). *The managed health care handbook* (2nd ed.). Gaithersburg, MD: Aspen Publishers.

Lewin-VHI, Inc. (1993, January 27). *Managed care: Does it work?* (Report prepared by R. Atlas, D. Kennell, D. Sockel, & L. Lewin). Chicago: American Hospital Association.

Marion Merrell Dow, Inc. (1994). *Managed care digest, update edition: HMO cost analysis and midyear enrollment update, 1994.* Kansas City, : Kansas City, MO: Author.

National Committee on Quality Assurance. (1993). *Health Plan Employer Data Information Set and users' manual, version 2.0.*

Nighswander, A. (1994). *Integrated health care delivery: A blueprint for action.* St. Paul, MN: Interstudy.

Satinsky, M. A. (1995). *An executive guide to case management strategies.* Chicago: American Hospital Publishing.

Senge, P. M. (1990). *The fifth discipline: The art and practice of the learning organization.* New York: Doubleday.

Shortell, S. M. (1993). Creating organized delivery systems: The barriers and facilitators. *Journal of the Foundation of the American College of Healthcare Executives, 38*(4), 447–466.

Solovy, A. (1994). New power strategies (the battle for control). *Hospitals and Health Networks, 68*(24), 24–34.

Somerville, J. (1995, February 13). Tennessee's new governor orders review of TennCare. *American Medical News, 38*(6), 5–6.

Work, M., & Mackevicius, N. K. (1995). Information systems' key role in healthcare change. *Journal of Healthcare Resource Management, 13*(1), 23–26.

10

Collaboration and Advanced Practice Nursing

Kathleen B. King ■ *Kathleen M. Parrinello* ■ *Judith G. Baggs*

Much of what has been written about collaborative practice can be divided into the literature focused on collaboration between staff nurses and physicians, often resident physicians, or on collaboration between primary care nurse practitioners and attending physicians in private practice. Until recently, there has been considerably less attention focused on collaborative practice involving the acute-care nurse practitioner (ACNP). This chapter first gives a general definition of collaborative practice and follows with a review of the literature on collaboration in acute care and primary care. Next, the authors discuss a framework for how the concept of collaboration can be operationalized in advanced practice nursing for acute and primary care. Specific suggestions are given for structuring the system to support the ACNP in a collaborative practice model.

DEFINITION OF COLLABORATION

Collaboration is "nurses and physicians cooperatively working together, sharing responsibility for solving problems and making decisions to formulate and carry out plans for patient care" (Baggs & Schmitt, 1988, p. 145). Collaboration combines the activities of cooperation, or concern for another's interests, with assertiveness, or concern for one's own interests (Thomas, 1976). The interests considered in nurse–physician collaboration are professional, that is, concerns for the nursing or medical care of patients and for patient outcome, rather than the provider's personal interest.

The purpose of collaboration among healthcare professionals is to enhance quality of care and improve patient outcomes that "could not be offered in practices organized differently" (Kitzman, 1986, p. 141). Although patient needs are the primary focus, collaboration also is defined as a synergistic alliance that optimizes the contributions of each professional participant (Weiss & Davis, 1985). The end result is that patient care is enhanced and professional satisfaction is achieved.

Hickey JV: ADVANCED PRACTICE NURSING: Changing Roles and Clinical Applications © 1996 Lippincott–Raven Publishers

COLLABORATION IN CLINICAL PRACTICE

The current interest in development of collaborative practice models between nurses and physicians began with work in the early 1970s. In 1971, the American Medical Association and the American Nurses' Association founded the National Joint Practice Commission (NJPC), a group composed of an equal number of physicians and nurses. The group's goal was to "make recommendations concerning the roles of the physician and the nurse in providing high quality health care" (NJPC, 1981, p. 1).

By 1977 the NJPC had developed guidelines for collaborative practice and, with funding from the W.K. Kellogg Foundation, implemented model collaborative care units in four hospitals. In 1981, the NJPC published a description of collaboration results in the model units along with guidelines for establishing collaborative practice units (NJPC, 1981).

The NJPC focused on hospital care, as that was where they believed the majority of nurses and physicians practiced and were associated with each other. The NJPC used the terms *joint practice* and *collaborative practice* interchangeably, and were concerned with collaboration of staff nurses and physicians. In describing what such practice was like, the commissioners used terms such as "jointly determined relationship," "integrated care regimens," a "climate of trust and respect," "explicitly and jointly defined, mutually complementary roles," and "shared responsibility" (NJPC, 1981, p. 3). The five clinical elements they identified for establishing collaborative hospital care were encouragement of nurses' individual clinical decision making, primary nursing, integrated patient records, a joint practice committee, and joint patient care record review (NJPC, 1981, p. 4).

Although most physicians and nurses in the model units believed patient care had improved, the data consisted primarily of subjective participants' opinions. The NJPC concluded that collaboration resulted in increased quality of care, patient and care provider satisfaction, and decreased length of stay (Devereux, 1981a, 1981b, 1981c; NJPC, 1981).

Nurse–Physician Interactions

Beginning in the late 1960s, a number of authors addressed nurse–physician interactions and issues that could divide the professions. Pellegrino (1966) wrote of two separate cultures. Stein (1967) wrote of what he called the *doctor–nurse game,* a form of communication between the two groups in which the nurse must make recommendations while appearing passive, so that the physician could appear to be the instigator of decisions about care. Lynaugh and Bates (1973) also addressed communication, believing that the existence of completely separate educations for the two groups led to failure to communicate, decreased cooperation, and poor performance. In an earlier study comparing nurses and physicians, Bates (1966) found differing values that could block collaboration in care. As an example of such differences, physicians viewed nurses positively if they assisted skillfully, followed orders, and were willing to deviate from policy. Nurses rated physicians positively for conserving nursing resources and honoring policy. Kalish and Kalish (1977) associated the pattern Stein had identified of physician dominance and nurse deference with impaired communication. Sheard (1980) discussed differences in ways the two professions structure their work, leading to miscommunication and misunderstandings. McLain (1988a, 1988b), in a study of primary care teams, found both nurses and physicians contributed to conditions that blocked collaboration.

Several studies demonstrated a disparity in interactions between the two professions. Two were qualitative studies that considered the ways inequity in authority and status between nurses and physicians are demonstrated (Katzman & Roberts, 1988; Tellis-Nayak & Tellis-Nayak, 1984). In a quantitative study of interpersonal distance, researchers found that each profession interacted more frequently and more closely with its own members than with the other profession (Kerr, 1986).

In addition, a number of studies from different types of practice sites have demonstrated that collaboration is not the usual mode of interaction between nurses and physicians. Lamb and Napodano (1984) studied two physician and nurse primary care teams. They rated only 5 of the 22 interactions that occurred as collaborative, although participants thought they were collaborating in 13 of the interactions. Prescott and Bowen (1985) investigated how disagreements are handled between nurses and physicians in medical, surgical, intensive care, and medical–surgical specialty care units in 15 metropolitan acute-care hospitals. They found competition to be the most common mode of handling disputes. Only 14% of physicians and 7% of nurses reported using collaborative problem solving.

Although many authors have stressed differences between the professions, a number of authors in addition to the NJPC have articulated the benefits of more collaborative interactions and have made suggestions for interventions to promote collaboration. Bates (1970) believed that the common goal of physicians and nurses in delivering patient care provides a basis for shared decision making and better care. Aradine and Pridham (1973) discussed the unique capabilities and knowledge of each profession, so vital to share in a time of rapidly expanding knowledge and technology.

Support for Collaborative Practice

Collaboration has been identified as the appropriate interaction mode between practicing nurses and physicians in many official publications, such as the American Nurses' Association (1980) *Nursing: A Social Policy Statement*. The American Association of Critical-Care Nurses and the Society for Critical Care Medicine (1982) published a document supporting collaboration between nurses and physicians in intensive care units (ICUs), both at the staff and leadership levels. Support for collaborative care has also come from the Institute of Medicine (1983), National Commission on Nursing (1981), and Secretary's Commission on Nursing (1988). Christensen and Larson (1993) supported collaboration as a method for individuals with varying roles, status, and information access to maximize sharing and integrating the different knowledge that each has in order to improve decision making.

In addition to the empirical data from the NJPC (1981) studies, other research studies have demonstrated positive outcomes related to collaborative practice. One group of studies concerned ICUs; another, interdisciplinary team care; and one study was conducted on a general unit in an acute-care hospital. The focus of the studies was on collaboration between staff nurses and physicians—in most cases, resident physicians.

Studies in Intensive Care Units

Knaus, Draper, Wagner, and Zimmerman (1986) studied 13 ICUs across the United States and established that some of the units differed significantly from the others in an actual mortality/predicted mortality ratio, controlling for severity of illness. They found that none of their measured variables, such as teaching versus nonteaching hospital, capacity to provide one-to-one nursing coverage, technical capabilities, or level of administration, predicted patient outcome. They concluded that staff interaction, communication, and coordination (collaboration) was the critical independent variable. However, in more recent work (Zimmerman et al., 1993), this group has been unable to link structural and organizational characteristics with patient mortality.

Mitchell, Armstrong, Simpson, and Lentz (1989) studied an ICU that was said to embody five elements of organizational structure and process critical to excellence in care. These elements were nurse–physician collaboration, staff of all registered nurses, critical care certification of nursing staff, participative management, and use of the American Association of Critical-Care Nurses standards of critical care nursing. Patient mortality was less than what would have been predicted by the patients' severity of illness.

Baggs, Ryan, Phelps, Richeson, and Johnson (1992) studied the decision to transfer patients out of an ICU. The more collaboration that nurses reported had occurred between nurses and physicians in making a transfer decision, the lower the patient's risk of death or readmission to the ICU during that same hospital stay.

Team Studies

Interdisciplinary team care is a form of institutionalized collaborative practice. Studies of such care have been generally positive. Wood-Dauphinee and colleagues (1984) randomly assigned stroke patients to team or traditional care and found a trend toward higher survival among the team patients. Rubenstein and colleagues (1984) randomly assigned frail elderly patients to a geriatric evaluation unit for team care or to the regular unit and found significantly better health outcomes for the team care patients.

In one quasi-experimental study, patients were randomly assigned to one of four teams or to usual care (Feiger & Schmitt, 1979; Schmitt, Watson, Feiger, & Williams, 1982). Videotaped team meetings were rated for degree of collegial interaction. Patients who had received team care had better outcomes than those who had received usual care. In addition, the rank order of teams for collegiality was the same as their rank order for success in patient outcomes.

The only acute-care, non–ICU study of collaboration reported in the literature was conducted by Koerner and colleagues (Koerner & Armstrong, 1983; Koerner & Armstrong, 1984; Koerner, Cohen, & Armstrong, 1985). They studied two medical units. The experimental unit incorporated the five clinical elements described as collaborative by the NJPC. The control unit provided usual care. The experimental unit had lower costs and increased patient satisfaction compared with the control unit. No differences were found in length of stay, numbers of cardiac arrests, transfers to the ICU, or deaths.

Overall, collaborative practice has been advocated by both nursing and medicine as a method to enhance patient care and patient outcomes. In general, research to date supports this approach, although the studies in acute care have exclusively focused on collaboration between staff nurses and physicians.

Collaboration in Advanced Practice Nursing

A multitude of studies have examined and supported the efficacy of care delivered by primary care nurse practitioners compared with physicians (for reviews, see Feldman, Ventura, & Crosby, 1987; Safriet, 1992; and Brown & Grimes, 1993). Fewer studies in the literature have examined the process of collaboration between advanced practice nurses (APNs) and physicians, and much of the research that has been done has focused on primary care (Ames & Perrin, 1980; Aradine & Hansen, 1970; Clawson & Osterweis, 1993; Lamb, 1991; Lamb & Napodano, 1984; Roueche, 1977). However, even in early discussions about advanced practice nursing, it is apparent that the acute-care setting was attracting nurses with advanced education (Ford, 1979; Kitzman, 1983). Two books about collaborative practice for nurses (England, 1986; Steel, 1986) considered the value of collaboration with physicians at all levels in nursing, from staff nurse to doctorally prepared clinician. A recent description of a collaborative clinical nurse specialist role included managing complex care for inpatients as well as providing ambulatory care, functions that have traditionally been considered "practitioner" activities (Walton, Jakobowski, & Barnsteiner, 1993).

One of the difficulties in tracking literature about collaboration for advanced practice nursing is terminology. There is a long-standing tradition to refer to any acute-care inpatient practitioner as a clinical nurse specialist. Concomitantly, the term *nurse practitioner* has long been construed as referring only to the primary care nurse practitioner. Terms such as *acute care nurse practitioner* (Davitt & Jensen, 1981), *tertiary nurse practitioner* (Keane &

Richmond, 1993) and *nurses in advanced clinical practice* (Mirr, 1994) have been proposed to identify those nurses who combine the skills traditionally used by primary care nurse practitioners and clinical nurse specialists.

The fusion of traditional nurse practitioner and clinical specialist education programs has been advocated by many, including one of the original developers of the practitioner role (Ford, 1992). Forbes, Rafson, Spross, and Kozlowski (1990) studied 359 graduate programs preparing practitioners or clinical specialists. Many more similarities than differences were found comparing the two types of educational programs. Similarly, Elder and Bullough (1990) found many similarities comparing the roles of practicing clinical specialists and nurse practitioners. Forbes and colleagues were early advocates for combining the American Nurses' Association Council of Clinical Nurse Specialists and Council of Primary Health Care Nurse Practitioners, a move that was accomplished. This new joint council has been incorporated into the most recent American Nurses' Association restructuring as the Council for Advance Practice Nursing.

As new roles and titles continue to develop, there is a need to distinguish between skills and functions generic to all advanced practice roles and those specific to different types of practice. Collaboration is one function that is generic to all advanced practice roles. However, the way in which it is operationalized in acute care and primary care is different and is the topic of the following section.

APPLICATION OF COLLABORATION IN ADVANCED PRACTICE NURSING

Although there is growing agreement on the philosophical definition of collaboration and its efficacy in patient care delivery, the rationale set forth for its operationalization differs depending on patient care needs and setting. Different interpretations about how collaboration is applied can lead to confusion in understanding models of care. The following are views proposed in the literature regarding the application of collaboration to advanced practice nursing and a framework for using its appropriate application in different types of practice.

A rationale for using a collaborative practice model in primary care is based on studies that have asserted that, although the nurse practitioner can safely and effectively deliver 70% to 80% of primary care, for 20% to 30% of patient encounters, the nurse practitioner must have a collaborator (physician) as backup (Mundinger, 1994). This argument has asserted that it is not 70% to 80% of patients per se, but 70% to 80% of patient encounters in which care can be fully provided by a nurse practitioner. Thus, the contention is that any one patient will require either physician consultation or physician care at some point (DeAngelis, 1994). This application also assumes that, for a relatively high number of primary care functions—that is, 70% to 80%—the nurse practitioner can substitute for the physician, and vice versa. Although the nurse practitioner and the physician may use different approaches in the delivery of care, the outcome for the patient would be similar (Griffith, 1984). For example, either a nurse practitioner or physician would be equally effective in diagnosing and treating a patient with otitis media.

The preceding application of collaboration to primary care uses a population-based rationale. That is, any *group* of patients will have access to the services of either the primary care nurse practitioner or physician, depending on the patient need at a given time (DeAngelis, 1994; Mundinger, 1994). The nurse practitioner has authority and responsibility to manage independently the care of a patient within his or her scope of practice. Collaboration of the nurse practitioner with the physician occurs for those patient needs that are not within the nurse practitioner's scope of practice. Conversely, collaboration of the physician with the nurse practitioner occurs for those patient needs that are not within the physician's scope of practice.

Collaboration in this context is viewed as independent practice with interdisciplinary consultation and referral.[1]

In contrast, the rationale for using a collaborative practice model in acute care is based on the idea (in that there are no research findings) that the patient's needs are such that he or she requires the services of different types of providers simultaneously *for each encounter* or hospital admission. Different providers, or types of providers, make unique contributions in affecting the outcome of the patient's problem. Thus, for a relatively high number of functions, one type provider cannot substitute for another team member. If one provider did substitute for another and try to provide for the unique functions of the other, the outcome would be different. An example of nonsubstitution would be that the surgeon has ultimate authority and responsibility for the patient in the operating room, whereas the ACNP has ultimate authority and responsibility regarding patient teaching, discharge planning, and the decision to discharge the patient (Norsen, Opladen, & Quinn, 1995).

This application uses an individual based rationale, as contrasted to the population based rationale used for primary care. That is, any *individual* patient requires care from both types of providers—the ACNP and the physician—during the course of one acute-care encounter to effect a quality outcome. Although some functions may be performed by either provider, more cannot. Collaboration in this context is viewed as interdependent interdisciplinary practice.

Central to both applications of collaboration is that patient needs are the foremost priority in the provision of care (Chavigny, 1993; DeAngelis, 1994). Embedded is an emphasis on patient outcomes. To effect quality outcomes, professionals assume responsibility in the provision of care for which they are best prepared.

Confusion can occur in that collaboration may be played out differently by the primary care provider than by the acute-care provider. The primary care provider plays out collaboration with consultation and referral and applies collaboration to managing a group of patients. The acute-care provider plays out collaboration as interdependent practice and applies it to the management of every patient. If the way in which collaboration is played out is applied appropriately for each type of practice, each provider's scope of practice is used fully. The mix of providers contributing to a patient's care at any one time depends first on patient needs and then on the provider's scope of practice.

Figure 10-1 illustrates the interaction between APNs and physicians within different types of practice. This model is an adaptation of work by Griffith (1984). The circles represent patient needs or problems as well as the healthcare activities or functions that address the patient needs. The amount of overlap represents patient needs or problems that can be addressed in an equally effectively manner by either type of provider. The nonoverlapping part of the circles represents those patient needs or problems that are within the principal domain of one type of provider. These "principal domain" needs cannot be addressed as well (if at all) by another type of provider. The scope of practice of each type of provider is defined by his or her discipline and education.

There is no intention to imply that any need that fits into the overlapping portion of the circles would necessarily be addressed in the same manner by different types of providers. For some needs, different providers "perform the same general function but may approach it in different ways" (Griffith, 1984, p. 112). Thus, it is assumed that different providers would deliver care using different philosophical models of care depending on their discipline and education. However, for needs that can be addressed equally by either provider, the patient outcome should be similar.

---

[1]Lewis (1991) has distinguished between collaboration and consultation: collaboration is an ongoing process of working together and *consultation* is a short-term interaction. This chapter uses *collaboration* as an overarching term to describe the continuum of joint practice between nurse practitioners and physicians.

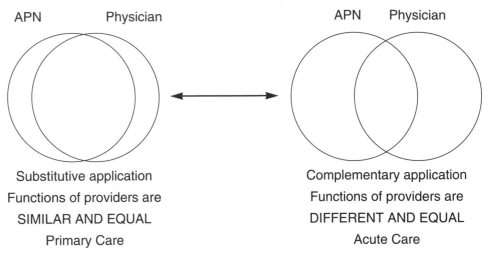

FIGURE 10–1. The application of collaboration along a continuum.

The authors of this chapter assert that the substitutive application is appropriate to primary care, whereas the complementary application is appropriate to acute care. Where a provider practices along the continuum depends on the needs of the patient or patient population with whom the practitioner works. A critical assumption in either application is that the core collaborative practice team is composed of APNs and physicians who have attained full professional status (Gleeson et al., 1990; Norsen et al., 1995). That is, each partner will have completed his or her basic education and postgraduate training. This element is essential for a collaborative practice team to take advantage of and use each partner's full scope of practice.

Applications of collaborative practice are good only to the extent that practitioners understand the context in which they are playing it out. Problems arise when an application to one type of practice is misapplied to another. One major problem is that confusion occurs regarding the role of each collaborator, often resulting in the nurse practitioner's being hindered from practicing to the full extent of his or her scope.

An unfortunate example is the application of the primary care substitutive approach to acute care (Mundinger, 1994). In this case, the nurse practitioner is regarded as a substitute for a medical or surgical resident. One disadvantage of this application is that the nurse practitioner's scope of practice is defined as only that part that overlaps with the attending physician's scope of practice (Fig. 10-2). Although it is appropriate to view the functions of a resident or trainee as part of the whole, it is inappropriate to view the functions of the nurse practitioner as only part of the whole. The full scope of advanced practice nursing is not recognized in that those functions unique to the nurse practitioner are truncated. In addition, the APN is put in the position of being supervised by the attending physician—he or she is equated with a trainee—rather than being viewed as a true complementary partner.

The resident replacement approach has gained increasing exposure in the acute-care setting where trainee positions in specialty care are being reduced or are threatened with reduction. As a result of this trend, many physicians and administrators have recognized—some for the first time—areas of overlap in physician practice and advanced nursing practice. Although recognition of the overlap is important in settings where the number of trainees is being reduced, it is imperative to recognize the areas of advanced nursing practice that are unique and independently contribute to desired patient outcomes. Failing to recognize the full scope of advanced nursing practice has the potential to promote undervaluing of APNs' contributions in the long run.

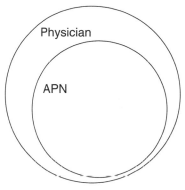

Substitutive application in acute care
(substituting APN for resident)

Functions of providers are

SIMILAR BUT *NOT* EQUAL

FIGURE 10–2. Misapplication of collaboration in acute care.

Establishing a collaborative practice in which the ACNP and attending physician comprise the core team has the advantage of providing for ongoing continuity and coordination of care (Davitt & Jensen, 1981; Norsen et al., 1995). Trainees, both nurse practitioner students and residents, are integrated into the team. In their trainee role, they are viewed as temporary team members who are accountable to both partners of the permanent team. The relationship among the ACNP, attending physician, and trainees is illustrated in Figure 10-3.

Correspondingly, the application of the complementary version of collaborative practice in primary care undervalues the primary care nurse practitioner's contribution. Problems arise because the full scope of advanced practice nursing in primary care is not acknowledged in that there is an expectation that the nurse practitioner will consult with the physician on all patient encounters. Again, this puts the nurse practitioner in a position of being supervised by the attending physician. In addition, healthcare costs may rise because of redundancy in the services delivered.

The paramount advantage of applying the substitutive version of collaborative practice to primary care and the complementary version to acute care is that patient care is enhanced, thereby helping the patient to achieve the best outcome possible. Applying the appropriate collaborative model necessitates making the distinction between the population-based rationale versus the individual-based rationale. This will clarify the type of practices in which a substitutive approach appropriately predominates and in which type of practice the complementary approach appropriately predominates.

ADMINISTRATIVE SUPPORTS FOR ACUTE-CARE NURSE PRACTITIONERS

Institutions can create supportive environments that facilitate and enhance collaborative practice among physicians, ACNPs, and other health team members. Important components of a supportive environment include organizational structure; effective administrative processes to guide clinical privileging and performance review; support for interdisciplinary teams with integration of clinical documentation, patient rounds, conferences, and interdisciplinary clinical research; and an organizational commitment to a model of shared governance and decision making embraced by senior clinical and administrative leadership.

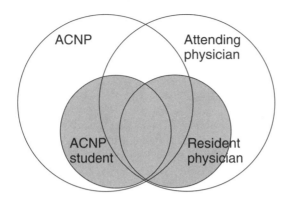

FIGURE 10–3. Collaborative practice model for acute care.

Organizational Structure

Institutions have adopted various organizational models to incorporate the role of nurses in advanced practice positions. Each model can be evaluated in terms of its role in fostering a collaborative work relationship between physicians and ACNPs.

One organizational model is perhaps the oldest and most traditional in design. It is the physician model in which the ACNP joins a physician group or individual practice and establishes a working relationship with physicians based on the individual ACNP's ability to negotiate role and responsibilities. The ACNP reports administratively to a physician director. The ACNP's clinical responsibilities typically involve the evaluation of patients referred to the specialty practice as well as the care and management of inpatients including discharge planning and postdischarge follow-up.

The physician model can be advantageous in that the ACNP's clinical practice can be readily interwoven into that of the medical staff. Disadvantages of the model include the potential tension resulting from differences in how the relationship is perceived, that is, collaborative versus supervisory, and in how the physician's role as team member is perceived. For example, the physician may perceive himself or herself as supervisory, that is, having ultimate authority over all aspects of patient care and all aspects of the ACNP role. These issues have the potential to interfere with the formation of a collaborative practice in which authority and accountability for patient care management and decision making rest on competence, not on historical medical dominance. In this organizational structure, the substitutive application is likely to predominate, because the ACNP role is directed by the physician, and the part of the role that overlaps with the physician's role (see Fig. 10-2) is of primary interest, particularly if physician resources are stretched thin. In addition, this organizational model has the potential to result in isolation of the ACNP from nursing colleagues and in a loss of credibility among nursing staff in the clinical setting.

Another model is the nursing model in which ACNPs report administratively to nursing directors and are assigned to work with physicians in managing patient care and addressing clinical issues. The model represents the traditional clinical nurse specialist model. There is potential, however, for decreased collaboration with physicians if the ACNP is perceived as having a primary responsibility to a nursing division with a parallel responsibility for patient care, as opposed to an interdependent relationship with other patient care team members. In the model, ACNP practice can become separated from the physician practice with differences in the roles emphasized over commonalities.

The joint-practice model of collaborative practice is emerging. In the model, the ACNP and physician provide care to patients as a team and share authority equally for providing care within their respective scopes of practice. A cohesive physician–nurse clinical care delivery model is cultivated and the communication structure between physicians and ACNPs is formalized. Reporting relationships reflect a matrix management model in which the ACNP is responsible to a physician director for patient outcomes related to the medical management of patients and to a nursing director for issues relating to professional practice, program development, and systems improvement. The ACNP maintains identity with and involvement in the nursing organization of the institution and maintains parity with physician team members who also report to the physician director. The concept of interdependency is emphasized in the model, with the complementary application of roles predominating. The goal is to achieve coordination of care and integration of services within a complex institutional setting. In the healthcare environment of today with its many complexities and potential for fragmentation, it is imperative to establish organizational structures that reflect the professional interdependence required to deliver high-quality and cost-effective healthcare services.

Administrative Processes for Clinical Privileging and Performance Review

The ACNP role at the University of Rochester/Strong Memorial Hospital (URSMH) was developed in 1979 with the appointment of an ACNP assigned to the cardiac surgery service (Davitt & Jensen, 1981). This advanced practice role has evolved into a nationally recognized prototype for advanced nursing practice in the acute-care setting. ACNPs have graduate degrees in clinical nursing and are recognized through certification or licensure to practice in an expanded capacity involving the diagnosis and treatment of healthcare conditions. At the URSMH, the ACNP's role encompasses comprehensive direct patient care and scholarly practice and conforms to professional practice standards. The ACNP's direct care responsibilities at the URSMH include gathering patient health histories and performing complete physical exams, ordering and performing diagnostic testing and screening, diagnosing illness, prescribing both pharmacologic and other treatments for patients, and providing health maintenance and promotion interventions such as patient and family education and counseling. In addition, the ACNP assumes accountability for indirect care responsibilities that support patient care. These responsibilities include staff and student education, clinical research, program development, and quality improvement activities.

Table 10-1 depicts a condensed version of the scope of practice and professional practice standards developed by the ACNPs and nursing leadership at the URSMH. The *scope of practice,* a statement of expectation regarding practice responsibilities, outlines in broad terms those elements that define advanced nursing practice (Norsen et al., 1995). The scope of practice is unique to each practitioner in a collaborative arrangement and has legal implications in defining the clinical practice activities of each member of the interdisciplinary healthcare team. The specific responsibilities of each practitioner for patient care must be determined within the guidelines outlined by the scope of practice. Although most elements of the scope of practice are particular to the type of practitioner, there are areas of overlap between medical practice and advanced nursing practice that should be negotiated between the physician and ACNP to eliminate duplication and redundancy in services provided to patients cared for by the team.

Practice standards, an operationalization of the scope of practice, are clear and specific statements outlining activities or behaviors that constitute daily practice (Norsen et al., 1995). At the URSMH, the standards developed for the ACNP provide a delineation of both direct and indirect care domains. The condensed version of the six practice standards developed for the surgical ACNP group also are contained in Table 10-1. The practice standards serve as the basis for outcome measurement and performance evaluation of the ACNP. Performance criteria for the ACNP are presented in Table 10-2. These criteria reflect the practice standards for the ACNP and support the ACNP role being placed at the highest level in the clinical track of the career advancement system (Clements & Parrinello, in press). Many institutions are devel-

TABLE 10-1 **University of Rochester/Strong Memorial Hospital Surgical Nursing Practice Acute Care Nurse Practitioner Professional Practice Standards**

Scope of Practice

The ACNP is an advanced practice nurse who functions in an expanded nursing role in a collaborative practice model. The ACNP has completed graduate education in nursing science and demonstrates a comprehensive knowledge base in a specialty practice area exhibiting a high level of clinical competence in caring for acutely ill patients. The ACNP provides patient care using advanced assessment skills and a sound knowledge of clinical therapeutics. The ACNP provides indirect patient care services to support patient care, promote professional education, and advance knowledge through research and scholarly activities. All duties and responsibilities of the ACNP conform to professional practice standards, hospital guidelines, and are in accordance with a written practice agreement with a physician member of the medical staff at the University of Rochester/Strong Memorial Hospital.

	Standard	Rationale
I. Entry into acute care	The ACNP facilitates entry of the patient into the acute-care system at the first contact	Effective entry into the acute care system ensures the identification and management of the presenting concern and establishes a mechanism for anticipating and dealing with future patient care needs that may arise during the episode of acute care
II. Comprehensive care	The ACNP provides direct care that is comprehensive, continuous, coordinated, and accessible throughout hospitalization and after discharge The ACNP provides indirect care that supports care delivery systems, promotes education, and advances scholarly practice	Comprehensive, care includes timely assessment and intervention, and promotes quality outcomes for the patient while decreasing costs of health care
III. Interdisciplinary practice	The ACNP collaborates with other health care providers in caring for patients within a given specialty population	Interdisciplinary practice utilizes the expertise of all healthcare professionals to ensure delivery of quality care
IV. Continuing competence	The ACNP assumes responsibility for maintaining competence in a specialty area	Theory and knowledge of healthcare and disease management increases at a rapid rate. Because technology advances continuously, the skills necessary to practice safely and effectively must be reviewed and updated regularly
V. Quality assessment and improvement	The ACNP provides leadership in quality assessment and quality improvement activities in the acute care setting	Participation in quality improvement activities promotes excellence in the delivery of patient care in the acute-care setting
VI. Research/scholarly practice	The ACNP supports scholarly practice by integrating research into practice, by providing leadership in a specialty area, and by educating students	Scholarly practice enhances professional growth and quality patient outcomes

(From University of Rochester, Nursing Practice. Reproduced with permission.)

oping internal systems of credential review for APNs to assure that practitioners are qualified to provide patient care that meets the practice standards set forth by the institution, accrediting agencies, and professional organizations (Quigley, Hixon, & Jangen, 1991; Smith, 1991).

Key points and steps of the review process for credentialing ACNPs at the URSMH are as follows. The ACNP initiates a request for practice privileges and submits it to the clinical nursing chief of the service for which privileges are requested. The ACNP also submits letters of recommendation, his or her curriculum vita, proof of licensure as a registered nurse, and

TABLE 10-2   University of Rochester/Strong Memorial Hospital Surgical Nursing Practice Performance Criteria for Acute Care Nurse Practitioners

		Performance Criteria
Professional practice	Professional involvement in group activity	A. Influences the direction and outcome of group activities at the unit/service level
		B. Actively participates in professional organizations
	Scholarly activities	A. Facilitates clinical research through collaboration with others in investigations, analysis of practice problems to generate researchable questions, and enabling access to clients and data
		B. Assists others in applying scientific knowledge to nursing practice and clinical decision-making
		C. Disseminates nursing knowledge through presentation or publication at the local-regional level
	Role development	A. Maintains a current knowledge base in area of specialization
		B. Develops and implements plan for professional growth and development
	Professional image interpersonal skills	A. Enhances care delivery by serving as a mentor for others
		B. Promotes nursing and quality patient care when interacting with other professionals, patients families, and the public
		C. Represents nursing positively in recruitment and retention activities
Care delivery	Direct/indirect care	A. Assesses the quality and effectiveness of nursing care delivery system in assigned specialty area
		B. Delivers direct care and coordinates interdisciplinary plan of care for patients requiring the expertise of an advanced practitioner
		C. Provides leadership in the development, implementation, and evaluation of standards of practice, policies, and procedures
		D. Facilitates the process of ethical decision making in clinical practice
	Consultation	Serves as a consultant in improving patient care and nursing practice based on expertise in area of specialization.
Clinical coordination	Education	A. Applies teaching/learning theory to patient, family, community, and professional education as a means to influence patient outcomes
		B. Identifies learning needs of various populations and contributes to the development of educational programs/resources
		C. Serves as a formal educator and clinical preceptor for students, staff, or others
		D. Participates in school of nursing activities as negotiated
	Quality improvement-critical analysis	A. Identifies system-specific problems requiring evaluation or change
		B. Participates in strategic planning for the practice area/service
		C. Provides direction for and participates in unit/service quality improvement programs
		D. Evaluates impact of changes in clinical practice and formulates recommendations regarding appropriateness and cost-effectiveness
	Program development	Actively participates in the development, implementation, and evaluation of practice-related programs in collaboration with nursing leadership

(From University of Rochester, Nursing Practice. Reproduced with permission.)

advanced practice certification documentation. The practitioner also submits a scope of practice statement with the practice standards along with a listing of proposed procedures and skills to be performed. In New York State, nurse practitioners are certified by the state only after submitting a written practice agreement with a physician that contains broadly defined practice protocols on which practice will be based. A copy of this practice agreement is also included as part of the credentials review process.

The nursing chief of service and medical chief of service collaboratively conduct the formal review of required documentation. A standing committee of the professional nursing organization reviews and endorses all candidates. The Hospital Patient Care Policy Committee conducts the final review of all endorsed candidates and formally confers practice privileges to the ACNP. Privileges are reviewed 1 year following initial appointment and every 2 years thereafter (Parrinello, 1995). Performance in the role is measured using the ACNP performance criteria. ACNP and physician team members conduct a quarterly review of patient records in which adherence to and compliance with the practice standards are evaluated. Renewal of practice privileges is contingent on documentation of satisfactory performance in the role.

Interdisciplinary Teams and the Integration of Clinical Documentation, Patient Rounds, Conferences, and Clinical Research

An essential structure for operationalizing collaborative practice is the interdisciplinary healthcare team. The mission and goals of the institution, which are embraced by the team members, determine the composition of the team. Optimally, the organization that wishes to facilitate and enhance collaborative practice has made a commitment to patient-centered care in which the center of the healthcare team is the patient and family. In this context, the focus of goal setting revolves around assessment and validation of patient and family care needs. Depending on the typical needs of the specialty patient population, the collaborative team may include other healthcare professionals, such as nursing staff or specialists, physical therapists, occupational therapists, dietitians, social workers, and other specialty-based physicians. Although it may be unnecessary for each team member to participate in the care of every patient on the team, it is important that team members are consistently a part of the team. An identified professional should be assigned to be a part of the team, not just any therapist, nurse, or social worker who is available to meet a patient care need on a given day. A cohesive and effective interdisciplinary team relies on participants who gain familiarity with each other and are committed as individuals to the group effort required of the team. Underlying the theme of collaboration is mutual regard and interest about other team members' perspectives and roles.

Supporting collaborative team practice are the format, policies, and procedures relating to clinical documentation of patient care. An integrated medical record in which clinical documentation from all team members is included and reviewed by other team members is essential. Optimally, patient clinical data are collected in a systematic and ongoing fashion and are inclusive of all appropriate health team members' assessments. Wherever possible, forms used in documentation should consolidate medical and nursing information to improve efficiency, reduce redundancy, and focus further assessments. In addition, institutional policies for order writing including laboratory testing, therapeutic interventions, medications, and consult requests must be developed to enable the ACNP to perform in the advanced practice role consistent with the established scope of practice.

Interdisciplinary patient rounds represent an essential clinical process in an effective collaborative practice team. During rounds, the team establishes, evaluates, and continuously updates the patient's care plan. This assures timely communication among practitioners and between practitioners and the patient and family, facilitating proactive modifications to the care plan, which include input from the patient and result in a more efficient use of healthcare resources.

Routine interdisciplinary clinical conferences represent another important marker of collaborative practice teams. The focus of conferences can be on individual patient case presentations or systems issues affecting patient groups. They also can be project driven, based on activities of team members. Administrative support for the time, space, and resources to meet on a regular basis is essential, if collaborative practice teams are to thrive and achieve optimal levels of performance. Interdisciplinary conferences provide the setting necessary to formalize peer review and outcome assessment. Evaluating patient outcomes in an interdisciplinary setting encourages practitioners to examine care critically and to critique standards of care, systems for providing care, conventional thinking regarding care delivery, practice patterns, and clinical routines (Pike, McHugh, & Canney, 1993). These activities provide the framework for innovation and proactive changes in practice to better meet the needs of patients and their families.

Interdisciplinary clinical research represents the highest level of collaborative practice, resulting in an intermingling of science from two distinct but related professional bodies of knowledge. The purpose of interdisciplinary clinical research is to improve patient care. Interventional studies in which the effect of specific clinical strategies are identified and tested are particularly useful in designing optimal care delivery approaches. Organizational support for interdisciplinary clinical research is essential for the success of such efforts in today's busy clinical settings, where practitioners get pulled in many directions and the demands of patient care are great. At the URSMH, the establishment of the small grants program Innovations in Patient Care is an example of the effort of one institution to support clinical research of an interdisciplinary nature. This program is clearly designed to scientifically evaluate clinical interventions in an effort to identify the best practice to assure optimal patient outcome and efficiency in resource use (Franklin, Panzer, Brideau, & Griner, 1990).

Organizational Commitment to Shared Governance and Decision Making

Collaborative practice teams are facilitated in organizations that have adopted a philosophy of shared governance and have decentralized decision making to the point of service. It is essential to have a "bottom-up" management style that emphasizes the primacy of patient care within the organization and encourages care providers to become empowered to solve systems problems as well as to address clinical management issues.

Hamilton (1993) proposed a team-based organizational design as an alternative to the traditional functional, hierarchical organizational model found in so many healthcare institutions. A team-based organizational model offers the more flexible and dynamic structure needed in today's proactive healthcare organization. Characteristics of the model that make it particularly conducive to supporting collaborative practice teams are as follows:

1. Management layers are replaced with team leaders who facilitate and coach rather than direct and control.
2. Authority and responsibility for decision making are vested in team members.
3. Teams are empowered to directly communicate with other teams, including customers, suppliers, and executive management.
4. Emphasis is on broadening each team member's vision of the entire array of services provided by the organization to promote continuity and coordination of services.

Interteam cooperation replaces traditional turf protection in this type of organizational structure. In addition, reward systems support organizational and individual success by incorporating team rewards with individual professional development opportunities. Healthcare executives who recognize that care providers are their greatest asset will strive to match the basic organizational structure with the emerging operational realities associated with delivering healthcare services in a continually changing environment. Institutions that support the establishment and ongoing development of collaborative practice relationships between physicians, ACNPs, and other care providers are investing in a future in which the approach to clinical accountability and authority will shift from an individual orientation to a team orientation. In today's complex healthcare environment, it is essential that organizational strategies aimed at enhancing continuity, reducing redundancy, and eliminating fragmentation in care delivery are adopted and nurtured if patients are to experience a seamless interface between their care requirements and our care delivery systems.

References

American Association of Critical-Care Nurses and the Society for Critical Care Medicine. (1982). *Collaborative practice model: The organization of human resources in critical care units.* Newport Beach, CA: Author.

American Nurses' Association. (1980). *Nursing: A social policy statement.* Kansas City, MO: Author.

Ames, A., & Perrin, J. M. (1980). Collaborative practice: The joining of two professions. *Journal of the Tennessee Medical Association, 73,* 557–560.

Aradine, C. R., & Hansen, M. F. (1970). Interdisciplinary teamwork in family health care. *Nursing Clinics of North America, 5,* 211–222.

Aradine, C. R., & Pridham, K. F. (1973). Model for collaboration. *Nursing Outlook, 21,* 655–657.

Baggs, J. G., Ryan, S. A., Phelps, C. E., Richeson, J. F., & Johnson, J. E. (1992). The association between interdisciplinary collaboration and patient outcomes in a medical intensive care unit. *Heart and Lung, 21,* 18–24.

Baggs, J. G., & Schmitt, M. H. (1988). Collaboration between nurses and physicians. *Image: The Journal of Nursing Scholarship, 20,* 145–149.

Bates, B. (1966). Nurse–physician teamwork. *Medical Care, 4,* 69–80.

Bates, B. (1970). Doctor and nurse: Changing roles and relations. *New England Journal of Medicine, 283,* 129–134.

Brown, S. A., & Grimes, D. E. (1993). *Nurse practitioner and certified nurse–midwives: A meta-analysis of studies on nurses in primary care roles.* Washington, DC: American Nursing Publishing.

Chavigny, K. H. (1993). AMA's policies and nursing's role in emerging systems. *Nursing Management, 24*(12), 30–34.

Christensen, C., & Larson, J. R. (1993). Collaborative medical decision making. *Medical Decision Making, 13,* 339–346.

Clawson, D. K., & Osterweis, M. (Eds.). (1993). *The roles of physician assistants and nurse practitioners in primary care.* Washington, DC: Association of Academic Health Centers.

Clements, J., & Parrinello, K. (in press). Career advancement for the nurse in advanced practice. *Nursing Management.*

Davitt, P. A., & Jensen, L. A. (1981). The role of the acute care nurse practitioner in cardiac surgery. *Nursing Administration Quarterly, 6*(1), 16–19.

DeAngelis, C. D. (1994). Nurse practitioner redux. *JAMA, 271*(11), 868–871.

Devereux, P. M. (1981a). Does joint practice work? *Journal of Nursing Administration, 11*(6), 39–43.

Devereux, P. M. (1981b). Essential elements of nurse–physician collaboration. *Journal of Nursing Administration, 11*(5), 19–23.

Devereux, P. M. (1981c). Nurse/physician collaboration: Nursing practice considerations. *Journal of Nursing Administration, 11*(9), 37–39.

Elder, R. G., & Bullough, B. (1990). Nurse practitioners and clinical nurse specialists: Are the roles merging? *Clinical Nurse Specialist, 4*(2), 78–84.

England, D. A. (Ed.). (1986). *Collaboration in nursing.* Rockville, MD: Aspen Publishers.

Feiger, S. M., & Schmitt, M. H. (1979). Collegiality in interdisciplinary health teams: Its measurement and its effects. *Social Science and Medicine, 13A,* 217–229.

Feldman, M. J., Ventura, M. R., & Crosby, F. (1987). Studies of nurse practitioner effectiveness. *Nursing Research, 36,* 303–308.

Forbes, K. E., Rafson, J., Spross, J. A., & Kozlowski, D. (1990). Clinical nurse specialist and nurse practitioner core curricula survey results. *Nurse Practitioner, 15*(4), 43, 46–48.

Ford, L. (1979). A nurse for all settings: The nurse practitioner. *Nursing Outlook, 27,* 516–521.

Ford, L. C. (1992). Advanced nursing practice: Future of the nurse practitioner. In L.H. Aiken & C.M. Fagin (Eds.), *Charting nursing's future: Agenda for the 1990s* (pp. 287–299). Philadelphia: J.B. Lippincott.

Franklin, P. D., Panzer, R. J., Brideau, L. P., & Griner, P. F. (1990). Innovations in clinical practice through hospital-funded grants. *Academic Medicine, 65,* 355–360.

Griffith, H. (1984). Nursing practice: Substitute or complement according to economic theory. *Nursing Economic$, 2,* 105–112.

Gleeson, R. M., McIlvain-Simpson, G., Boos, M. L., Sweet, E., Trzcinski, K. M., Solberg, C. A., & Doughty, R. A. (1990). Advanced practice nursing: A model of collaborative care. *MCN: American Journal of Maternal–Child Nursing, 15,* 9–12.

Hamilton, J. (1993, January 5). Toppling the power of the pyramid. *Hospitals and Health Networks, 67*(1), 38, 40–41.

Institute of Medicine. (1983). *Nursing and nursing education.* Washington DC: National Academy Press.

Kalish, B. J., & Kalish, P. A. (1977). An analysis of the sources of physician–nurse conflict. *Journal of Nursing Administration, 7*(1), 51–57.

Katzman, E. M., & Roberts, J. I. (1988). Nurse–physician conflicts as barriers to the enactment of nursing roles. *Western Journal of Nursing Research, 10*(5), 576–590.

Keane, A., & Richmond, T. (1993). Tertiary nurse practitioners. *Image: The Journal of Nursing Scholarship, 25*(4), 281–284.

Kerr, J.A.C. (1986). Interpersonal distance of hospital staff. *Western Journal of Nursing Research, 8*(3), 350–364.

Kitzman, H. (1983). The CNS and the nurse practitioner. In A. B. Hamric & J. Spross (Eds.), *The clinical nurse specialist in theory and practice* (pp. 275–290). New York: Grune & Stratton.

Kitzman, H. (1986). Education in nursing. In J. E. Steel (Ed.), *Issues in collaborative practice* (pp. 139–159). Orlando: Grune & Stratton.

Knaus, W. A., Draper, E. A., Wagner, D. P., & Zimmerman, J. E. (1986). An evaluation of outcome from intensive care in major medical centers. *Annals of Internal Medicine, 104,* 410–418.

Koerner, B. L., & Armstrong, D. A. (1983). Collaborative practice at Hartford Hospital. *Nursing Administration Quarterly, 7*(4), 72–81.

Koerner, B., & Armstrong, D. (1984). Collaborative practice cuts cost of patient care: Study. *Hospitals, 58*(10), 52–54.

Koerner, B. L., Cohen, J. R., & Armstrong, D. (1985). Collaborative practice and patient satisfaction. *Evaluation and the Health Professions, 8,* 299–321.

Lamb, G. S. (1991). Two explanations of nurse practitioner interactions and participatory decision making with physicians. *Research in Nursing and Health, 14,* 379–386.

Lamb, G. S., & Napodano, R. J. (1984). Physician–nurse practitioner interaction patterns in primary care practices. *American Journal of Public Health, 74,* 26–29.

Lewis, F. M. (1991). Consultation and collaboration among health care providers. In S. B. Baird, R. McCorkle, & M. Grant (Eds.), *Cancer nursing* (pp. 957–964). Philadelphia, W.B. Saunders.

Lynaugh, J. E., & Bates, B. (1973). The two languages of nursing and medicine. *American Journal of Nursing, 73,* 66–69.

McLain, B. R. (1988a). Collaborative practice: A critical theory perspective. *Research in Nursing and Health, 11,* 391–398.

McLain, B. R. (1988b). Collaborative practice: The nurse practitioner's role in its success or failure. *Nurse Practitioner, 13*(5), 31–38.

Mirr, M. P. (1994). Advanced clinical practice: A reconceptualized role. *AACN Clinical Issues, 4,* 599–602.

Mitchell, P. H., Armstrong, S., Simpson, T. F., & Lentz, M. (1989). AACN demonstration project. *Heart and Lung, 18,* 219–237.

Mundinger, M. O. (1994). Advanced-practice nursing: Good medicine for physicians? *New England Journal of Medicine, 330,* 211–214.

National Commission on Nursing. (1981). *Initial report and preliminary recommendations.* Chicago: American Hospital Association.

National Joint Practice Commission. (1981). *Guidelines for establishing joint or collaborative practice in hospitals.* Chicago: Author.

Norsen, L., Opladen, J., & Quinn, J. (1995). Practice model: collaborative practice. *Critical Care Nursing Clinics of North America, 7*(1), 43-52.

Parrinello, K. (1995). Advanced practice nursing: Administrative perspective. *Critical Care Nursing Clinics of North America, 7*(1), 9-16.

Pellegrino, E. D. (1966). What's wrong with the nurse–physician relationship in today's hospitals? *Hospitals, 40*(24), 70–80.

Pike, A. W., McHugh, M., & Canney, K. (1993). A new architecture for quality assurance: Nurse–physician collaboration. *Journal of Nursing Care Quality, 7,*(3), 1–8.

Prescott, P. A., & Bowen, S. A. (1985). Physician–nurse relationships. *Annals of Internal Medicine, 103,* 127–133.

Quigley, P., Hixon, A., & Jangen, S. (1991). Promoting autonomy and professional practice: A program of clinical privileging. *Journal of Nursing Quality Assurance, 5*(3), 27–32.

Roueche, B. (Ed.). (1977). *Together: A casebook of joint practices in primary care.* Chicago: National Joint Practice Commission.

Rubenstein, L. Z., Josephson, K. R., Wieland, G. D., English, P. A., Sayre, J. A., & Kane, R. L. (1984). Effectiveness of a geriatric evaluation unit. *New England Journal of Medicine, 311,* 1664–1670.

Safriet, B. J. (1992). Health care dollars and regulatory sense: The role of advanced practice nursing. *Yale Journal on Regulation, 9*(2), 417–488.

Schmitt, M. H., Watson, N. M., Feiger, S. M., & Williams, T. F. (1982). Conceptualizing and measuring outcomes of interdisciplinary team care for a group of long-term, chronically ill, institutionalized patients. In J. E. Bachman (Ed.), *Proceedings of the Third Annual Interdisciplinary Team Care Conference: Interdisciplinary health care* (pp. 169–182). Kalamazoo: Center for Human Services, Western Michigan University.

Secretary's Commission on Nursing. (1988). *Final report: National Center for Healthcare Research and Technology.* Washington, DC: U.S. Department of Health and Human Services.

Sheard, T. (1980). The structure of conflict in nurse–physicians relations. *Supervisor Nurse, 11*(8), 14–18.

Smith, T. (1991). A structured process to credential nurses with advanced practice skills. *Journal of Nursing Quality Assurance, 5*(3), 40–51.

Steel, J. E. (Ed.). (1986). *Issues in collaborative practice.* Orlando: Grune & Stratton.

Stein, L. I. (1967). The doctor–nurse game. *Archives of General Psychiatry, 16,* 699–703.

Tellis-Nayak, M., & Tellis-Nayak, V. (1984). Games that professionals play: The social psychology of physician–nurse interaction. *Social Science Medicine, 18*(12), 1063–1069.

Thomas, K. (1976). Conflict and conflict management. In M. D. Dunnette (Ed.), *Handbook of industrial and organizational psychology* (pp. 889–935). Chicago: Rand McNally College Publishing.

Walton, M. K., Jakobowski, D. S., & Barnsteiner, J. H. (1993). A collaborative practice model for the clinical nurse specialist. *Journal of Nursing Administration, 23*(2), 55–59.

Weiss, S. J., & Davis, H. P. (1985). Validity and reliability of the colloborative practice scale. *Nursing Research, 34,* 299–305.

Wood-Dauphinee, S., Shapiro, S., Bass, E., Fletcher, C., Georges, P., Hensby, V., & Mendelsohn, B. (1984). A randomized trial of team care following stroke. *Stroke, 15,* 864–872.

Zimmerman, J. E., Shortell, S. M., Rousseau, D. M., Duffy, J., Gillies, R. R., Knaus, W. A., Devers, K., Wagner, D. P., & Draper, E. A. (1993). Improving intensive care: Observations based on organizational case studies in nine intensive care units: A prospective, multicenter study. *Critical Care Medicine, 21,* 1443–1451.

Issues Related to Advanced Practice Nursing

Introduction: Sandra L. Venegoni

Throughout the course of history, professional issues have been studied along with the art and science of nursing. Every period of civilization contains certain philosophical thoughts, ideas, and situations that are pertinent not only to the time but that affect future events. So, too, with the chapters in Section III, which develop major issues affecting the present and future role of the advanced practice nurse (APN). Issues pertinent to the individual APN role include accountability, state regulatory processes, empowerment, and use of research to improve practice. General issues affecting all APNs are economic and healthcare financing issues and cost containment initiatives.

In Chapter 11, Accountability: The Covenant Between Patient and Nurse Practitioner, Strumpf and Asimos focus attention on the pivotal element of the advanced practitioner's relationship with the patient: the concept of individual accountability. Like all clinicians, the APN is responsible, both legally and ethically, for the quality of care provided—care that must be satisfying to the patient and conducted with efficient use of resources. The APN is accountable not only to the patient, family, and community but also to legal authorities and professional peers and colleagues.

In Chapter 12, Licensure, Certification, and Credentialing, Porcher clarifies regulatory information pertinent to the APN role, that is, the regulation, licensure, certification, and credentialing process. Although she compares the regulatory differences between individual states, she also traces national trends. It will behoove APNs to become more knowledgeable in these matters and to become involved at the state and national level to make legislative changes necessary for the role.

In Chapter 13, Economics and Healthcare Financing, Buerhaus traces the economic forces during the past several decades that are responsible for the price competition in the healthcare marketplace. With an understanding of the information presented, APNs will be better prepared to determine future pricing for services and the consequences of their decisions. Factors related to healthcare economics and financing will continue to be two of the most significant forces in the ongoing healthcare reform.

In Chapter 14, Empowerment: Activism in Professional Practice, Conway-Welch discusses two essential ingredients needed by APNs to become more empowered and, thus, increase control over their professional lives. One ingredient is the increased use of data as the foundation for their arguments and decision making. The other ingredient, improvement knowledge, compliments the APN's professional knowledge. Examples of improvement knowledge include systems theory, variation theories, psychological theories, and learning theories. The increased knowledge and use of data will serve to not only empower APNs but to assist them as they become politically active.

In Chapter 15, Research Use in Advanced Practice Nursing, Champagne, Tornquist, and Funk promote a research-based practice for APNs, define benefits and barriers to this type of practice, and describe ways to improve individual and organizational use of research findings. Two models, the Stettler/Marram and Iowa models, are presented to enhance the use of research in practice.

In Chapter 16, Cost-Containment Initiatives: Analysis of Clinical Resource Use, Rutledge and Bennett familiarize readers with information needed to become more involved with cost-containment initiatives, including a discussion of trends related to external causal factors, the infrastructure of healthcare costs, and definitions associated with quality management and outcomes assessment. The authors also discuss the role and functions of the acute-care nurse practitioner as a member of a joint-practice model of care and as a future project coordinator.

Each of the authors in Section III presents an overview of a pertinent issue related to the APN role. During the transition to the 21st century, the issues will continue along similar pathways so that, historically, knowing now as much as one can about each issue will better prepare an individual for the future. The need for the APN to possess a solid, foundational knowledge base about professional issues is illustrated in the remaining sections of the book. In the exemplars, APNs and clinical experts present their narratives about how they carried out their role in a unique situation. In reading their stories, note how they apply their own knowledge base and how they understand the issues affecting their situation and the future. In this sense, they indeed give testimony to the similarity of the past, present, and future APN—how the APN must understand professional issues to provide the healthcare needed by patients.

CHAPTER

11

Accountability: The Covenant Between Patient and Nurse Practitioner

Neville E. Strumpf ■ *Kristie Asimos*

Accountability, the covenant that exists between nurse and patient, is the yardstick by which nurses measure themselves professionally. Subsumed within it are the expectations of patients, other colleagues, and society. Most important, accountability is a deeply held value intimately related to personal expectations about professional worth, responsibility for care, and meaning in one's work. As nursing evolves, and particularly as healthcare services undergo enormous transformation, this is an ideal moment to reconsider the numerous facets of accountability for practice.

Accountability can simply be defined as "responsibility" or "answerability" (Creasia & Parker, 1991, p. 152). This definition fails, however, to capture the essence or full scope of professional practice. Neither *responsibility* nor *answerability* addresses the essentialness of accountability as an integral part of nursing or the importance of the mutual nature of a relationship between nurse and patient. Any definition of accountability must include the broad roles of providers in diverse settings, as well as possible regulatory or legal limits to authority or practice.

A finite definition of accountability is unlikely given the complexities and changes in provider–patient relationships, legal and regulatory issues, and subtle interplays created by culture, education, training, collaboration with other professionals, and work settings. In their own way, these factors influence the nature of accountability and its articulation to patients, colleagues, and self. In this chapter, we explore various meanings and interpretations of accountability. Like the profession itself, accountability also evolves to fit with the circumstances of increasingly complex care needs and systems for delivering care, especially in an era of managed care.

The themes of relationship and caring are pervasive in the historical, educational, and clinical literature, and are integral to the concept of accountability in nursing. To understand

Hickey JV: ADVANCED PRACTICE NURSING: Changing Roles
and Clinical Applications © 1996 Lippincott–Raven Publishers

accountability, one must first consider its historical roots as an early foundation for professional nursing practice. In addition, external, as well as self-regulatory, influences on definitions of nursing and accountability have emerged in recent years and must be explored. This chapter provides a brief history of emerging ideas about accountability in nursing and discusses the effect of external and self-regulatory measures on perceived accountability. Existing research, barriers to accountable practice, and current understanding of accountability are addressed. The most fundamental aspect of accountability—*caring*—also is examined using available literature on the subject and material collected during interviews with advanced practice nurses (APNs).

HISTORICAL EVOLUTION OF ACCOUNTABILITY

Early discussions of accountability in nursing emphasized moral and ethical standards and the nurse–patient relationship. These have remained as core concepts in the educational preparation of nurses. Especially early in the development of the profession, devotion, veracity, confidentiality, and loyalty permeated the literature and influenced education and practice.

Florence Nightingale (1859/1992) in *Notes on Nursing: What It Is and What It Is Not*, published in 1859, understood moral and ethical principles as inherent to nursing. Nightingale's emphasis on accountability and preventive care assumed advocacy, veracity, dignity, empathy, and confidentiality. According to Nightingale, nursing was more than "administration of medicines and the application of poultices" (p. 6). Nursing must "put the patient in the best condition for nature to act upon him" (p. 75). Nursing ought "to signify proper use of fresh air, light, warmth, cleanliness, quiet, and the proper selection and administration of diet" (p. 6). Nightingale specifically mentioned important moral concepts as truthfulness (p. 22), trust (p. 55), confidentiality (p. 70), duty (p. 59), and responsibility (p. 24).

In describing the notion of respect for and duty to the patient, Isabel Hampton Robb wrote in 1901 that the "nurse should always make it her rule to think of every patient as an individual sick human-being, whose wishes, fancies, and peculiarities call for all the consideration possible at her hands" (p. 214). Robb later added that "confidences should always be held sacred and inviolable" (p. 234) and

> [the] whole conduct of the nurse should be such as to assure the patient that a moment of weakness will never be blazoned abroad. None of the privacies of personal or domestic life, no infirmity of disposition or little flaw of character, observed while caring for a patient, should ever be divulged by the nurse. . . . (p. 234)

Similarly, Amy Pope (Pope & Young, 1934) echoed these moral and ethical aspects of accountability in a 1934 text, noting that the nurse's responsibility was to maintain "high ethical and professional standards" (p. 3). She also emphasized that it was the professional nurse's duty to practice with "conscientiousness" (p. 3) and in a manner that demonstrated the nurse's respect of patient dignity and privacy.

The moral and ethical themes identified by Nightingale, Robb, and Pope were given more immediate application in Bertha Harmer's (1925) *Text-book of the Principles and Practice of Nursing*. Harmer noted that moral and ethical values such as reliability and trustworthiness inspired confidence in relationships with patients and contributed to the healing process. She viewed prevention as a crucial aspect of nursing and understood the work of nursing as holistic in nature.

> Nursing is rooted in the needs of humanity and is founded on the ideal of service. Its object is not only to cure the sick and heal the wounded but to bring health and ease, rest and comfort to mind and body, to shelter, nourish and protect and to minister to all those who are helpless or handicapped, young, aged, or immature. Its object is to prevent disease and to preserve health. (p. 3)

Virginia Henderson attributed her ethically based humanistic approach to nursing to her teacher, Annie W. Goodrich, Dean of the Army School of Nursing at Walter Reed Hospital, Washington, DC. Henderson (1966) described visits by Goodrich to the unit as moments when sights were lifted "above techniques and routines. . . . She never failed to infect us with the ethical significance of nursing" (p. 7). Henderson's now classic description of the nature of nursing considered holistic care of the patient as an explicit outcome of the relationship between patient and nurse. Henderson saw the nurse as a

> substitute for what the patient lacks to make him 'complete, whole, or independent' . . . 'in mind and body'. . . . She is temporarily the consciousness of the unconscious, the love of life for the suicidal, the leg of the amputee, the eyes of the newly blind, a means of locomotion for the infant, knowledge and confidence for the young mother, the "mouthpiece" for those too weak or withdrawn to speak. (pp. 15–16)

Accountability is implied in complete obligation to the patient and in the relationship between nurse and patient. Contemporaneous with Henderson, Gertrude Ujhely (1968) described general agreement in the nursing literature that the "main concern of nursing is, or should be . . . care of the whole patient" (p. 86). Doris Schwartz, a leader in public health and an advocate of advanced practice nursing in geriatrics, urged that the humanistic, moral, and ethical values inherent in comprehensive patient care never be relinquished, regardless of setting and diversity of role, or of sophistication in technology (Schwartz, 1988).

In contrast to these more philosophical explications, accountability was also defined in a program review report under provisions established by the U.S. Public Health Service in the federal Nurse Training Act of 1964 (U.S. Department of Health, Education, and Welfare, 1967). In the report, it was "for the care of patients that nursing is accountable to society" (p. 15). The report sought to determine the "nature of nursing practice . . . what it is today and what it will be tomorrow" (p. 15). Reflecting a continuum of greater complexity in nursing and in the healthcare environment, the statement concerning professional accountability extended beyond traditional moral or ethical and medical models. It emphasized the concept, first alluded to by Florence Nightingale, that professional practice in nursing is theory oriented more than technique oriented and is founded on a body of knowledge derived from scientific investigation. The role of the nurse was described as "doing for the patient what temporarily cannot be done alone" and helping "to develop and use physical and emotional resources effectively to move toward being well" (p. 16). These statements echo and expand on the sentiments of early nurse educators that nursing accountability involves a holistic sense of caring.

Today, schools of nursing uniformly emphasize caring and empathy as foundational aspects of professional practice at all levels. Separate courses or integration of content related to nursing ethics and values are required components of the curriculum, and students are evaluated clinically on care provision that demonstrates accountability to patients, peers, and self. This accountability refers to the "sense of overriding concern for the whole process of nursing care" including concepts of duty, autonomy, service, competence, authority, and commitment (Claus & Bailey cited in Omerod, 1993, p. 730).

Definitions of nursing have traditionally recognized patients' physical as well as emotional needs and have viewed both as essential to quality care. Despite the growth and evolution of more technical and scientifically based practice, meeting the basic physical and emotional needs of patients remains a paramount desire in nursing.

SCOPE AND STANDARDS OF PRACTICE

Although early nurse educators addressed ethical and moral values, technical skill, and holistic approaches to care as components of professional nursing, tremendous variability nevertheless existed in the early years of nursing in training, education, and skill. Those people with varied backgrounds who cared for sick persons were referred to as "nurses," regardless of the quality of the programs from which they had graduated. In time, the need for consistency in nursing education and skill became apparent.

Self-Regulation

With the formation of permanent American schools of nursing in the 1870s, nursing was legitimized as a vocation, and the movement toward regulation began (Goodnow, 1943). Regulatory efforts were clearly a response to extreme needs for trained nurses with standardized skills who could minister to sick people, as well as for better conditions in late 19th and early 20th century hospitals, where "nurses" could still be relatively unsupervised workers waiting on patients (Goodnow, 1943).

As nursing care of hospitalized patients improved, hospitals proliferated along with the schools of nursing frequently associated with them. Nurses increasingly wished to define the mission of a growing profession and to organize and communicate with one another.

The first national meeting of nurses in the United States was at the Chicago World's Fair in 1893 (Goodnow, 1943). It resulted in the formation of the American Society of Superintendents of Training Schools, a name that was later changed to the National League of Nursing Education (Goodnow, 1943). At about the same time, in 1896, with Isabel Hampton Robb as its first president, a general society of graduate nurses was formed: the Nurses' Associated Alumnae of the United States and Canada. The name was changed in 1912 to the American Nurses' Association (ANA)(Goodnow, 1943). The ANA, in 1897, stated its purpose as follows: "(1) to establish and maintain a code of ethics, (2) to elevate the standards of nursing education, and (3) to promote the usefulness and honor, the financial and other interests of the nursing profession" (Nurses' Association Alumni of the US and Canada, 1897).

By 1920, every state had an association of nursing that, in addition to setting standards and identifying scope of practice in association with the ANA, was given responsibility to secure registration laws. Over time, the functions of registration and regulation of practice increasingly shifted toward external regulation by the states.

Today, the profession still establishes standards and scope of practice for its members. Standards, which are continually revised and evaluated, commonly exceed minimum state guidelines. In addition to the profession's code of ethics for nurses, more than 20 other ANA publications describe nursing standards and scope of practice in various practice settings and are a gold standard by which educators, clinicians, and consumers can measure accountability in practice.

In addition to the setting forth of standards and scope of practice, to which all nurses hold themselves accountable, the profession also sets specific criteria for certification in advanced practice in a specialty. Almost all certification for advanced practice by the various credentialing bodies prescribes specific educational criteria, usually a master's degree in nursing from an accredited college or university. One such certifying body, the American Nurses Credentialing Center (1994), offers certification examinations in 12 generalist, five nurse practitioner, five clinical specialist, and two nursing administration specialties. An increasingly common requirement for employment in advanced practice roles is some form of certification based on a credentialing process (usually an examination) by a professional association.

External Regulation

Along with optimal standards set through self-regulation by the profession, legislative and regulatory bodies have increasingly played a role in establishing at least minimal standards for professional practice. As mentioned, the trend toward external regulation began in 1920, when requirements for registration as a professional nurse were set forth in state law. In 1944, a few states administered the first uniform multistate nursing board examination; this was followed by the development of State Board Pool tests, which have been used in all states since 1950 (Deloughery, 1977). These examinations provide consistent and uniform testing of knowledge essential to performance as an entry-level professional nurse.

Health professions, including nursing, are regulated by means of state rules for licensure and practice. Licensure controls admittance into the profession, whereas practice acts define scope of practice for licensed practitioners. This protection issues from the legislature, which speaks for the state, with authority often delegated to a state board of nursing. Functions of the board include determining eligibility requirements for initial licensure of professional and practical nurses, approving and supervising educational institutions of nursing, developing rules and regulations concerning practice, and enforcing restrictions (Deloughery, 1977). In determining licensure and practice, these regulatory boards have contributed to current understanding of accountability.

Although each state has fairly consistent legislation regarding entry-level practice, regulation for advanced practice nursing varies from state to state, in sharp contrast to the professional guidelines for standards and scope of practice. The professional guidelines for standards and scope of practice are consistent for each specialization and clearly transcend the discrepancies in role or authority that may be prescribed at the state level. Among many possible criteria for advanced practice, a state board of nursing may accept professional certification as sufficient to meet advanced practice regulations, may determine which schools have acceptable curricula for advanced practice, or may have additional requirements (e.g., specific continuing education programs and various tests of competency). In addition, the parameters of practice on a state-by-state basis can also vary widely, especially regarding prescriptive privileges and practice protocols (Pearson, 1994). Although opponents of broadened practice guidelines have charged that public health would be jeopardized if nurse practitioners were allowed to prescribe drugs, studies have showed that nurse practitioners make appropriate decisions when prescribing medications (Mahoney, 1994).

Balancing Internal/External Regulation

The current trend toward advanced practice nursing is clearly a response to profound changes in needs for healthcare and systems for delivering services. Consistency between the profession's standards and scope of practice and state regulations is essential if the skills of APNs are to be used.

Accountability in advanced practice nursing is measured against established professional standards for education and expertise. Thus, the educational base for advanced practice, assuming it is uniform throughout the profession for a particular specialty, should mean that any APN is accountable to provide similar care regardless of the state where he or she practices (Pearson, 1994).

Barriers to practice depending on state regulations contribute greatly to the uncertainty of consumers and other professionals concerning expanded nursing roles. Guidelines developed by the ANA or other professional organizations need to be more fully used by legislative and regulatory bodies charged with redefining the legal parameters of advanced practice, including accountability and authority.

Truly accountable practice, which requires and incorporates both internally and externally imposed standards and regulations, must also extend beyond them. Katims (1993) described nursing as holding two primary values: caring and excellence. These values shape nursing actions in significant ways. Although caring is foundational to the nurse–patient relationship, excellence addresses particular skills, moral or ethical obligations, and professional standards. Understandably, the nursing profession adheres to standards that exceed the requirements imposed by state regulations. As the skills of advanced practice and practice "privileges" come under greater legal scrutiny, the profession must strengthen its commitment to the caring relationship as integral to all accountable practice.

Nurse–Patient Relationship

Much of nursing literature and nursing research has been concerned with the nurse–patient relationship.

> 'Each time a nurse encounters a patient, something happens. The meeting is never a neutral event. It is the power of the nurse–patient relationship that makes nursing exciting and . . . not a series of automatic performances. The . . . nurse must understand that every patient encounter is meaningful, that it always has impact, that it always affects both the patient and the nurse.' The effect may be subtle or dramatic 'but something— either positive or negative—always occurs.' (Kenner et al cited in Jurchak, 1990, p. 456)

Indeed, one bond uniting nurses, regardless of diversity in backgrounds, experiences, and roles is attention to the nurse–patient relationship. "The essence of nursing is the caring connection that transcends time and culture" (Rawnsley, 1994, p. 189).

Growing concerns about dehumanization in the healthcare encounter (Carper, 1979) have led to greater interest in caring. *Compassion,* the genuine capacity to feel and to "share in . . . pain and anguish, . . . understanding . . . what sickness means, . . . together with a readiness to help and to see the situation as the patient does" (Pellegrino, cited in Carper, 1979, p. 18), is necessary to an authentic sense of caring. Such authenticity by healthcare professionals is frequently perceived by patients as an important factor in the quality of healthcare (Carper, 1979). As technology and specialization contribute to a greater sense of depersonalization, caring behaviors—patience, trust, honesty, humility, hope, compassion, courage, knowledge, and flexibility—are increasingly desired by consumers.

In an essay recalling his personal experiences as a physician, Schnabel (1983) described "medicine's art" as "a skillful manipulation of the relationship between doctor and patient, which when combined with the logical use of medicine's science, leads to the best kind of patient care" (Schnabel, 1983, p. 1259). This view is congruent with the values of excellence and caring inherent in nursing as described by Katims (1993). Like Carper (1979), Schnabel worried that increased specialization and frequency of referrals to specialists would negatively affect continuity and the relationship between primary provider and patient. Relationship and continuity between provider and patient might actually be lost in the trade-off between more personalized versus more specialized care. Schnabel boldly suggested that the provider–patient relationship may affect outcomes of care and contribute to the "cure" of the patient. He warned of the potential harm to patients if the "art" of healthcare were lost. More research aimed at defining and describing this core facet of accountable practice is definitely needed.

Mitchell (1982) described two approaches to practice: the "medical model structured from the top down to carry out the mission of curing, healing, and saving patients' lives [and] the sensitivity model structured from base up to meet the multiple needs of patients" (p. 174). Cassel (1986) pointed out that the medical model strongly emphasizes cure, but that dramatic cure in some populations (e.g., elderly people) is unusual. Nurses may have a more realistic sense of the problems associated with illness, especially chronic disease, the accompanying ethical issues, and patient desires. Because nurse practitioners often have "curing" as well as "caring" functions, conflict can exist for APNs confronted with these two approaches to healthcare. Nurses' familiarity with the realities of managing more troublesome aspects of continuous or chronic care may be an advantage, and one leading to improved patient outcomes.

The importance of relationship is increasingly evident in the current healthcare environment in which emphasis is shifting to greater collaboration between patients and providers, with both working jointly to determine goals and weigh alternative courses of action and approaches to healthcare (Kasch, 1986). Consumers appear to value in their healthcare providers the fusion of curing and caring and the inclusion of clinical excellence as well as healing art. Patients are no longer content to be passive recipients of healthcare. These changing perceptions of patients must be considered in any definition of holistic and accountable practice.

Managed care will no doubt intensify concerns about provider–patient relationships. Choice, communication, competence, compassion, and continuity will be essential (Emanuel, Mezey, & Dubler, 1993). Compassionate delivery of competent and effective primary healthcare is fundamental to accountable practice in care of the whole patient. With accountability comes a sense of responsibility for providing continuity that exceeds a set time or a set problem.

Ethical Base for Accountability

The conceptual framework and moral dimensions of accountability for nursing practice are based on certain ethical principles and are integral to education and practice. The traditional principles of nonmaleficence, beneficence, autonomy, justice, and veracity can be expanded to include concepts such as advocacy, loyalty, care or caring, compassion, and human dignity (Creasia & Parker, 1991; Strumpf & Paier, 1993). These concepts are frequently discussed in the nursing literature as intrinsically connected to nursing's work. Although critical to the concept of accountability, such "caring" concepts are difficult to measure and to quantify.

In nursing, much of the covenant between patient and nurse is unspoken and based on an understanding of traditional nursing values and ethics (e.g., caring and empathy). Much of what is viewed as responsibility and accountability to and for patients is intimately associated with a caring relationship. Although elements of the relationship and the accompanying ethical values are felt by patient and nurse, they are not easily defined; rather, they are understood. Patients consistently describe this relationship as essential to responsive practice and care by a nurse, although "caring, the essence of nursing, defies measurement" (Baer, 1993, p. 109).

Research Related to the Nurse–Patient Relationship

In available studies of patient outcomes, findings to date have pointed to the importance of relationship and indirectly to accountability in practice. Much more investigation, however, is needed to tease out the effect of the nurse–patient relationship on outcomes of care. This type of research is hampered by numerous methodologic problems, among them defining specific nursing interventions and using measures that truly capture outcomes of care.

In the narratives of nurses in 88 caring situations, Astrom and colleagues (Astrom, Norberg, Hallberg, & Jansson, 1993) sought to interpret the meaning and effect of caring actions on patients, from both the patients' and the nurses' points of view. Consistently, patients and nurses agreed on which caring actions made a difference. Typically, these situations involved a well-developed nurse–patient relationship characterized by empathy from the nurse, along with knowledge of the patient's personality and preferences.

Ongoing research concerning comprehensive discharge planning for hospitalized elderly patients has shown the positive effect of advanced practice nursing on patient outcomes following discharge. In one randomized clinical trial conducted at a large medical center (Naylor et al., 1994), 276 patients and 125 caregivers were assigned randomly to intervention and control groups. Patients in the control group received the routine hospital discharge plan, whereas those assigned to the intervention group received, in addition to the routine hospital plan, a comprehensive, individualized discharge plan designed specifically for elderly patients and implemented by gerontologic nurse specialists. Patients in the intervention group were seen by a nurse specialist within 24 hours to 48 hours of admission and every 48 hours thereafter to revise and implement the discharge plan. The last hospital visit was made within 24 hours of discharge. Following discharge, the nurse specialist made home visits and was available by telephone for 2 weeks postdischarge. From the initial hospitalization until 6 weeks after discharge, patients in the intervention group had fewer readmissions, fewer total days rehospitalized, lower readmission charges, and lower charges for healthcare services after discharge. The results of this study suggested the importance of a relationship with the nurse, of continuity and trust, and of individualization of care.

In another study of 87 people infected with human immunodeficiency virus (Aiken et al., 1993), patients' perceptions of clinical care by nurse practitioners compared with physicians were explored. Patients were assigned to either nurse practitioners or physicians for their periodic visits. Those patients followed by the nurse practitioners experienced greater satisfaction with their healthcare as evidenced by significantly fewer reports of problems with their care providers. Although patients in both groups experienced symptoms between visits, patients were more likely to report these symptoms to the nurse practitioners. These findings suggested the importance of a trusting provider–patient relationship in acquiring information and achieving optimal healthcare.

Although limited in number, such studies have linked nurses' approaches to healthcare, and their relationship to patients and others in the healthcare system, to patient outcomes. They represent a preliminary effort to quantify the significance of a caring relationship.

BARRIERS TO ACCOUNTABLE PRACTICE

Barriers to Caring

Caring, what should serve as a unifying concept for healthcare providers, is unfortunately an undervalued commodity. Reasons for this devaluation are complex. Certainly the explosion of science and technology are contributing factors, but perhaps more important, the changes wrought by these advances on the relationships between patients and providers have had a significant and probably detrimental effect on perceptions of caring.

The historical progression of "nursing care," as described by Susan Reverby (1987) in *Ordered To Care: The Dilemma of American Nursing, 1850–1945*, illustrates the myriad factors contributing to the undervaluation of caring. Reverby suggested that a crucial dilemma exists in contemporary American nursing: "the order to care in a society that has refused to value caring" (Reverby, 1987, p. 1). Nursing developed within a set of cultural expectations about caring as part of women's duties to family and community. When training for nursing was introduced in the late 19th century, it was based on this understanding of women's duty, but not of women's rights (Reverby, 1987).

Unquestioning subservience and acceptance of orders under the watchful control of hospitals and physicians became increasingly unacceptable as trained nurses gained knowledge and a sense of advocacy and independent accountability to patients. Conflict soon developed among physicians, nurses, and others over the appropriate role of the nurse (Reverby, 1987, p. 202). Despite desires for increasing autonomy and accountability, nurses often had little of either as the economic and cultural power of hospitals and physicians increased throughout much of the 20th century. Nursing's "educational philosophy, ideological underpinnings, and structural position made it difficult to create the circumstances from which to gain a recognized claim of rights" based on caring (Reverby, 1987, p. 203).

More recently, social, political, and economic conditions have permitted greater autonomy in decisions regarding practice. Increased technical expertise has given nurses more "ability to integrate and synthesize volumes of differentiated knowledge in order to translate that knowledge into coordinated, safe patient care" (Reverby, 1987, p. 204). Moreover, the increasing acceptance of women's rights has enhanced respect for the role of women in society and in the professional world. What still remains, however, are potent barriers to the valuing of much of women's work, especially that related to nurturance and care. As already discussed, these are essential elements of accountable practice, and challenge nursing professionals who struggle to deliver both technically proficient and humane care.

Barriers Imposed by Healthcare System Constraints

In addition to the undervaluation of caring, or perhaps associated with it, the healthcare system itself can impede accountable practice. System constraints such as time, access, reimbursement, and models of care are often complicating factors. All can negatively affect fundamental elements of the ideal provider–patient relationship and, hence, patient satisfaction and optimal healthcare.

Both managed care and reimbursement issues potentially threaten choice in healthcare. In managed care plans, decisions may be and often are determined to a great extent by insurers or case managers. Limits on reimbursement for specific diagnostic and treatment alternatives can affect choices in providers, facilities, and options for care. Although there is much to applaud in reforming healthcare to include more integration of services and providers, greater continuity, and curtailment of unnecessary costs, these changes represent remarkable departures from the ways in which healthcare has been delivered for nearly a century. Such changes will inevitably and dramatically affect the practices and decisions of all providers, including physicians and nurse practitioners.

In a recent letter to the *New York Times,* Becker (1994) illustrated several constraints under which healthcare providers must currently operate in some managed care organizations, including predetermined number and length for office or clinic visits and management decisions influenced by reimbursement. An example given is that of the depressed, suicidal patient covered in a managed care agreement with limited mental health services. Because of the potential risks associated with the outcomes of inadequate care (e.g., complications associated with delayed treatment, or even suicide), many providers worry about accountability and malpractice. Given the access and care issues inherent in the existing health delivery system, one is reluctant to dismiss the changes now occurring; however, many questions are raised for providers about practice in accountable and caring ways in these highly cost-driven systems. Regardless of changes already here, or yet to come, one hopes that financial considerations will not eliminate compassion in clinical decision making.

Barriers to Collaboration

Historically, nurses were viewed as "helpers and agents of physicians; not co-workers or colleagues" (Reverby, 1987, p. 131); thus, collaboration, even with APNs, remains difficult for many physicians to embrace. In providing care for the "whole" person, nursing has accepted accountability for aspects of care that overlap with the accountability and authority of other professions (Ujhely, 1968), especially physicians. Overlaps in professional accountability frequently cause confusion regarding authority and responsibility, cause feelings of competition, and further inhibit the collaborative efforts necessary in accountable healthcare.

It is not surprising that these issues stemming from historical antecedents in nurse–physician relationships have also contributed to inconsistency from state to state regarding practice roles and privileging. From these political and competitive pressures, often driven by the medical and nursing associations, a feeling of resentment and reluctance to collaborate has developed and has been difficult to overcome.

In their book *Nurse Physician Collaboration: Care of Adults and the Elderly,* Eugenia Siegler and Fay Whitney (1994) referred to their frustrations in promoting and maintaining collaborative practice in settings that are often indifferent and occasionally hostile. Physicians and nurses receive different educations and thus think differently. But both disciplines must cope with "expanding knowledge bases, rapid technological changes, increasing complexity of patient care inside and outside of the hospital, and difficult fiscal management and policy issues" (p. 19). Paradoxically, the need to collaborate "grows exponentially" as the system becomes more complex, but the priority to teach principles of collaboration "falls in the wake of the pressure to disseminate new knowledge" (p. 19). Thus, those professionals who do practice collaboratively must overcome many barriers at professional, institutional, and legislative levels. Collaborative practice, although largely misunderstood, rarely valued by academic institutions, and currently not compensated by third-party payers, is a necessary ingredient in accountable advanced nursing practice and for solutions to America's continuing healthcare crisis.

CASE VIGNETTES

The following three vignettes by nurse practitioners in home care, a community-based family health center, and an emergency room, respectively, are based on interviews by one of the authors (Asimos) and illustrate many of the themes discussed in this review of accountability.

Vignette 1

M. Catherine Wollman, MSN, RN, Gerontological Nurse Practitioner in Discharge Planning, School of Nursing, University of Pennsylvania

Wollman is part of the staff for the research project Comprehensive Discharge Planning for the Elderly (Naylor et al., 1994) described in the section Research Related to the Nurse–Patient Relationship. The setting for her work is a large tertiary medical center and the surrounding community. The focus is acutely ill elderly patients, mainly those with respiratory, cardiovascular, or orthopedic problems (both medical and surgical). All are selected because of "high risk" due to multiple chronic conditions, age (older than 80 years), and frequent or recent hospitalizations.

A major goal of the comprehensive discharge planning protocol is maintenance of function during and after hospitalization. This goal is accomplished by careful monitoring and evaluation throughout hospitalization and follow-up at home as often as necessary for 1 month after discharge (in the original study, for 2 weeks). During home visits, nurse practitioners manage acute problems as they arise, assess and resolve a wide range of concerns about function, and respond to caregiver concerns. Referrals are made as necessary, and a close relationship is maintained with several home care agencies to which patients have been assigned.

Key to success of the intervention is development of a trusting relationship with clear communications, one that permits understanding of personal preferences, assessment of needs, and determination of realistic outcomes mutually agreeable to patients and their families. Each case requires individualized care planning and much creativity. Among the varied problems that can arise are the need to follow specific drug regimens, to overcome environmental barriers, or to cope with acuity associated with rapid discharge from the hospital (e.g., patients undergoing coronary artery bypass surgery may be discharged in 5 days).

In this unusual role, the barriers to practice faced by Wollman often center on explaining to colleagues from all disciplines the nature of her role, gaining trust, and obtaining cooperation in implementing necessary interventions. Bridging the gaps from hospital to home and maintaining continuity of care can be exceedingly challenging. Wollman believes that one of the most urgent changes needed in healthcare is greater accountability by hospital staff for discharge planning and greater responsibility for outcomes posthospitalization. Collaboration with physicians, many of whom do not know the nurse practitioners or are unfamiliar with the skills of APNs or the project, can be difficult. For the nurse practitioners who so clearly understand patients' needs and experience so intimately the barriers created by the system of care, frustration can be intense.

Nevertheless, this role provides an opportunity for the nurse practitioner to establish a care plan with the patient and caregiver and to bring it to fruition. Each encounter reinforces the need for a model of services based on transitional care, and findings from the study have increasingly documented that such services performed by an APN produce positive, cost-effective outcomes (Naylor et al., 1994). In addition, the need for reimbursement or managed care arrangements for these services is clearly evident.

Accountability to the patient is 24 hours a day, 7 days a week. It requires collaboration with other providers and commitment to improved function, reduction in complications, and avoidance of rehospitalization. Wollman has described the extraordinary sense of responsibility that accompanies management aimed at achieving these goals with frail elderly patients in the community. Conditions faced by the nurse practitioners are rarely ideal, as the following examples attest, but the rewards are often great.

One case involved an 80-year-old male, alone at home following serious abdominal surgery. He refused short-term placement in a nursing home or rehabilitation facility; despite the risks, his only desire was to be in his own home. With a hospital bed on the first floor, and visits from home health aides and family members coordinated by the nurse practitioner, the patient did improve over time. For this man, the nurse practitioner's accountability included not only assessment and monitoring, but also ethical commitment to honor a wish to be at home.

Even more challenging was the case of J, a 66-year-old male hospitalized for 18 days with congestive heart failure complicated by diabetes, renal disease, and asthma. J was poor and illiterate, and many assumptions were made about his capacity, and that of his wife, to provide care. Of greatest concern to J was management of his medication regime, something no one believed that J and his wife were capable of doing. The nurse practitioner never succeeded in teaching the wife to use a medication compliance aid, but, undaunted, spent many hours helping J learn to recognize the first letters of the days of the week and the times so that he could use the aid correctly. Humor provided some essential common ground during this difficult and potentially humiliating process. Once J had mastered use of the compliance aid and could take his medications properly, his sense of self-esteem and personal accountability increased considerably. This extraordinary accomplishment was attributed to the "beautiful nurse who cared for him." Wollman viewed her accountability to J as believing in him, making no judgments about capacity or willingness to comply, and working through numerous system constraints to get the supplies and equipment needed for self-sufficiency.

Vignette 2

Melinda Jenkins, PhD, RN, Family Nurse Practitioner, Abbotsford Community Health Center, Philadelphia

Abbotsford, a nurse-managed center located in a public housing complex, provides family healthcare to residents in one of Philadelphia's poorest neighborhoods. Nurse practitioners see patients of all ages, including prenatal, pediatric, adult, and elder care. Jenkins has characterized accountability for care at the center, and responsibility of the nurse practitioners, as congruent with the ANA (1980) social policy statement: the profession of nursing serves the public and, in so doing, contributes to the good of society. Relationships between a committed tenant counsel and staff of the center are strong, and there is a sense of shared accountability for services rendered and received.

Currently, nurse practitioners at the center find themselves in a complex struggle over interpretation of rules governing Medicaid contracts to health maintenance organizations in Pennsylvania. Although the nurse practitioners have been following patients covered by two managed care contracts for several years, and have been reimbursed, a stringent reinterpretation of the rules could in the future prevent nurse practitioners from serving as primary providers to Medicaid patients and receiving direct reimbursement. In the balance of this decision are 500 Abbotsford patients who have a trusting relationship with their nurse practitioners, a coherent service successfully meeting community needs, and survival of the center itself. The situation, which undoubtedly will be repeated elsewhere, illustrates continuing, and as yet unresolved, barriers to accountable advanced practice—regulations on scope of practice and issues of reimbursement. What happens when providers must tell patients that their insurance plan no longer covers the care they have been receiving, or that they must change plans or providers to receive care? The irony, of course, is that nurse practitioners, especially in managed care arrangements serving similar populations, are best able to respond to changing incentives for delivering services—namely, health promotion and disease prevention aimed at reducing expensive hospital care.

An example of such services is the case of a woman in her early 20s followed by Jenkins for prenatal care. Following the delivery of a healthy baby, B came in for routine pediatric care only. One day, just as the center was about to close, she called Jenkins in great alarm over the extreme fatigue and sudden 30-lb weight loss of her fiancé. The man was obviously reluctant to seek care, but because B trusted the nurse practitioners at the center, he agreed to see Jenkins, who also felt it was an emergency. A quick history and examination revealed 4+ glucose in the urine and a random blood glucose of 400. Hospitalization for a diabetic crisis was prevented. Jenkins is convinced that this successful outcome depended greatly on a sense of accountability for care and the relationship with patient and community.

Vignette 3

Michael Clark, MSN, RN, Nurse Practitioner in Emergency Services, Hospital of the University of Pennsylvania

As part of emergency services provided by the Hospital of the University of Pennsylvania, a walk-in clinic staffed by nurse practitioners (with physician backup) has been established for people requiring less emergent care. Protocols help delineate practice parameters, but it is experience gained over time and the ability and confidence "to think on one's feet" that most define what the practitioners do. In this setting, the dialogue between nurse practitioners and physicians concerning collaboration and decision making is an ongoing one.

First and foremost, the nurse practitioners view their primary obligation and accountability to patients. Frequently, this takes the form of advocacy, especially with a patient population that has problems accessing more appropriate primary care services. Most clinic patients have Medicaid coverage or its equivalent; helping them overcome barriers experienced in obtaining care is often the focus of interventions by the nurse practitioners. Thus, Clark queries all patients the reasons they are in the emergency room and not somewhere else. Often, it is "last straw" phenomena—long-standing dissatisfaction with providers, enormity of healthcare problems, exhaustion and frustration, or declining resources (personal and financial)—that precipitate visits to the emergency room.

Although patients struggle with barriers related to access, nurse practitioners work against numerous time and volume constraints to maximize what is likely to be a single patient encounter. For practice to be truly responsive to the public, Clark believes that patients coming to the walk-in clinic must be empowered with information to care for themselves. Although these patients can benefit from services and expertise unique to an academic medical center, it is translation of that knowledge, quickly and in pragmatic terms, that is essential. Many factors must be considered as to which interventions will be useful, feasible, and cost-effective.

Clark related the story of an older couple who arrived in the triage area. The wife was immaculately groomed and refined in her manner; the husband was extremely agitated and demanded that his wife "be tested for drugs." Immediately, the nurse practitioner made a decision to separate the couple for purposes of assessment and possible admission to the hospital. In eliciting a history from the wife, the nurse practitioner learned that her husband had been physically assaultive for the past few weeks. Psychiatric consultation was arranged for the couple, which ultimately led to resolution of some family stresses and problems. This story represents the kind of situation that could easily be dismissed in an emergency room as bizarre and a waste of time. In this case, however, commitment to look beyond superficial behavior and appearance, and to gather additional data, made a difference in quality of life for the couple and potentially prevented serious injury.

Each example of advanced clinical practice is shaped by setting, characteristics of and constraints on particular practices, and perceptions of accountability and responsibility. Whether care is acute and episodic, or continuous over time, a consistent theme emerges: the focus of the nurse practitioners is holistic and devoted to principles of primary care. Accountability is understood in terms of ethical commitments to honor and respect individuals and their needs, to remain nonjudgmental, to empower through information sharing and advocacy, and to be true to community and societal expectations and trust.

SUMMARY AND CONCLUSIONS

The covenant between nurse practitioner and patient is rooted in the profession's moral and ethical foundations and its abiding commitment to people in need. As healthcare has changed and as nursing has advanced its knowledge base, the boundaries of practice have expanded considerably. Practice is influenced by professional standards, as well as external regulations designed to protect the public. These forces have served both to facilitate and to constrain practice, and undoubtedly will continue to evolve over time.

In its statement of graduate outcomes for primary care nurse practitioners, the National Organization of Nurse Practitioner Faculties (1993) identified as critical competencies caring, advocacy, support, relationships, therapeutic communication, interpersonal skills, and ethics.

Similar to this chapter, the statement of graduate outcomes also included professional and legal standards, collaboration and consultation with others, and maintenance of certification as part of accountable practice.

What permeates every aspect of accountability, however, is responsible, excellent care, essentiality of the caring relationship, and commitment to the outcomes produced by caring for individuals and for society. Nurse practitioners will be challenged daily by complexities in patient care and barriers to practice, but among their rewards will be the satisfaction that comes from truly accountable care. The essence of that accountability, so beautifully illustrated in the case vignettes, is eloquently captured in a single, simple sentence from Doris Schwartz's personal story of 50 years in nursing: "Caring *about* a patient can be as important as providing care *for* the patient" (Schwartz, 1995, pp. 213–214).

References

Aiken, L. H., Lake, E. T., Semaan, S., Lehman, H. P., O'Hare, P. A., Cole, C. S., Dunbar, D., & Frank, I. (1993). Nurse practitioner managed care for persons with HIV infection. *Image: The Journal of Nursing Scholarship, 25*(3), 172–177.

American Nurses' Association. (1980). *Nursing: A social policy statement.* Kansas City, MO: Author.

American Nurses Credentialing Center. (1994). *Certification catalog* (brochure). Washington, DC: American Nurses Credentialing Center.

Astrom, G., Norberg, A., Hallberg, I. R., & Jansson, L. (1993). Experienced and skilled nurses' narratives of situations where caring action made a difference to the patient. *Scholarly Inquiry for Nursing Practice, 7*(3), 183–193.

Baer, E. D. (1993). Philosophical and historical bases of primary care nursing. In M. D. Mezey & D. O. McGivern (Eds.), *Nurses, nurse practitioners: Evolution to advanced practice* (pp. 102–118). New York: Springer.

Becker, E. A. (1994, December 25). Doctors bear all risks [Letter to the editor]. *The New York Times,* p. 8.

Carper, B. A. (1979). The ethics of caring. *Advances in Nursing Science, 1*(3), 11–19.

Cassel, C. K. (1986). The meaning of health care in old age. In T. Cole & S. Gadow (Eds.), *What does it mean to grow old* (pp. 179–198). Durham, NC: Duke University Press.

Creasia, J. L., & Parker, B. (Eds.). (1991). *Conceptual foundations of professional nursing practice.* Philadelphia: C.V. Mosby.

Deloughery, G. L. (1977). *History and trends of professional nursing* (8th ed.). St. Louis, MO: C.V. Mosby.

Emanuel, E. J., Mezey, M. D., & Dubler, N. N. (1993). *The provider patient relationship under the new health care system.* Unpublished manuscript.

Goodnow, M. (1943). *Nursing history in brief* (rev. ed.). Philadelphia: W.B. Saunders.

Harmer, B. (1925). *Text-book of the principles and practice of nursing.* New York: Macmillan.

Henderson, V. (1966). *The nature of nursing: A definition and its implications for practice, research, and education.* New York: Macmillan.

Jurchak, M. (1990). Competence and the nurse–patient relationship. *Critical Care Nursing Clinics of North America, 2*(3), 453–459.

Kasch, C. R. (1986). Establishing a collaborative nurse–patient relationship: A distinct focus of nursing action in primary care. *Image: The Journal of Nursing Scholarship, 18*(2), 44–47.

Katims, I. (1993). Nursing as aesthetic experience and the notion of practice. *Scholarly Inquiry for Nursing Practice, 7*(4), 269–278.

Mahoney, D. F. (1994). Appropriateness of geriatric prescribing decisions made by nurse practitioners and physicians. *Image: The Journal of Nursing Scholarship, 26*(1), 41–46.

Mitchell, C. (1982). Integrity in interprofessional relationships. In G. J. Agich (Ed.), *Responsibility in health care* (pp. 163–184). Dordrecht, Holland: Reidel.

National Organization of Nurse Practitioner Faculties. (1993, November). *Primary care nurse practitioner graduate outcomes.* National Organization of Nurse Practitioner Faculties Education Committee, Washington, DC.

Naylor, M., Brooten, D., Jones, R., Lavizzo-Mourey, R., Mezey, M., & Pauly, M. (1994). Comprehensive discharge planning for the hospitalized elderly: A randomized clinical trial. *Annals of Internal Medicine, 120*(12), 999–1006.

Nightingale, F. (1992). *Notes on nursing: What it is and what it is not* (commemorative ed.). Philadelphia: J.B. Lippincott. (Original work published 1859)

Nurses' Association Alumni of the US and Canada, "Constitution," 1897, updated in ANA 1985, Code for Nurses with Interpretive Statements, Kansas, MO, author.

Omerod, J. A. (1993). Accountability in nurse education. *British Journal of Nursing, 2*(14), 730–733.

Pearson, L. J. (1994). Annual update of how each state stands on legislative issues affecting advanced nursing practice. *Nurse Practitioner, 19*(1), 11–21.

Pope, A. E., & Young, V. M. (1934). *The art and principles of nursing.* New York: G.P. Putnam's Sons.

Rawnsley, M. M. (1994). Response to "The nurse–patient relationship reconsidered: An expanded research agenda." *Scholarly Inquiry for Nursing Practice, 8*(2), 185–190.

Reverby, S. M. (1987). *Ordered to care: The dilemma of American nursing, 1850–1945.* Cambridge, MA: Cambridge University Press.

Robb, I. H. (1901). *Nursing ethics: For hospital and private use.* Cleveland: J.B. Savage.

Schnabel, T. G. (1983). Is medicine still an art? *New England Journal of Medicine, 309*(20), 1258–1261.

Schwartz, D. R. (1988). In T. M. Schorr & A. Zimmerman (Eds.), *Making choices, taking chances: Nurse leaders tell their stories* (pp. 311–320). Washington, DC: C.V. Mosby.

Schwartz, D. (1995). *Give us to go blithely: My fifty years of nursing.* New York: Springer.

Siegler, E. L., & Whitney, F. W. (1994). *Nurse–physician collaboration: Care of adults and the elderly.* New York: Springer.

Strumpf, N. E., & Paier, G. (1993). Meeting the health care needs of older adults. In M. D. Mezey & D. O. McGivern (Eds.). *Nurses, nurse practitioners: Evolution to advanced practice* (pp. 208–231). New York: Springer.

Ujhely, G. B. (1968). *Determinants of the nurse–patient relationship.* New York: Springer.

U.S. Department of Health, Education, and Welfare. (1967). *Nurse Training Act of 1964: Program review report* (USDHEW Public Health Service Publication No. 1740). Washington, DC: Author.

12

Licensure, Certification, and Credentialing

Frances K. Porcher

All states have statutes relating to nursing that contain at least a definition of nursing, criteria for licensure and endorsement of those nurses who are licensed in other states, and rules and regulations governing licensure processes. Some state statutes contain more specific and often more restrictive regulatory information. It is the definition of nursing, however, that frames scope of practice. The definition of nursing is especially important for advanced practice nurses (APNs), whose practice combines both medical and nursing components. This chapter examines regulatory aspects of the APN role, including methods of regulation, licensure, certification, and credentialing.

METHODS OF REGULATION

The purpose for legal regulation of nursing practice is the protection of public health, safety, and welfare. Regulatory criteria should reflect minimum requirements for safe and competent nursing practice. Legal regulation of nursing practice is the joint responsibility of state legislators and boards of nursing.

The first and least restrictive level of regulation is designation/recognition (National Council of State Boards of Nursing [NCSBN], 1992). Advanced practice nurses with state-recognized credentials are granted permission from the state board of nursing to represent themselves with those specific credentials: NP (nurse practitioner), CNS (clinical nurse specialist), or CNM (certified nurse-midwife). This approach does not involve any inquiry into competence and accordingly offers the least protection in terms of public health, safety, and welfare. The right of any APN to practice is not limited.

The second level of regulation, registration, requires APNs to list their names on an official roster maintained by the state board of nursing (NCSBN, 1992). Again, there is no inquiry into competence and usually scope of practice is not defined.

The third level of regulation, certification (NCSBN, 1992), should not be confused with the meaning adopted by nongovernmental agencies or professional associations to recognize

Hickey JV: ADVANCED PRACTICE NURSING: Changing Roles and Clinical Applications © 1996 Lippincott–Raven Publishers

professional competence. In the regulatory sense, certification indicates that individuals have met specified requirements and are therefore "certified." These requirements may vary among states. Boards of nursing often use the professional association certification as a substitute for regulatory certification.

The fourth and most restrictive level of regulation is licensure (NCSBN, 1992). People having met predetermined qualifications to engage in a particular profession to the exclusion of others may be granted a license by a regulatory agency or body such as the state board of nursing. Rules and regulations define the qualifications, scope of practice, and use of title. Unique to this level of regulation is a high level of accountability and intent to protect public health, safety, and welfare.

In 1986, the NCSBN adopted a position paper on advanced clinical nursing practice, concluding that designation/recognition (level 1) was the preferable method of regulating APNs (NCSBN, 1992). Additionally, educational preparation of APNs was to be at least a master's degree in nursing. Significant changes in healthcare, nursing, and society since the mid-1980s prompted the NCSBN to review this position, resulting in a proposed position paper that recommends licensure (level 4) as the preferred method of regulation for advanced nursing practice (NCSBN, 1992). According to the position paper, care activities of APNs are complex, require specialized knowledge and skill, great proficiency, and independent decision making. The potential of harm to the public is great unless there is a high level of accountability such as is expected with licensure. *Advanced practice registered nursing* is defined as "practice based on the knowledge and skills acquired in a basic nursing education, through licensure as a registered nurse, and in graduate education and experience, including advanced nursing theory, physical and psycho-social assessment, and treatment of illness" (NCSBN, 1992, p. 6). Skills and abilities for safe APN practice are listed in Table 12-1.

LICENSURE

Nurse practice acts have evolved through four distinct phases. In the early 1900s, the first nursing statutes were actually nurse registration acts. A designated board examined the applicant's competency to hold a "certificate of registration," thereby allowing the nurse to use the title "R.N." (registered nurse). The practice of nursing was not defined. North Carolina was the first state to pass a Nurse Registration Act in 1903, followed shortly by New York, New Jersey, and Virginia. By 1923, all states had passed nurse registration acts.

The passage of the mandatory practice act in New York in 1938 marked the start of the second licensure phase. The New York practice act legally defined nursing by defining scope

---

TABLE 12-1 **Skills and Abilities of APNs**

- Advanced assessment skills
- Advanced ability to synthesize and analyze data
- Advanced ability to apply nursing principles
- Ability to provide expert guidance and teaching
- Ability to work with clients, their families, and other healthcare workers
- Ability to manage client's health–illness status
- Ability to recognize practice limits
- Ability to use abstract thinking and conceptualization
- Ability to make decisions independently
- Ability to diagnose and prescribe
- Ability to consult with or refer to other healthcare workers

(Adapted from National Council of State Boards of Nursing. (1992, May. *National Council of State Boards of Nursing position paper on the licensure of advanced nursing practice*. Chicago: Author.)

of practice, specifying the education or training necessary for licensure, and prohibiting the practice of nursing without a license (Bullough, 1976). Nursing was narrowly defined to acknowledge dependent care activities pursuant to physician supervision.

This dependent nursing role predominated in nursing practice acts until the American Nurses' Association (ANA) proposed the following model definition of nursing in 1955:

> The practice of professional nursing means the performance for compensation of any act in the observation, care, and counsel of the ill, injured, or infirm, or in the maintenance of health or prevention of illness of others . . . the foregoing shall not be deemed to include acts of diagnosis or prescription of therapeutic or corrective measures. (Kelly, 1974, p. 1314)

Although this definition modified requirements for physician supervision for all nursing functions, nurses were specifically prohibited from diagnosing and prescribing.

A decade of change followed in the 1960s, marked by the birth of Medicaid and Medicare, a growing shortage of primary care physicians, the start of the first formal nurse practitioner and physician's assistant programs, the Vietnam War, and the emerging women's movement. All of these events contributed to the growing recognition that nursing practice was significantly restricted by state laws.

In 1971, Idaho became the first state to amend the nurse practice act to provide recognition for advanced practice nursing (phase 3). Idaho added a qualifying statement to the portion of the nurse practice act that prohibited nurses from diagnosing and treating patients to allow nurses to diagnose and treat as authorized jointly by the board of nursing and the board of medicine. Although this was a significant step, advanced practice nursing was still defined by nursing and medicine.

In 1982, the NCSBN published a new model nursing practice act that defined the practice of nursing to include diagnosis, planning, implementation, and evaluation of care and treatment.

Following publication of this definition, several states modified their nurse practice act to define both advanced practice nursing as well as who holds regulatory responsibility for advanced practice nursing (nursing versus medicine, or a combination of both). As of 1994, at least 38 states had specific regulations in their nurse practice act that identified regulation of advanced practice nursing as belonging to the state board of nursing (Pearson, 1995). Several states are in the process of revising their nurse practice acts to update the definition of advanced practice nursing and the regulatory mechanisms of such practice, still others maintain restrictive practice acts for APNs.

In 1992, the NCSBN recommended that the preferred method of regulation for advanced practice nursing be licensure rather than designation/recognition. That significant change hallmarks phase 4 of licensure. According to the position statement, advanced practice nursing should be based on graduate nursing education and boards of nursing should regulate advanced nursing practice by licensure because the risk of harm from unsafe or incompetent clinicians at this complex level of care is quite high.

According to a 1992 survey of NCSBN members, 50 boards of nursing have language in their practice acts that addresses advanced nursing practice and 22 boards issue a state certificate to APNs. Nineteen boards have other means of APN recognition such as issuance of a letter of authority. Additionally, 26 boards authorize APNs to prescribe and nine more have other methods that allow APNs to select, order, furnish, or otherwise authorize use of medications. Boards of nursing in 42 states hold regulatory control for advanced nursing practice; 36 states have sole regulatory responsibility for at least one APN category, 13 share regulatory responsibility with boards of medicine, and one state shares responsibility with medicine and pharmacy. In two states, the board of medicine has sole regulatory responsibility for advanced nursing practice, and four states identified other agencies such as the state department of education with regulatory responsibility and control (NCSBN, 1993).

The 1992 model identified an umbrella classification for advanced practice licensure for the purpose of regulation only. The classification is not intended to be used as a title, per se. Licensure at this level is designated as Advanced Practice Registered Nurse in one of the following four categories: nurse practitioner, certified registered nurse anesthetist, certified nurse-midwife, or clinical nurse specialist. The NCSBN believes that consistent titling and uniform use of terminology will improve public understanding of the roles, ensure safe advanced nursing practice, and provide a basis for regulating advanced practice.

Not all nurses support the concept of second licensure as a means to differentiate nurse generalists from nurse specialists. Not all nurses believe that differentiation is necessary. The 1992 NCSBN model legislation has been criticized for not addressing issues of clinical competency, mastery of skills, or validation of specific advanced practice knowledge (Hardy Havens, 1992). Rather, some critics believe the law should identify only the generic category of nurses and not specialists or advanced nurses. Some nurses believe that a rational, comprehensible system of credentialing needs to be established (Styles, 1990).

The ongoing debate about titling is directly related to the licensure issue in that prescriptive authority has traditionally been afforded only to nurse practitioners. As the scope of practice for other APNs such as clinical nurse specialists expands, prescriptive authority becomes an increasingly more important necessity to the role. Nurse practice acts are beginning to change to reflect the need for non–nurse-practitioner APNs, such as clinical nurse specialists, to obtain prescriptive authority without having to meet licensure requirements as a nurse practitioner in addition to those for clinical nurse specialist.

There is a growing interest among nurse educators in merging the roles of clinical nurse specialist and nurse practitioner. Titles found in the literature addressing the combined clinical nurse specialist/nurse practitioner role include *advanced nurse practitioner* (Calkin, 1984), *advanced registered nurse practitioner* (Sparacino, Cooper, & Minarik, 1990), and *advanced practice nurse* (Safriet, 1992). Supporters of a merger claim that many similarities already exist in the educational preparation and clinical roles and in the practice settings for both APNs, which are expanding and overlapping. Furthermore, supporters have suggested that professional unity would lead to greater power in activities with legislators, administrators, and consumers. Opponents of a merger assert that the scope of practice is quite different, graduate programs would need to be lengthened, and the legal entanglements outweigh the benefits of a merger (Soehren & Schumann, 1994). Full discussion of this issue is beyond the scope of this chapter.

Phase 4, second licensure for APNs, reflects the many internal and external forces acting on the nursing profession. The healthcare reform movement of the 1990s is forcing the nursing profession to increase professional accountability and to set national practice standards, particularly at the advanced practice level. Changes in state nurse practice acts, including advanced practice licensure, represent responses by the profession to an increasing public demand for comprehensive, quality healthcare.

CERTIFICATION

Certification is a process by which a nongovernmental agency or association attests that an individual licensed to practice a profession has met certain predetermined standards specified by that profession. In response to a proliferation of specialties in nursing and a growing emphasis on quality care in the health professions, the ANA initiated a national certification program in 1974 to recognize excellence in nursing practice. The certification process was voluntary, and initially 191 nurses were certified. In 1978, the purpose of the certification process had expanded to include assurance of quality beyond basic registered nurse licensure, identification of nurses who may be eligible for direct reimbursement for services, and recognition of professional achievement and quality of practice (Hawkins & Thibodeau, 1993).

Ten generalist and specialty certification examinations were available in 1978. Three more specialty examinations were added in 1979. By 1993, more than 93,000 nurses had achieved ANA certification in 24 categories consisting of 21 clinical areas, two administrative areas, and one staff development area.

In 1980, the Nurses' Association of the American College of Obstetricians and Gynecologists assumed responsibility for certification of obstetric/gynecologic nurse practitioners, neonatal intensive care nurses, and inpatient obstetric nurses. In 1993, the name of the group was changed to National Certification Corporation for the Obstetric, Gynecologic, and Neonatal Nursing Specialties, and five other area-related certification examinations were added.

Although the ANA served as a leader in the development of national certification examinations for nurses, several professional organizations or associations offer APN certification processes. For example, the American College of Nurse Midwives certifies nurse-midwives, the American Association of Nurse Anesthetists certifies nurse anesthetists, and the National Certification Board of Pediatric Nurse Practitioners and Nurses certifies pediatric nurse practitioners. In 1993, the American Academy of Nurse Practitioners (AANP) began to offer national certification examinations for family and adult nurse practitioners. See Tables 12-2, 12-

---

TABLE 12-2 **ANA Certification**

Specialty areas

Nurse practitioner:	*Clinical specialist*:
Adult	Medical surgical nursing
Family	Gerontologic nursing
School	Community health nursing
Pediatric	Adult psychiatric and mental health nursing
Gerontologic	Child adolescent psychiatric and mental health nursing

Eligibility requirement

Contact agency for details; most exams require an active RN license, a master's degree or higher in nursing, formal academic preparation in specialty area, and a minimum number of specialty-specific clinical practice hours

Exam date(s)

Every October and every other June (in conjunction with ANA biennial convention)

Application date(s)

Usually April preceding October exam
Usually March preceding June exam

Cost (1994 rates)

Application fee:	$30 (member),	$60 (nonmember)
Exam fee:	$90 (member),	$200 (nonmember)
Certificate fee:	$18 (member),	$18 (nonmember)

Credential

RN: CS (registered nurse, certified specialist)

More information

Marketing Services
American Nurses Credentialing Center
P.O. Box 2244
Waldorf, MD 20602
(800-284-CERT)

TABLE 12-3 AANP Certification

Specialty areas

Family nurse practitioner

Adult nurse practitioner

Eligibility requirements

Contact agency for details; generally require completion of a master's level family or adult nurse practitioner program; American Nurses' Credentialing Center–certified family nurse practitioners or adult nurse practitioners eligible to apply for reciprocity without examination

Exam date(s)

Usually November and June (in conjunction with AANP annual conference)

Application date(s)

Usually July preceding November exam

Usually February preceding June exam

Cost (1994 rates)

Examination:	$185 (member),	$270 (nonmember)
Renewal:	$95 (member),	$195 (nonmember)
Reciprocity:	$95 (member),	$195 (nonmember)

Credential

NP–C (nurse practitioner–certified)

More information

American Academy of Nurse Practitioners
Capitol Station, LBJ Building
P.O. Box 12846
Austin, TX 78711
(512-442-4262)

3, and 12-4 for detailed information on select certification processes for APNs. A number of certification review courses and guidebooks are available. Information can be obtained by contacting either the specialty organization or Health Leadership Associates, Potomac, Maryland (301-983-2405).

Certification of APNs serves to protect the public by assuring that an individual titled as an APN has mastered a certain body of knowledge and acquired a particular set of specialized skills. Specialists are expected to have expert competence, and certification serves as one means to verify the knowledge and skills of nurses who claim competence at a certain level. Certification of nursing specialists represents a judgment made by the nursing profession about an individual's credentials. Many nurses are certified in more than one area.

Because several specialty groups offer certification, much variability exists in the certification processes. In the past, attempts to standardize certification processes have not been successful for several reasons, one being the intense concern of specialty organizations to maintain control of their specialty practice. For example, in the late 1970s, following 3 years of extensive study, an ANA committee on credentialing recommended that a separate national credentialing center be established (Hawkins & Thibodeau, 1993). The intent was to have one national credentialing center that would be responsible for certification for all nursing specialty groups. Although a national center was never established, the ANA did establish its own

TABLE 12-4   **National Certification Board of Pediatric Nurse Practitioners/Nurses**

Specialty area

Pediatric nurse practitioner

Eligibility requirements

Contact agency for details; current licensure as an RN, completion of a pediatric nurse practitioner program approved by the National certification Board of Pediatric Nurse Practitioners/Nurses, a master's degree in nursing or completion of a post-master's pediatric nurse practitioner program approved by the National certification Board of Pediatric Nurse Practitioners/Nurses

Exam date

Every October

Application date

Usually July preceding October exam

Cost (1994 rates)

$300

Credential

CPNP (certified pediatric nurse practitioner)

More information

National Certification Board of Pediatric Nurse Practitioners/Nurses
416 Hungerford Drive
Suite 222
Rockville, MD 20850-4127
(301-340-8213)

---

credentialing center, which now offers 24 certification exams for nurses. Two other national nursing organizations that are also intensely concerned about certification include the National Federation of Specialty Nursing Organizations and the Nursing Organization Liaison Forum.

Specialty designation and national certification also play a central role in both state licensure and in reimbursement for specialty nursing services. Several states now require national specialty certification as a requirement for APN licensure. Furthermore, Medicaid reimburses only certified family and pediatric nurse practitioners for their services. These activities mandate that professional organizations address the certification issue. What does certification mean in the 1990s? Should certification be linked to professional licensure or third-party reimbursement? Who should set the standards for certification?

Regarding the growing need for appropriate credentialing of acute-care nurse practitioners, some nursing leaders apparently believe that the available specialty certification examinations for nurse practitioners are inappropriate for these specialists because the examinations are based on nationally recognized standards of nursing practice for primary care. Yet several states require national certification for licensure as an APN. Efforts are underway at the national level to address this need through planned meetings involving representatives of the ANA Credentialing Center, the NCSBN, and various nationally renowned nurse practitioner and clinical nurse specialist faculty. A major focus of the discussions involves the difficulty in making a clear distinction between acute care and primary care relative to advanced nursing practice. The potential effect of these discussions and decisions on advanced practice nursing education is tremendous.

A recent trend involves the requirement by individual states of state-specific certification for APN licensure. Currently, three states (California, Florida, and New York) require state certification for APN licensure (Pearson, 1995). In addition to providing documentation of formal educational preparation as an APN, applicants must also meet other statutory requirements such as written protocols or supervisory agreements with a physician. The state certification may or may not be designated on the license. Some states recognize national certification in lieu of state certification.

CREDENTIALING

Credentialing refers to the validation of required education, licensure, and certification. Credentialing of APNs is necessary not only to assure the public of safe healthcare provided by qualified individuals but also to assure compliance with federal and state laws relating to nursing practice. Legal regulation provides clear authority for qualified APNs to provide advanced nursing care including certain aspects of healthcare such as diagnosing and prescribing. Credentialing acknowledges the APN's advanced scope of practice. Credentialing mandates accountability. Individual APNs must be held accountable for the quality of healthcare they provide as well as their continued professional growth. Credentialing systems must be accountable to the public by providing appropriate avenues for public or individual practice complaints. Credentialing allows the profession to be accountable to the public and its members by enforcing professional standards for practice.

A number of disturbing problems are evident in the nursing profession's current credentialing system for advanced practice nursing. Because the requirements for the various certification examinations vary widely, the term *certification* lacks uniform meaning (Hawkins & Thibodeau, 1993). In some states, the scope of advanced practice nursing is so severely restricted that the financial cost and time investment to become appropriately credentialed outweigh the benefits. This is particularly true if the employment situation also fails to recognize the significance of credentialing.

Currently, the issue of titling or name designation is also somewhat controversial. To most nurses, the particular advanced practice designation seems to signify certain professional accomplishments and some political advantages or disadvantages. In this era of healthcare reform, both legislators and the public are confused by nursing's many titles. What exactly is a *nurse practitioner,* or a *clinical nurse specialist,* or a *certified specialist?* Clarification through simplification of the APN title will foster professional unity and ultimately facilitate and cement the APN role in healthcare reform.

CONCLUSION

The healthcare reform movement of the 1990s has provided nursing with an opportunity to reevaluate the regulatory aspects of the APN role. At the state level, there seems to be an increasing trend toward more physician involvement in regulation of advanced practice nursing. Many states require joint regulation of APNs by the board of nursing and the board of medicine. Many require restrictive controls such as protocols or detailed written practice agreements between the APN and physician. Yet other states legally acknowledge the professional contribution of the APN to healthcare through regulation by the board of nursing only. There is also a trend to specify in state statutes that a master's degree in nursing be the mandatory minimum educational requirement for the APN role and that national certification serve as a requirement for APN licensure.

On the national level, the most significant trend is toward standardization and uniformity. APN licensure is being proposed as the most effective method of self-regulation. It is postulated that second licensure will facilitate mobility among states and increase professional accountability. Current trends also include use of national certification as a credentialing mechanism rather than as a voluntary measure of competence. Nationally there is a growing need to set practice standards and monitor APN educational programs relative to these standards. It is definitely an exciting yet challenging time to be an APN.

References

Bullough, B. (1976). Influence on role expansion. *American Journal of Nursing, 76,* 1476–1481.

Calkin, J. D. (1984). A model for advanced nursing practice. *Journal of Nursing Administration, 14*(1), 24–30.

Hardy Havens, D. (1992). Licensure for advanced practice: Be informed, be alert. *Pediatric Nursing, 18,* 540.

Hawkins, J. W., & Thibodeau, J. A. (1993). *The advanced practitioner: Current practice issues* (3rd ed.). New York: Tiresias Press.

Kelly, L. Y. (1974). Nursing practice acts. *American Journal of Nursing, 74,* 1310–1319.

National Council of State Boards of Nursing. (1982). *The model nursing practice act.* Chicago: Author.

National Council of State Boards of Nursing. (1992, May). *National Council of State Boards of Nursing position paper on the licensure of advanced nursing practice.* Chicago: Author.

National Council of State Boards of Nursing. (1993, July). *Advanced nursing practice* [fact sheet]. Chicago: Author.

Pearson, L. J. (1995). Annual update of how each state stands on legislative issues affecting advanced nursing practice. *Nurse Practitioner, 20*(1), 13–51.

Safriet, B. J. (1992). Health care dollars and regulatory sense: The role of advanced practice nursing. *Yale Journal on Regulation, 9*(2), 117–187.

Soehren, P. M., & Schumann, L. L. (1994). Enhanced role opportunities available to the CNS/nurse practitioner. *Clinical Nurse Specialist, 8*(3), 123–127.

Sparacino, P.S.A., Cooper, D. M., & Minarik, P. A. (1990). *The clinical nurse specialist: Implementation and impact.* Norwalk, CT: Appleton-Lange.

Styles, M. M. (1990). Nurse practitioners creating new horizons for the 1990s. *Nurse Practitioner, 15*(2), 48–57.

13

Economics and Healthcare Financing

Peter I. Buerhaus

Over the course of the 1980s and early 1990s, the convergence of certain economic forces has stimulated the development of price competition among healthcare providers in a growing number of areas of the country. These same forces have substantially influenced the content of healthcare reform proposals developed thus far, and will continue to shape the political and ideological dynamics that ultimately will decide the outcome of the drawn-out national debate over health system reform. The economic forces that have stimulated the development of market competition in healthcare have built up enough momentum so that the nature and direction of fundamental change in the economic incentives that guide the organization and delivery of healthcare services are already established. The changes underway are likely to continue in the same direction, regardless of whether health reform proposals are implemented incrementally or all at once and even if it turns out that no substantive health reform legislation is enacted during the Clinton administration. Although the "details" and timing of healthcare reform certainly matter, they are likely to matter far less than the competitive forces that are fueling the growth of managed care and the beginning formation of integrated healthcare systems. The evolution of price competition and growth of managed care are transforming the way society receives healthcare services, defining new roles for providers, reshaping the attitudes of leaders of healthcare organizations, and changing policymakers' notions about the delivery of healthcare in contemporary American society.

If advanced practice nurses (APNs) are to compete successfully in a price-competitive environment, then they must understand the forces that have led to its emergence, anticipate the expected consequences of price competition, and implement strategies to take advantage of the many opportunities it will create in the years ahead. Thus, this chapter begins by discussing the development and evolution of key forces that are expected to guide the future economic activity of the healthcare delivery system. The chapter also summarizes the economic concepts and relationships underpinning price competition and discusses the sources of costs that APNs in solo or independent group practice will have to consider carefully when making decisions on the price to charge for their services. Following this is an economic analysis

Hickey JV: ADVANCED PRACTICE NURSING: Changing Roles and Clinical Applications © 1996 Lippincott–Raven Publishers

showing how APNs' pricing decisions can positively affect their own capacity to thrive, as well as the expected economic effects of their practice on physicians and consumers. The chapter concludes by identifying and discussing opportunities and challenges that APNs in prepaid capitated healthcare firms are expected to face.

ECONOMIC FORCES SHAPING HEALTHCARE

The dominant forces presently guiding the economic activity of the healthcare system emerged in the early 1980s and, as they evolved throughout the decade, steadily applied economic pressure on federal and state governments, hospitals, physicians, and insurers. These forces are expected to intensify during the remainder of the 1990s and exert even greater influence in the 21st century. Consequently, they will create many of the opportunities and challenges that APNs will face in the years ahead. To appreciate the significance of these forces and anticipate their expected consequences to APNs, their history and evolution are described.

Exploding Federal Budget Deficits

During the 1980s the federal government began to run up annual budget deficits in excess of $200 billion. As the amount of the national debt grew rapidly, a greater portion of the federal government budget each year was required to pay interest on the debt, which, in turn, reduced the amount of dollars available for other discretionary spending. At the same time that annual budget deficits were accumulating, however, the rate of escalation in federal government spending on healthcare was showing no sign of slowing down from the torrid pace experienced throughout the 1970s. Indeed, from 1966 to 1980, the federal government spent almost $2 trillion (in 1991 dollars) on healthcare, and during the 1980s, spent another $1.6 trillion. During the same periods, the states spent a total of $1 trillion and $1.4 trillion, respectively. Since the beginning of the Medicare and Medicaid programs in 1966, total public spending on healthcare increased 40-fold and reached approximately $400 billion in 1994 (Center for Health Economics Research, 1994).

As worrisome as the sustained high annual rate of increase in healthcare expenditures was becoming to many policymakers, nevertheless, it was an unpleasant shock when, during the latter half of the 1980s, the rate of annual increase in the national debt surpassed the rate of growth in federal healthcare spending (Prospective Payment Assessment Commission, 1991). More and more members of the media, financial community, and even politicians became alarmed at the potential negative effect of the combination of steadily growing federal budget deficits and healthcare spending on the future economic prosperity of the United States. Because the Executive Office is responsible for overseeing the administration of federal agencies and preparing the federal government budget, it is in the President's best political interests to limit spending and reduce budget deficits. Given the effect of federal healthcare spending on budget deficits, the Executive Office and Congress realized that, during the latter half of the 1980s, neither could consider health policy initiatives without carefully examining the effect on federal spending and the deficit. Budget policy was becoming the principal determinant of public policy with regard to healthcare. Moreover, the political difficulty associated with cutting spending on other entitlement programs, such as social security, meant that politicians had little choice but to target healthcare spending as a primary area for achieving significant future budget savings.

As long as sizable budget deficits continue in the 1990s, as is expected, APNs can anticipate that much of the federal government's effort to reform the healthcare system will be driven by its overriding interest in reducing budget deficits. Thus, to the extent that budget considerations cause healthcare policymakers to emphasize primary care and preventative health measures more seriously in an effort to help contain healthcare costs and reduce future government health expenditures, these budgetary pressures should create economic conditions that increase the demand for APN services.

Increasingly Tough Medicare Regulations To Contain Hospital Costs

The 1980s also saw the intensification of federal regulatory initiatives to control the rate of hospital cost increases and forestall the then impending bankruptcy of the Medicare Hospital Trust Fund. The major federal initiative was the introduction of a prospective payment system (PPS) based on inpatient diagnosis-related groups (DRGs) for acute care provided to Medicare beneficiaries. Although for a few years in the mid-1980s the annual growth rate in hospital Medicare-related inpatient operating costs slowed, costs began to increase in the latter part of the 1980s and, at the same time, Medicare lowered the amount of PPS payments to hospitals.

As a result of the subsequent shortfall between hospital operating costs and Medicare payments, and of technological advances, hospitals shifted more patient care to outpatient settings where payment rates were relatively better. Additionally, hospitals increased the price of services provided to patients covered by private health insurers and health maintenance organizations (HMOs)—a concept known as *cost shifting*. Consequently, these purchasers of hospital care reacted by increasing the prices they charged employers and consumers in the form of higher health insurance premiums. Thus, although Medicare payment policies certainly had a positive effect on lowering Medicare spending, they also played an important role in fueling the inflation of non–Medicare hospital operating costs, promoting cost shifting, and thereby helping to push up the price of health insurance premiums. Unfortunately, as premiums rose, the ability to purchase health insurance became increasingly out of reach for more Americans, which only aggravated problems related to access to healthcare.

Assuming that comprehensive healthcare reform is enacted, then depending on the outcome of the debate over how it will be financed—some proposals would finance reform by drastically reducing Medicare spending—Medicare expenditures for inpatient hospital care could be ratcheted down even further during the remaining years of the 1990s. Moreover, by the end of the 1990s, the Medicare program is expected to implement a PPS for beneficiaries receiving care in both outpatient facilities and ambulatory care settings. Once these payment systems are fully implemented (along with new physician fee schedules), the federal government will have established price controls on virtually all Medicare Part A and Part B spending. However, unlike the 1980s and early 1990s when the private sector allowed hospitals to shift a large portion of Medicare payment shortfalls onto them, the health insurance market has become more competitive and, therefore, insurers and HMOs are much less willing to absorb these costs and pass them along in the form of premium increases. Such behavior could quickly lead to an insurer's economic demise. Thus, it can be expected that hospitals will have to absorb Medicare shortfalls fully, which in turn will stimulate them to explore new ways to reduce their costs. To the extent that Medicare reduces payments to teaching hospitals for direct and indirect costs of graduate medical education, the size of hospital budgets will inevitably shrink and the financial stability of more hospitals will be threatened.

These changes will mean that APNs who practice predominantly in hospital-based settings can anticipate having fewer resources and making adjustments similar to those required of their inpatient nurse colleagues when diagnosis-related groups were implemented in the inpatient setting in the 1980s. However, as teaching hospitals respond to graduate medical education and PPS payment decreases, reduced capacity to shift costs, and deteriorating financial health, some are bound to reduce the number of interns and residents in their education programs. As a result, APNs employed in teaching hospitals may be increasingly used as substitutes for interns and residents, which could lead to further increases in demand for APNs. Such changes would present significant clinical opportunities and challenges, especially if the provision of more *medical* care is shifted onto them.

New Medicare Payment Policies Affecting Physicians

In 1996, the federal government is expected to complete the 4-year phase-in of its Resource-Based Relative Value Scales (RBRVS) payment system for physicians under Part B of the Medicare program. Although the program seems to be accomplishing one of its primary objectives—to transfer payments away from tests and procedures and apply them toward evaluation and management services—physicians are experiencing a number of dissatisfactions with the program. More important, the Physician Payment Review Commission (1994), which monitors the implementation of the fee schedule, has expressed strong concern that low Medicare RBRVS payments may negatively affect beneficiaries' access to physicians. Results from other studies (Cohen, 1993; Lee & Gillis, 1993) have shown that low Medicaid fees hamper access to office-based physicians and encourage use of hospital outpatient departments and emergency rooms, which only reinforce Physician Payment Review Commission concerns about the link between physician payments and decreased access to care. However, should federal budget deficit pressures result in prolonging inadequate RBRVS payments (approximately 75% of Medicare physician payments are financed using general tax dollars) and physicians respond by reducing the medical care provided to an increasing number of Medicare beneficiaries, then additional demand for APNs could develop. Advanced practice nurses may be called on to address access gaps and provide needed primary care, health education, preventative services, and management of chronic care conditions.

Private Sector Adoption of Government Cost-Containment Efforts

As a major buyer of healthcare services, federal and state governments exercise significant monopsony power over providers. Thus, it is not surprising that, as the size of state Medicaid populations grew rapidly and expenditures on healthcare escalated strikingly during the 1980s, more states began to adopt PPSs to pay for hospital and physician care. As these payment systems developed, however, payment shortfalls to providers increased. Indeed, Schramm (1994) estimated the size of Medicare and Medicaid payment shortfalls during the 1980s at $135 billion for physicians and $100 billion for hospitals. But, as physicians and hospitals shifted public sector payment shortfalls onto private sector payers, especially charge-based payers, insurers began to counter this development by embracing government payment policies and implementing other actions to pressure providers to lower their costs.

Moreover, in recent years, insurance companies have encountered much negative publicity and even the threat of a single-payer health reform proposal that, if enacted, would eliminate the insurance industry altogether. These public pressures have added to insurers' motivation to adopt more stringent payment policies and act vigorously to force hospitals and HMOs to lower their costs. Unlike federal and state policies that pertain to Medicare (the aged population) and Medicaid (the poor population), the actions of private insurers are directed at the rest of the population younger than age 65 years who have insurance. The net effect is to reinforce price control payment policies imposed by federal and state governments.

These changes suggest that HMOs, hospitals, and physicians will experience steadily rising economic pressures as more insurance companies and self-insured businesses exert their purchasing power and develop other programs to lower healthcare expenditures. In turn, providers will have to take further actions to lower their costs, especially as opportunities to shift costs all but disappear. However, to the extent that APNs are perceived as lower cost substitutes for much of the care that generalist physicians and medical interns and residents can provide, these economic pressures on traditional providers should result in further increases in the demand for services provided by APNs.

Expanded Health Services Research

In the latter part of the 1980s, the National Center for Health Services Research was revitalized and transformed into the Agency for Health Care Policy and Research (AHCPR). Subsequently, the agency launched a multifaceted intramural and extramural research agenda. This agenda included the development and dissemination of practice guidelines for treating various medical conditions and numerous large-scale studies to determine the appropriateness and cost-effectiveness of medical procedures and interventions and to investigate issues related to health education, prevention, assessment, quality of healthcare, and primary care.

In the future, the outcomes of the agency's research agenda and its work on guidelines are expected to play an increasingly important role in determining federal government policies regarding the procedures for which it will pay. Moreover, the agency will be heavily involved in developing the indicators that will be monitored as part of a quality assessment and reporting process that is anticipated to be included in national healthcare reform. Therefore, in the years ahead, federally funded researchers will devote far more attention to determining the impact of APNs on patient outcomes, quality and cost of care, effectiveness and appropriateness of inpatient and outpatient health services, increased access to healthcare, development of financing models, and impact of guidelines. Researchers will also be interested in exploring the degree to which and the circumstances in which APNs can substitute for physicians.

Other Precursors to Economic Competition

At the beginning of the 1980s, several private and public sector initiatives sprang forth and acted both independently and together to stimulate the beginning of economic competition among hospitals and physicians. The first of these initiatives occurred as a result of several events: American businesses were struck by double-digit inflation during the Carter administration, followed by a sharp economic recession during the Reagan administration, and during both of these jolts, the volume of lower priced imported goods rose substantially as did competition from Japan and other countries. For the first time, many American businesses became aware of and concerned about the effects of steadily rising healthcare premiums, which were increasing the costs of labor. In turn, many employers started to fear that, if left unchecked, rising healthcare costs could thwart the ability to price their products competitively in a global market. Thus, some companies began to form business coalitions or collect data; others actively tried to reduce costly inpatient hospital stays by beginning programs that mandated prehospital testing and screening, starting utilization review, requiring second opinions for surgical procedures, and pressuring insurance companies to cover the provision of less costly outpatient settings. Even before Medicare implemented diagnosis-related groups, these private sector actions were causing a decline in hospital occupancy rates and number of admissions (Feldstein, 1993).

Another precursor of competition in healthcare was the increasing realization that the various federal and state regulatory efforts developed in the 1970s to constrain healthcare expenditures had failed to contain costs. These efforts included certificate of need, voluntary and state health systems planning, professional standards peer review, hospital rate setting, and other programs that were part of numerous health systems, planning laws. As a result, many policymakers and academicians began to question the reliance on a predominantly regulatory-driven policy to constrain healthcare costs, and health planning legislation was significantly scaled back during the 1980s.

Furthermore, despite the strong opposition by organized medicine, several state and Supreme Court rulings decided that antitrust laws applied to healthcare, thereby removing real and perceived legal barriers to economic competition. Another precursor to the development of competition was the substantial excess in hospital capacity (ie, too many unfilled beds, which regulations failed to remove) and the rising supply of physicians. In addition, the

Medicare program became a more prudent buyer of healthcare by replacing its inflationary, cost-based reimbursement system with a PPS based on diagnosis-related groups.

Over time, the cumulation of these and other developments resulted in a surge in the growth rate of Americans enrolled in HMOs and the onset of what has become known as managed care. By the late 1980s, some observers of the healthcare market and many actual participants were beginning to talk about the spread of competition in healthcare.

Development of Price Competition in the 1990s

Although the development of economic competition in healthcare and implications for nurses and APNs are discussed in detail elsewhere (Buerhaus, 1992, 1994a, 1994b, 1994c), this chapter clarifies the meaning of competition in an economic sense. This is best explained by contrasting price competition with nonprice competition. *Nonprice competition* refers to activities such as those that hospitals have undertaken to attract physicians to join their medical staffs, thereby expanding hospital access to patients and keeping beds occupied. To compete for physicians, hospitals have paid off physician loans, provided rent-free office buildings, built new facilities, added services, and acquired the latest technology for physician use, even though, in many cases, these efforts were duplicative, usually very expensive, marginally effective, and underused. But these forms of nonprice competition are not what is meant by competition in the sense that economists use the term.

To an economist, *economic competition* is based on the price and quality of the products and services that are sold in the marketplace; most of the nation's economic activity is organized around economic competition. By competing on the basis of price, firms (suppliers) are given incentives to produce products using the least costly combination of labor and capital (buildings and equipment). By keeping production costs low, a firm can price its products below or roughly equal to the price of similar products offered by rival firms and thus sell more and earn higher profits. If the firm fails to keep its production costs low, then it will be unable to price its products competitively, with the result that it will sell less, have to make adjustments in its production processes, switch to producing a different product, or go out of business. Because firms in competitive industries face such harsh and impersonal incentives, society's resources, for the most part, are used in the best possible way. If some firms use methods of production that are too costly and wasteful, then their price will be too high and they will go out of business, thereby freeing up resources that can be used more efficiently by other producers.

Because purchasers (demanders) consider the quality of the products and services they buy, in addition to the price they are charged, firms must keep a sharp focus on the quality of their products. If the firm should achieve a reputation for poor quality, then it will be unable to sell its products and services and, unless it makes changes, will ultimately go out of business. Thus, firms invest considerably in marketing activities in an effort to discover the needs of potential purchasers and the consumer's evaluation of the quality of their products. Additionally, firms place advertisements and undertake promotional activities aimed at pointing out the various qualitative attributes of their products, especially those that distinguish them from competitors. Successful firms combine such information with improvements and innovations in production processes so that they can keep costs low, quality high, and remain competitive in an environment characterized by rapid development of new technologies and constantly changing consumer tastes and preferences.

However, when thinking about these economic incentives in relation to the production and consumption of personal healthcare services, it is apparent that little economic competition has existed among providers on the basis of price or quality (with the exception of Minneapolis-St. Paul, southern California, San Francisco Bay Area, and perhaps a few others). For reasons described elsewhere (Buerhaus, 1994a), hospitals and physicians have resisted the development of price competition, and large employers and labor unions have knowingly—or in some cases unwittingly—retarded its development among healthcare providers. Certain government regulations demanded by those threatened by the development of economic competition have erected barriers to its development. However, with the cumulative effects of public and private sector forces that evolved over the 1980s, the development of economic competition in healthcare was inevitable. Most important, the managed competition approach to reforming the healthcare system articulated by Enthoven (1993; Enthoven & Kronick, 1989a, 1989b, 1991) raised the intellectual level of the debate over the virtues and drawbacks of price competition, focused the attention of policymakers and employers on the barriers to its development and how the barriers can be overcome, and offered practical solutions. These solutions included a defined, if not controversial, role for government and business to deal with the potentially negative outcomes of price competition (i.e., how to prevent adverse risk selection in which some HMOs would be saddled with a disproportionate share of more acutely ill people who consume more resources and thereby increase the average costs per enrollee relative to other HMOs). Consequently, many members of Congress and the Clinton administration adopted elements of managed competition in formulating proposals to reform the nation's healthcare system.

Thus, for organizations and professionals who provide healthcare services, Wall Street financiers and investors, federal and state governments, and essentially all who make their living by either buying or selling products or services in the healthcare industry (one-seventh of the nation's economy), the 1990s is becoming the decade in which providers will increasingly compete more on the basis of price and quality. These developments will be reinforced by the strengthening of existing federal and state Medicare and Medicaid payment regulations, promulgation of new regulations to fold in PPS payments covering outpatient and ambulatory care, persistent federal budget deficits that require large annual interest payments paid for by tax dollars, steady elimination of providers' capacity to shift costs, eradication of costly excess capacity, growing influence of scientifically obtained knowledge on outcomes and the quality of healthcare, and continued growth in the number of people enrolled in HMOs and other managed care firms. The healthcare system is evolving in ways that should enable society to obtain greater value (more per dollar) from the resources it allocates to healthcare. This transformation means that APNs and the nursing profession will constantly confront new opportunities and challenges. Advanced practice nurses will have to consider carefully how they price their services if they are to compete successfully and thrive in the future. The remaining sections of this chapter address the economic concepts that APNs should consider when contemplating their responses to increasingly cost-conscious healthcare purchasers who are demanding greater value for their dollar.

PRICING SERVICES PROVIDED BY ADVANCED PRACTICE NURSES

To an economist, the meaning of the term *price* is probably comparable in depth and breadth to what *health* means to nurses: both are so vital and fundamental to their respective disciplines yet neither will probably ever be adequately or fully explained. For example, at a global conceptual level, the price system can be thought of in terms of how it operates to enable a society's economic system to perform four basic tasks: allocate resources among competing uses, determine how to combine and process these resources in such a way as to produce the desired amount of goods and services, determine how the various goods and services that will be produced are distributed among society's members, and determine what provisions are required for future economic growth (Mansfield, 1982). Entire books, theoretical and applied courses, and even Nobel Prizes have been awarded to economists for their contributions to understanding how the price system works to influence the behavior of firms, individuals, and governments to accomplish these tasks. However, when considering the issues involved in determining the price of APN services, it is necessary to step down the ladder of abstraction and examine a number of concrete factors that influence this calculation. Even then, the issues involved are neither simple nor straightforward. After reviewing the determinants of the price of APNs, it then is possible to examine how APNs' pricing decisions will ultimately determine their chances of surviving and growing in a more price-competitive marketplace.

Factors Advanced Practice Nurses Must Consider When Determining Price of Services

As the economic environment of healthcare becomes increasingly price competitive and hence more open to APNs who have a comparative cost advantage over physicians, a significant number of APNs are likely to decide to practice independently or form group practice arrangements that may or may not collaborate with physicians or other health professionals. Advanced practice nurses might establish contracts with a large employer, HMO, or insurance company to provide a defined set of health services. Alternatively, other APNs may become employees of managed care firms, but because these entities receive prepaid capitated payments, APNs will not have to make pricing-related decisions. This does not mean that APNs will be exempt from competitive risks—quite the opposite. However, these threats will be considered later; the discussion that follows is confined to the sources of costs that APNs in independent practice must consider in setting their prices.

Costs of Producing Services

Advanced practice nurses need to estimate the costs associated with overhead (e.g., rent, maintenance, utilities, office equipment, and insurance for fire, theft, and accidents); malpractice insurance; personal health insurance; the number of employees required and their wages; employee benefits; special equipment or supplies; individual and practice licenses and other fees; payment of principal and interest on loans; and other expenses or financial obligations. Advanced practice nurses must also decide the amount to reserve for contingency or emergency expenditures and determine whether there will be any bonus or incentive pay to employees or to other members of the practice. For the practice to be profitable, the total costs of the practice must be exceeded by the revenues that are generated by providing services.

Unit of Service

Advanced practice nurses will need to decide if they are going to price each service separately or bundle services together and price them as a package. Undoubtedly, payers' payment policies will influence this decision. If an APN firm anticipates providing care to consumers who pay out of pocket, then it will have to determine the costs of administration and bookkeeping that are involved in the billing and collection for individual versus bundled services, and compare these costs to the revenues that can be realistically received by either method.

Market Demand Characteristics

Advanced practice nurses need to understand the characteristics of the market (i.e., know what clinically related services are needed by whom and by how many people). Advanced practice nurses should analyze the geographical area where they intend to practice by determining the number of potential consumers, their healthcare needs, age and income distribution, and other community- and individual-level health deficits that they can address. The objective of such an analysis is to determine if there are enough people with the type of health problems, incomes, and health insurance that pays for APN services such that it is economically feasible for people to purchase appropriate care from APNs.

Structural Barriers

Advanced practice nurses must also ascertain if there are any structural barriers to their practice. These barriers could take the form of state practice acts that restrict APNs from performing certain activities that would be critical to the economic and clinical vitality of the practice or regulations or city codes that directly or indirectly raise the costs of the practice. Other barriers might include whether physicians are available who will collaborate with APNs and the existence of any social or culturally based customs or practices that might cause people to be unwilling to purchase care from APNs, regardless of economic circumstances. If barriers exist, then APNs must decide if the barriers can be removed and how much removal will cost in terms of time, effort, and dollars.

Presence of Competitors

It is essential that APNs understand who their competitors are, how many exist, where they are located, what services they offer, how much they charge, and how they are paid. Information on each of these points will tell APNs a great deal about what other providers have found seems to work (or not work), thereby sparing the APN practice from making time-consuming and costly mistakes. Knowing as much about the competition will also make it possible for APNs to determine how they can fill gaps in service, take advantage of market niches, and how they might do things differently and less costly.

Payment Amounts

Advanced practice nurses need to know who will pay for their services. If most of the likely consumers are covered through private or employer-provided insurance, it is essential to know whether insurers will pay for services provided by APNs, what services, how much, and how soon after submitting their bills they can expect to receive payment. However, if many people in the practice area are enrolled in HMOs, then APNs can expect that most will be unwilling to become clients because of the out-of-plan charges subscribers must pay. In that case, it would be wise to attempt to negotiate arrangements with each HMO to see if APNs can contract for certain services.

If the practice is locating in an underserved or low-income area, APNs need to understand the means by which providers are customarily paid for their services. Payment could involve accepting Medicaid payments that are less than the costs of providing services, small amounts of out-of-pocket cash, or in-kind services (e.g., snow shoveling, lawn care, maintenance, and so on) in exchange for healthcare services. An APN firm must decide the amount of uncompensated care it can provide, determine if cost shifting opportunities are available, and be aware of the amount of in-kind payments it can accept without harming the firm financially. Advanced practice nurses should also investigate opportunities through state, county, city, or private philanthropic organizations for grants and donations to help pay for care provided in underserved areas.

Advertising

For APNs to break into the market successfully and attract new clients, especially if there are existing provider–client relationships, advertising will be essential to inform potential consumers that APN services are available, where the office is located, and how much services cost. Information on the qualifications of practice members together with descriptions of the unique services, philosophy on health, and other attributes that can distinguish the firm from its competitors should be part of initial promotion efforts.

Undoubtedly, there are other sources of costs that need to be considered beyond those already identified. However, APNs must realize that the importance of many of these costs will change over time and will vary with an APN's practice pattern or location of the group or solo practice (e.g., rural, metropolitan, or inner city). Some of the costs could exert a great bearing at certain times. For example, if the price of malpractice insurance increases, an APN firm might have to consider raising prices, whereas other practice-related costs at different times may have little influence on the price charged. Unfortunately, there is no exact formula or precise way to calculate the price to charge for APN services; this is a complex decision that, in addition to the preceding information, involves a fair amount of guesswork and intuition, a strong set of nerves, and trial and error. Ultimately, however, the value that consumers attach to the service of APNs will indicate how much they are willing to pay. If they perceive that APN services are valuable, consumers will be more willing to pay a higher price and vice versa. To add further complexity, consumer preferences are constantly changing as well as their willingness to pay for APN services.

The bottom line is that, if APNs in either solo or group practice arrangements are to survive in a competitive market, then they will have to be alert, seek ways to innovate and keep their costs as low as possible, and be willing to make frequent adjustments to the quality of their services and how they price and market them. Although it is virtually impossible to specify the exact price that APNs should charge for their services, it is possible to recommend that APNs initially set their prices below the prevailing market price of services provided by physicians or their nearest competitor. Why this is so is explained next.

Economic Consequences of Advanced Practice Nurse Pricing Decisions

This section concentrates on the potential economic consequences of the pricing decisions of an APN group practice, including the anticipated effects on physicians and consumers. However, to explain these consequences adequately, it is necessary first to discuss the key economic terms and concepts that underpin the relationship between price and the firm's demand, amount of total revenues, profitability, and economic responses by physicians or consumers.

Price, Quantity Demanded and Sold, Total Revenue, and Price Elasticity of Demand

The total revenue (amount of dollars) that is earned by the APN practice is simply the product of the quantity of services sold multiplied by the price of each service. The quantity of services could be measured by the number of visits, billable procedures or treatments, number of minutes, or whatever unit of service the firm decides. Figure 13-1 shows the price of services on the *y*-axis and the quantity of services sold on the *x*-axis. Holding other things constant (e.g., consumers' incomes, prices of other services and goods, and so on), the relationship between the quantity sold and price is shown by a downward sloping line (D), which is the demand curve for the particular service provided by the APN firm. For example, at $50 per service, the firm could sell 20 units and generate revenue equal to $1000 ($50 × 20). Notice that as the price falls, to say $20, the practice can sell more services (35 units) and total revenue falls to $700 ($20 × 35). The firm's profitability is determined by calculating total revenues and subtracting total costs; what is left over is profit (or loss).

A critically important determinant of the amount of revenue obtained is the degree to which changes in the quantity of services sold are sensitive to changes in their price. Economists use the term *price elasticity of demand* to refer to the sensitivity or responsiveness in this relationship. For some goods or services, a small change in price will result in a large change in the quantity sold, whereas for other goods or services, a small change in price results in hardly any change in the quantity sold.

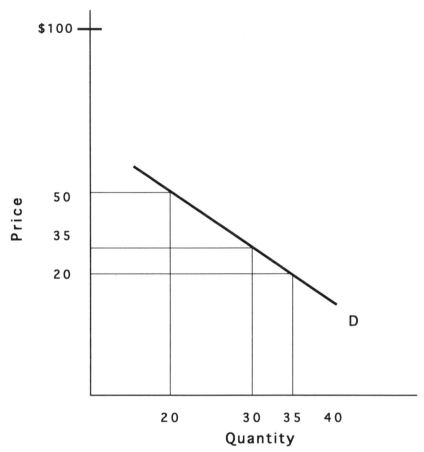

FIGURE 13-1 Price and quantity changes (D = demand).

The underlying relationship between quantity sold and price changes and the resultant effect on total revenues is illustrated in Figure 13-2. Once again, the price of the APN service is shown on the *y*-axis and the quantity sold is depicted along the *x*-axis. In Figure 13-2(a), notice that when the price is $35, the number of units sold is 30, and the corresponding revenue equals $1050. However, when the price increases to $40, the quantity sold decreases to 27, but note that revenue increases to $1080. Now consider Figure 13-2(b), which also shows that when the price is $35, 30 units are sold and total revenue is $1050. However, when the price is increased to $40, the amount sold decreases considerably, to only 10 units, and total revenue falls to $400. It should be clear that the same $5 increase in price, from $35 to $40 in Figure 13-2(a) and (b), results in vastly different decreases in the amount of the quantities sold and hence in the total revenue obtained ($1080 compared with $400).

These results should make clear that the sensitivity in the relationship between quantity sold and price—the price elasticity of demand—is a monumentally important determinant of the amount of the firm's total revenue and hence profitability. Graphically, when the relationship between quantity sold and price is like that depicted in the steeply sloped demand curve of Figure 13-2(a), the demand for the product or service is referred to as *inelastic*, which means that relationship is not very sensitive. The less steeply sloped demand curve shown in Figure 13-2(b) shows a much more responsive relationship between quantity and changes in price, and is referred to as an *elastic* demand curve. Because the degree of sensitivity in the

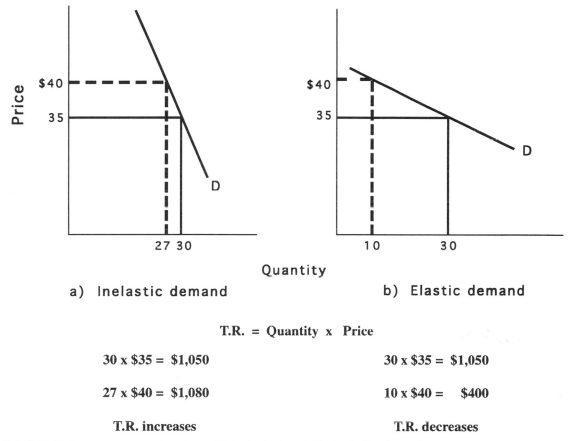

a) **Inelastic demand**   b) **Elastic demand**

T.R. = Quantity x Price

30 x $35 = $1,050   30 x $35 = $1,050

27 x $40 = $1,080   10 x $40 = $400

T.R. increases   **T.R. decreases**

FIGURE 13-2 Total revenue when demand is (a) inelastic and (b) elastic (D= demand).

relationship between quantity and price is a critically important determinant of total revenue, and hence the firm's profitability, it is important to consider what influences the underlying relationship to be sensitive or not very sensitive (or in economic terms, whether demand is elastic or inelastic).

Determinants of the Price Elasticity of Demand

The sensitivity of the relationship between price and quantity sold depends on three factors. First, and foremost, is the *number* and *closeness* of substitutes. The greater the number of close substitutes that are available for a particular good or service, the more its demand (quantity sold) is likely to be sensitive to changes in price. For example, if the price of a certain brand of television were to increase substantially, an individual would have an economic incentive to purchase a television produced by a different manufacturer. In this case, the demand for a particular television is likely to be sensitive to changes in price, as would be depicted by the relatively elastic demand curve in Figure 13-2(b). However, if there are few substitutes available for a particular good or the substitutes are not very close, a producer can raise the price of the good, and even though this will normally lead to a decrease in quantity sold, total revenues will not decrease—see the inelastic demand curve in Figure 13-2(a). In healthcare, there are few close substitutes to physicians and, consequently, their inelastic demand curve is an important reason why physicians have been able to raise prices without experiencing a decrease in total revenues and net incomes.

Second, the price elasticity of demand also depends on the importance of the commodity in a consumer's budget. To illustrate, the demand for commodities such as thumbtacks, salt, or pepper is likely to be quite inelastic (i.e., not very sensitive). Thus, if the price of salt goes up, then the consumption of salt is unlikely to fall much, if at all. But if an individual is buying a major appliance or an automobile, which would have a much greater effect on the person's budget, then the selection and purchase of the automobile are much more likely to be sensitive to price.

The third determinant of the sensitivity in the relationship between the quantity sold and price changes is the length of time over which the commodity is demanded by consumers. The longer the period, the easier it becomes for consumers or firms to substitute one good for another. Over a long period (versus a shorter period), there are few commodities that do not have substitutes, and the longer the commodity is being produced and sold, the easier it becomes for firms to find ways to produce new substitute goods and people to learn how to make substitutions by themselves. For example, in healthcare, consider how magnetic resonance imaging has substituted for computerized tomography, which has substituted for x-rays. Likewise, consider that cardiac catheterization can be a substitute for certain types of cardiac surgery, and lithotripsy can be a substitute for surgery to remove kidney stones and gallstones.

Effect of Advanced Practice Nurse Pricing Decisions on Physicians and Consumers

Effect on Physicians

To understand how price, quantity sold, total revenue, and the price elasticity of demand will ultimately determine the ability of APNs to successfully compete in a truly competitive environment, suppose that a number of APNs develop a formal group practice, and after considering all of the determinants of price discussed earlier, conclude that it is economically feasible to charge a lower price than that charged by physicians in the market for the same or similar services. Charging a lower price would be an economically rational decision because the relationship between the price charged and the quantity of APN services sold is likely to be quite sensitive, or elastic (after all, consumers view physicians as close and available substitutes to APNs). Given these circumstances, consumers need an economic incentive to purchase care from APNs, which would be provided by APNs who are charging a lower price than physicians. Moreover, charging a lower price will have important economic effects on APNs, physicians, and consumers. Consider Figure 13-3, which shows the two providers, APNs and a medical group, in a market competing for patients.

Assume that P_1 in Figures 13-3(a) and (b) is the existing market price for physician services. Advanced practice nurses can provide identical or nearly equivalent services (any differences are not significant to patients) but decide to charge a lower price, P_2, in Figure 13-3(a). Notice that the demand curve for APNs is relatively elastic, which reflects the influence of primary care physicians as available, close, and well-known substitutes. Consequently, the relationship between the quantity sold and price of APN services is quite sensitive. However, the physician's demand curve (D_1) in Figure 13-3(b) is less elastic (more steeply sloped), which reflects the assumption that most people in the market are less familiar with APNs and may not view them as close substitutes.

The fact that APNs offer their services at lower prices (P_2) than their medical competitors (P_1) will result in stimulating initial demand for their services. Provided that APNs attract additional consumers at this price, obtain a favorable reputation, and knowledge of their availability spreads through word-of-mouth and by advertising, more services will be sold (Q_2) and

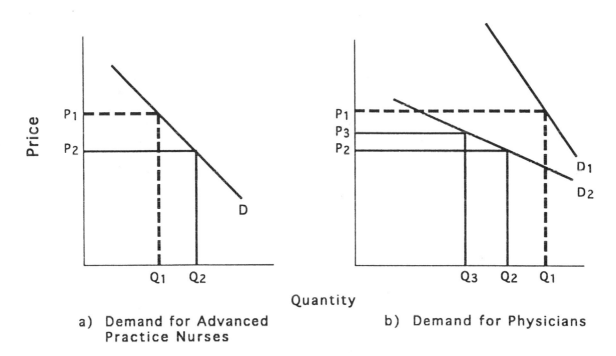

FIGURE 13-3 Effects of price change on demand for physicians (D = demand; P = price; Q = quantity).

APN revenues will expand to $P_2 \times Q_2$. If, however, APNs did not offer their services at a lower price, then they would not provide increasingly cost-conscious consumers or insurers an economic incentive to direct their subscribers to APNs, let alone give HMOs or large employers an incentive to selectively contract for a defined set of health services for their enrollees. Without consumers buying and payers purchasing APN services, the APN group will go out of business.

Assuming again that APNs initially charge a lower price (P_2) for the same or similar services that are offered by their competitors, this will create negative economic effects on physicians who are practicing in the same market. As more patients respond to the lower prices charged by APNs, the demand for physicians will fall (in microeconomics, this relationship between the change in price of one product and change in demand for another is referred to as a *positive cross-price elasticity of demand*). The reduction in demand for physician services is shown by the demand curve shifting inward and to the left (D_2). Notice that this decline in total demand is different from a change in the quantity demanded that results solely from a *price* change, in which case the movement in quantity sold would be along the stationary demand curve. The reduction in total demand to D_2 will exert two significant economic effects on physicians: (1) along the new demand curve, D_2, physicians will always sell less (see Q_2 or Q_3 in Fig. 13-3[b]), even if they lower their prices, compared with what they could have sold when demand was previously reflected by D_1, and (2) the reduction in quantity of services sold means that physicians' total revenues will be less, as will be net income.[1]

The presence of APNs in the market, and their use by consumers in response to lower prices, will exert an additional and important effect on the economic interests of physicians. Notice that not only does the demand curve shift inward and to the left (D_2), but the elasticity of the new demand curve increases, which means that there is greater sensitivity in the relationship between quantity demanded and price changes than what existed previously along D_1. As explained earlier with reference to Figure 13-2(*A*), physicians' relatively inelastic demand curve has long enabled them to increase the price of most services without diminishing total revenues (incidentally, to maximize total revenues, physicians in private practice have favored policies that would limit the supply of physicians or other competitors, thereby assuring that there would be an excess demand for their services). But as APNs become available and act as close substitutes for many of the services provided by physicians, physicians' comparatively inelastic demand curve will become more elastic. As demand becomes more elastic, physicians will find that if they increase their price to compensate for the loss in revenue, then they are likely to experience a substantial decrease in services sold and total revenues will decline even further. The lost revenues, however, will be gained by APNs as their lower prices attract patients who formerly purchased services from physicians.

From the perspective of physicians, the presence of close substitutes (APNs) in the market creates substantial negative changes in their economic position: demand is likely to increase, as will total revenues, and net income, and there will be greater sensitivity in the relationship between future quantity changes and price increases (i.e., physicians' demand curve would become more elastic). The expected *economic* response of physicians would be to lower their prices, increase advertising, and perhaps even improve the qualitative aspects of their medical practice. It is also conceivable that physicians might try predatory pricing, dropping their prices so low that APNs could not match the lower price and still remain in business. But because these changes would impose new costs to the medical practice, physicians perhaps would try less costly and more permanent solutions by trying to remove their competition by attempting to have the practice of APNs declared illegal; obtaining regulations that restrict the number or type of procedures and activities; blocking APNs from obtaining hospital admitting privileges (or removing them if they have them); boycotting insurance companies, HMOs, or other physicians who recognize or collaborate with APNs; or trying to influence payer policies toward APNs. Thus, as more APNs start group practice arrangements and the healthcare delivery system becomes more price competitive, APNs must anticipate these responses. Addressing these responses will take time and impose additional costs. For these and other reasons, it is essential that the antitrust provisions included in various health reform legislative proposals be modified specifically to include APNs and assure competition.

Effect on Consumers

With APNs successfully competing in the market, consumers benefit in at least three ways. First, the presence of APNs gives consumers new choices, and some are likely to find that they derive more satisfaction with the purchase of healthcare from APNs (e.g., consumers might find that APNs spend more time during visits, communicate better than physicians, and offer a different perspective about health). Second, consumers would be paying less for healthcare and hence have more of their income left to save, invest, or purchase other items that increase the satisfaction derived from using their money resources. Third, as the success (i.e., profitability) of more APNs provides an incentive for others to start independent practice

---

[1] When demand is strong, the practice is well established, and APNs are working close to full capacity, it would then be appropriate to consider increasing the price of their services.

arrangements, more price competition will develop and consequently the rate of future healthcare cost increases could be lower than would otherwise be the case.

The price of healthcare is likely to rise at a slower rate (even for patients seen by physicians), because if any one provider raises prices too much in a competitive market, then consumers, who can be expected to become more price sensitive as they steadily pay more out-of-pocket healthcare costs, are more likely to shop around and switch to a lower priced provider (assuming provider quality differences are not great). Such behavior would send a powerful and unmistakable message to all providers to keep their prices as low as possible. When summed over many providers and over time, the cumulative effect of price competition can be substantial, and the future rate of price increases is likely to be constrained.

ADVANCED PRACTICE NURSES IN PREPAID CAPITATED FIRMS

As much of the content of this chapter has attempted to convey, the forces that evolved in the 1980s and early 1990s and culminated in the development of price competition largely came about because it has become in the best economic interest of an increasing number of cost-conscious purchasers to obtain greater value for each dollar spent on healthcare. In the years ahead, APNs can expect that more of the clinical and economic forces that shape their practice and determine their personal income will be driven by impersonal and unambiguous incentives that govern price-competitive industries: providers and health professionals will be rewarded only to the extent that they keep their prices low and quality high.

The manifestation of a more competitive healthcare environment is expected to take the form of increasing enrollment in prepaid capitated healthcare firms, such as HMOs, and the formation of larger integrated systems. Their growth will be aided by continuing regulatory and market-based adjustments designed to ensure that providers compete fairly and on the basis of price and quality. The evolution of prepaid capitated firms, or the managed care industry, is a significant and positive development for APNs, whether they are employed by managed care firms or decide to compete independently as solo providers or in group practice arrangements. From the economic perspective of APNs, the major difference between practicing as an employee of an HMO or practicing independently is that, as an employee, the APN functions as an economic complement, whereas APNs in independent practice function largely as economic substitutes to an HMO or medical group practice. This section focuses on APNs as economic complements and briefly identifies some of the opportunities and challenges that many are likely to face as price competition develops among healthcare providers.

Advanced practice nurses are an economic complement if providing their services increases the productivity of the managed care firm and the profits of its owners. The complementary role is not unlike that of hospital-employed registered nurses, whose nursing practice functions to increase the productivity of physicians by allowing them both to treat inpatients and to maintain an office-based practice, thereby increasing physicians' revenues and net income. Because an HMO operates according to a prepaid capitated budget, it has an economic incentive to keep the total costs of providing healthcare as low as possible. In this way, any amount of unspent dollars can be retained as profit. Thus, HMOs have an economic interest to provide enrollees with more preventative care and health education so that they can reduce future consumption of HMO resources by treating fewer enrollees for preventable acute and chronic illness. Additionally, HMOs try to reduce admissions to costly hospitals, negotiate discounts on the purchase of pharmaceuticals and medical devices, and pursue other methods to reduce costs (including enrolling younger and more healthy people who are less likely to consume HMO resources and help lower overall costs).

A feature unique to HMOs is the use of primary care health professionals as gatekeepers. The economic objective of the gatekeeper is to ensure that the HMO uses its resources efficiently and hence keeps costs as low as possible. At the same time, gatekeepers must ensure that enrollees receive the appropriate kind and amount of healthcare, because if they do not, then HMO costs are likely to increase as treatable conditions and ailments worsen and eventually require additional resources. However, the gatekeeper, like other physicians and health professionals employed by the HMO, incurs costs that are associated with salary, benefits, and, in many cases, a year-end bonus or incentive pay. Because it has a strong economic incentive to keep its labor costs as low as possible, the HMO will want to find cheaper ways to fill gatekeeping roles and provide healthcare services.

Many of the clinical services that APNs provide can closely substitute for those provided by generalist physicians. But because APNs are less costly to an HMO in terms of salary and benefits requirements, they represent an economically attractive opportunity for an HMO to fill gatekeeping and other provider roles. As purchasers increasingly demand that HMOs lower the premiums charged per enrollee lest they induce their employees to enroll in a different and lower cost HMO, price competition among HMOs is expected to intensify significantly. Thus, HMOs will face even more pressure to keep their costs low, which should increase the demand for APNs even further. This does not mean, though, that APNs will totally replace generalist physicians, because physicians provide certain medical services that APNs cannot provide. The point is that the spread of price competition should materially increase HMO demand for APNs in the future. Moreover, because managed care firms will be increasingly motivated to keep their premiums competitively priced, it can be anticipated that they will develop new roles for APNs and experiment with delivery models that will be tailored extensively around APNs. The purpose would be to find new ways to lower costs while simultaneously increasing enrollees' satisfaction and attainment of desired clinical outcomes.

However, for at least two economic reasons, APNs must anticipate that primary care physicians and physician assistants will resist the increasing employment of APNs. First, as more APNs become available, the total supply of primary care health professionals will increase relative to the number of available managed care positions. Consequently, this will place downward pressure on the salaries that managed care firms are able to offer and still hire all the providers they want. As the supply of generalist physicians increases, specialty physicians become trained as primary care providers, and practicing medicine in managed care firms becomes increasingly acceptable to more members of the medical profession, additional physicians will be seeking employment in managed care firms and, therefore, competing for available positions with APNs who have a comparative cost advantage.

A second possible reason to expect physicians to resist the expansion of APNs in managed care is that many firms might adopt policies directing that APNs' caseloads comprise mostly the "less difficult cases." But by having to take care of the "difficult cases," primary care physicians may be unable to obtain appropriate outcomes or levels of patient satisfaction to qualify for a year-end bonus or incentive payments. Thus, APNs must understand that, although they present economic benefits to the owners of HMOs, they represent an increasingly visible economic threat to primary care and specialist physicians. For these reasons, it will be no surprise if organized medicine takes actions aimed at decreasing the supply of APNs in the same way, as mentioned earlier, that physicians may attempt to eliminate APNs in group practice from the marketplace to prevent price competition.

CONCLUSION

In contemplating the likelihood that the opportunities for APNs described in this chapter will actually materialize, it is important to reflect on the number and intensity of the economic forces discussed. These forces include effects of continuing federal budget deficits; the expansion of Medicare PPS to outpatient facilities and ambulatory settings; new and increasingly restrictive physician payment policies; the adoption of government regulatory efforts and other cost-containment innovations by the private sector; the growing resistance to cost shifting; effective use of purchasing power by more employers to stimulate price competition among managed care firms; and an invigorated health services research agenda.

These forces, together with the expectations raised over the healthcare reform debate, are compelling the development of true price competition in healthcare, serious and pervasive cost-control initiatives, and the beginnings of competition over quality and patient outcomes. As these forces grow, so too will the power and economic will to sweep away barriers that have existed in healthcare since the mid-1960s, barriers that have served all too well to protect the economic interests of traditional providers.

References

Buerhaus, P. I. (1992). Nursing, competition and quality. *Nursing Economic$, 10*(1), 21–29.

Buerhaus, P.I. (1994a). Economics of managed competition and consequences to nurses: Part I. *Nursing Economic$, 12*(1), 10–17.

Buerhaus, P.I. (1994b). Economics of managed competition and consequences to nurses: Part II. *Nursing Economic$, 12*(2), 75–80, 106.

Buerhaus, P.I. (1994c). Health care reform, managed competition, and critical issues facing nurses. *Nursing and Health Care, 15*(1), 22–26.

Center for Health Economics Research. (1994). *The nation's health care bill: Who bears the burden?* Waltham, MA: Author.

Cohen, J. W. (1993). Medicaid physician fees and use of physician and hospital services. *Inquiry, 30*(3), 281–292.

Enthoven, A. C. (1993). The history and principles of managed competition. *Health Affairs, 12* (Suppl. on Managed Competition: Health Reform American Style?), 24–48.

Enthoven, A. C., & Kronick, R. (1989a). A consumer choice health plan for the 1990s: Universal health insurance in a system designed to promote quality and economy. *New England Journal of Medicine, 320*(1), 29–37.

Enthoven, A. C., & Kronick, R. (1989b). A consumer choice health plan for the 1990s: Universal health insurance in a system designed to promote quality and economy. *New England Journal of Medicine, 320*(2), 94–101.

Enthoven, A. C., & Kronick, R. (1991). Universal health insurance through incentives reform. *JAMA, 265*(19), 2532–2536.

Feldstein, P. J. (1993). *Health care economics* (4th ed.). Albany, NY: Delmar Publishers.

Lee, D. W., & Gillis, K. D. (1993). Physician responses to Medicare physician payment reform: Preliminary results on access to care. *Inquiry, 30*(4), 417–428.

Mansfield, E. (1982). *Theory and applications* (4th ed.) New York: W.W. Norton.

Physician Payment Review Commission. (1994). *Physician Payment Review Commission annual report to Congress.* Washington, DC: Author.

Prospective Payment Assessment Commission. (1991) *Medicare and the American health care system. Report to the Congress.* Washington, DC: Author.

Schramm, C. J. (1994, May 24). What price controls wrought. *The Wall Street Journal*, p. A14.

14

Empowerment: Activism in Professional Practice

Colleen Conway-Welch

Nurses in today's constantly changing healthcare delivery system need to empower themselves, their registered nurse (RN) and non–RN staffs, and their patients by using nursing discipline–specific knowledge along with management knowledge to continuously improve work processes, the care system, and the nursing profession.

EMPOWERMENT DEFINED

Empowerment is a process aimed at changing the nature and distribution of power in a particular cultural context (Bookman & Morgan, 1988, p. 4). Empowerment enables people to recognize and feel their strengths, abilities, and personal power (Mason & Backer, et al., 1991, p. 6) through increased knowledge, control of practice, and command of resources (Nazarey, 1993, p. 7). Empowerment refers to "activities directed to increasing people's control over their lives" (Watson & Burkholder, 1990, p. 30).

The literature on nurses' acquisition and mobilization of power focuses on two general areas of concern. The first involves the concept of vertical, interpersonal power—defined as the influence one person has over another—and the ways in which individual power sources can be maximized. The second area of concern, which is the focus of this paper, is the need for changes in the nursing profession related to education, national organizations, knowledge, and socialization (Stuart, 1986).

For example, empowerment is compromised when the nursing profession weakens its power base by preparing too many nurses from too many educational levels (Diploma, ADN, BSN, MSN) to take the basic (N-CLEX) RN exam. As a result of the Flexner Report and medical licensing board policies, the number of physicians has been reduced substantially (Flexner, 1910). The nursing profession should consider the possible benefits of a similar strategy to reduce the number of nurses, along with the development of an organization to assess substitutability (of LPNs for RNs, diploma graduates for BSNs, and unlicensed personnel for LPNs or RNs) on the nursing subunit. Although this idea may be viewed as heresy by

Hickey JV: ADVANCED PRACTICE NURSING: Changing Roles and Clinical Applications © 1996 Lippincott–Raven Publishers

some, Stuart (1986) believed it warranted further study. Given the present climate of downsizing, nurse layoffs, and the paucity of jobs for newly graduated RNs without experience, it may be timely to revisit this issue. Credible data about downsizing and its effects on the nursing labor market are sorely needed.

EMPOWERMENT AND DATA-BASED DECISION MAKING

Data are absolutely essential to empowerment. Debates and arguments about nursing need to be based on data; without data and without a data set, the nursing profession will fail to resolve key issues and remain politically isolated from others, especially physicians and administrators, who have a stake in healthcare reform.

From a labor policy perspective, a national data bank of licensed RNs should be developed and maintained, and the data collected should be expanded to cover a wider range of current nursing policy issues. "Expansion of nursing into advanced areas of practice has stimulated a great deal of policy activity related to educational preparation, function and degree of independence of various nursing specialties" (Reichelt & Young, 1985, p. 167).

From a patient-care institutional perspective, nurse decision makers need accurate, timely, and retrievable information regarding 1) epidemiology and demography, referral patterns, and case mix of patients; 2) resource availability, allocation, and use; 3) performance measures, including output, outcome, quality, and patient feedback; 4) maintenance of staff skills; 5) monitoring and maintenance of morale; and 6) shaping and maintenance of a new organizational culture (Halloran, Sermens, & Barber, 1990, p. 24). There must also be an educational infrastructure that fosters skill development in these areas.

Discussion based on data allows systems, processes, and people to become more stable and predictable at all levels of communication. Stability and predictability are especially critical if one is attempting to influence a legislator or negotiate a raise. To understand the relationship between data and empowerment, it is essential that nursing educators and nursing administrators embrace a new body of knowledge—improvement knowledge—along with the traditional components of discipline-specific knowledge.

IMPROVEMENT KNOWLEDGE

Nurses educated only in discipline-specific knowledge will have difficulty seeing themselves as empowered to evaluate the systems within which they work and to improve processes that have gone amuck, since systems problems are rarely specific to nursing alone.

> Today a second body of knowledge [improvement knowledge] is available for use in the improvement of health care processes that enables us to use professional knowledge in a new way, to make more improvement of a different kind and faster than we have been able to do before—to engage in a continuing improvement of health care by adding improvement knowledge. (Batalden & Stoltz, 1993, p. 425)

What can be called "improvement knowledge," as opposed to discipline-specific or professional knowledge, includes four areas: systems theory, variation theories, psychological theories, and learning theories. W. Edwards Deming (1993) labeled these four areas of knowledge *systems of profound knowledge.* The combination of both professional and improvement knowledge will guide nurses on the journey to empowerment (Fig. 14-1).

Combining professional knowledge with improvement knowledge by collecting data and analyzing trends, predicting the impact of those trends, planning and preparing for the impact, identifying strategies to implement and assess progress, and then feeding this information into a feedback loop will empower nurses in practice (Batalden & Stoltz, 1993, p. 426). In addition, the quality of products (e.g., patient care, nursing education, and so forth) will become

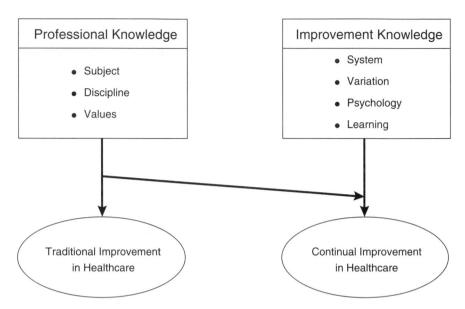

FIGURE 14-1 Traditional and continual improvement.

more consistent, and systems and processes will become more stable and predictable (Covey, 1991, p. 268).

To survive in a reengineered healthcare system, it is essential that nurses have not only professional, discipline-specific knowledge but also

- an understanding of the four areas of knowledge that will fuel their commitment to a program of continuous improvement in health service delivery
- the skills to apply improvement knowledge
- the ability to integrate the work of health professionals to meet individual and community health needs
- a professional ethic that supports such integrated work

To produce empowered nurses who can make major contributions to a reformed healthcare delivery system, the educational curriculum must devote more attention to the four areas necessary to build the improvement knowledge base. It is useful to examine the four areas of improvement knowledge and envision a curriculum that incorporates them without neglecting the professional, discipline-specific knowledge of nursing.[1]

Systems Theory

Empowered nurses can step back and look at a problem from a systems perspective—they are systems thinkers. They view the organization as a system of production—a group of interdependent people, items, processes, products, and services. This perspective is enhanced when the nurse asks, "How do we produce what we produce? Why do we produce what we produce? How do we improve what we produce?" Knowledge of systems helps nurses view healthcare reform as part of a broader economic issue and makes them much less tolerant of attempts to maintain the status quo (e.g., supporting a fixed RN/bed ratio).

---

[1] This chapter does not reconstruct the extensive details of Deming's (1993) proposal; rather, interested readers should review the Batalden and Stoltz (1993) article.

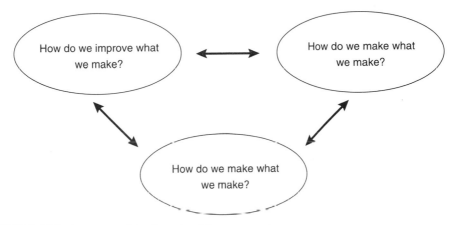

FIGURE 14-2 System capable of continual improvement.

Variation Theories

To improve work processes, knowledge of how to deal with point-to-point differences observed over time is crucial. The empowered nurse needs to be able to determine if a variation in a process reflects a common cause and is within common parameters (e.g., laundry delivery is 10 minutes late), and reflects a fairly stable system (e.g., the system can accept variation in laundry delivery to a unit within a 20-minute time frame), *or* if it is due to a special cause (e.g., laundry was 3 hours late because the delivery person called in sick).

Distinguishing the type of variation present (common cause versus special cause) is critical for improvement because special cause variation and common cause variation require different types of action. A process (laundry delivery) can be stabilized by removing a special cause (sick delivery person). Stabilizing a process by removing a special cause usually precedes changing a common cause as a means of improvement. Introducing fundamental change to a process that is reacting to a special cause variation wastes time and resources, and greatly diminishes the nurse's effectiveness; the system gets "tinkered with" rather than improved.

Psychological Theories

This area includes knowledge of work-related issues such as motivation, workplace design and culture, and the dynamics of change. "Managing change requires knowledge of change *within* [emphasis added] a system [first order change] which stabilizes the system. It also requires knowledge of change *on* [emphasis added] a system [second order change] which restructures [re-engineers] the system"(Batalden & Stoltz, 1993, p. 432).

Organizational policies, practices, activities, habits, and traditions frequently inhibit rather than facilitate performance. Barriers to intrinsic and extrinsic motivation must be removed. When people want to do well in their jobs, their motivation is more than financial reward. The nurse manager who understands this will be encouraged to review each organizational policy, practice, activity, habit, and tradition and to ask tough questions such as How do we do this? Why do we do this and what is the end result? How can we improve the end result? The nurse manager can then investigate and implement new reward systems that enhance success rather than count failures.

Learning or Problem-Solving Theories

Empowerment in the workplace requires the nurse to develop hypotheses about process problems and to take action. The two must be linked by way of small-scale pilot studies that attempt to test the hypotheses upon which actions or interventions are based. Empowerment occurs when "prediction and measurement of variation link theory and action" (Batalden & Stoltz, 1993, p.433).

OTHER SKILLS NECESSARY FOR EMPOWERMENT

In addition to the continuous use of improvement knowledge, empowerment requires skills in communication (the ability to deeply understand others and to be understood by others); organization (the ability to plan and act); and synergistic problem solving (the ability to arrive at an alternative solution).

Another important element of empowerment is the ability to delegate, bearing in mind that delegation involves the risk of having things done differently and sometimes wrong (Covey, 1991, p. 237). One way to ensure a win–win situation when delegating is to set up a win–win performance agreement with the delegatee based on the concept of "completed staff work," where staff correct problems *and* possible solutions (Covey, 1991, p. 237). Such an agreement should incorporate the following five points:

1. Provide a clear understanding of the desired results.
2. Give a clear sense of the level of initiative people have. Must they wait until told, seek permission, make recommendations, act and report immediately, or act and report periodically?
3. Clarify assumptions up front.
4. Provide those people charged to do completed staff work with as much time, resources, and access to the delegator as possible.
5. Set a time and place for presenting and reviewing the results of "completed staff work." Completed staff work gives more responsibility to the staff and increases their ability to respond wisely to different situations (Covey, 1991, p. 243).

A sixth step might be to never accept uncompleted staff work. Employees who "dump" problems into supervisors' laps without offering solutions are only disempowering themselves.

The current spirit of healthcare reform presents an opportunity to introduce new concepts that could lead to greater freedom and flexibility for nurses. Schools of nursing can empower their graduates by teaching

- expanded clinical skills
- strong business and financial expertise
- facility and systems thinking
- knowledge of social policy, network, legislation, and funding issues
- skills in outcome assessment, project management, and evaluation
- application of research to practice
- executive presentation techniques
- basic survival techniques including negotiation, delegation, team building, conflict management, and how to ensure completed staff work (Madden & Ponte, 1994).

IMPROVEMENT KNOWLEDGE AND POLITICS

Nurse empowerment is an evolutionary process that can be measured on a continuum. It is influenced by the evolving role of women, societal changes that increase people's involvement in decision-making processes, increases in educational levels, and economic factors that have forced the delegation of decision making to lower organizational levels (Schmieding, 1993).

A sense of empowerment and a strong educational exposure to improvement knowledge can lead nurses to a political agenda. A congruent linkage in politics occurs through vision, the structural components that involve nurse participation, and the use of a process of inquiry (Schmieding, 1993).

Nurses can use the *context, structure,* and *process* components [emphasis added] of empowerment to assess where they are on the empowerment continuum in their own practice as well as to assess their working and political environments (Schmieding, 1993).

> *Context* provides the connection that fosters unity in every situation. This contextual form of empowerment is actually a vision that represents an organizing principle. This concept is an example of *systems thinking* discussed earlier. In a particular situation, *vision* provides a focus for one's thoughts so that they are not fragmented but rather directed toward a single unity of purpose—a vision. Attention to context allows a person to view a situation not as a single event in isolation, but as an event that has *connection* [emphasis added] to the contextual whole. A vision of nursing as *connected* [emphasis added] is pivotal to all aspects of clinical and administrative decision-making. It provides the framework within which the other components of empowerment occur. (Schmieding, 1993, p. 240)

Structure is the second component needed to enhance the empowerment gained through this shared vision. Healthcare organizational structures have been notoriously bureaucratic, containing many hierarchical levels with centralized control of authority and decision making. Healthcare reform dictates the need to examine which structural elements facilitate and which impede the empowerment of nurses (Schmieding, 1993).

The third component of empowerment is *process,* in which nurses throughout the organization use a reflective process of inquiry in their contacts with patients, each other, and those people associated with patients (Schmieding, 1993). This component reflects a knowledge of systems, psychologic, variation, and learning theories.

Shifts in power within the nursing profession and the healthcare system raise questions as to how nursing will develop and use its power. Increasing nurses' political awareness and skills by refining their knowledge of the context, structure, and process components of empowerment is absolutely essential to bring about changes in the troubled healthcare system (Mason & Backer et al., 1991, p. 75).

Overall, the following poem seems to capture the essence of empowerment:

> *Alone, you can fight, you can refuse, but they roll over you. But two people, back to back, can keep each other sane, can give support, conviction, . . . hope*
> *Three people are a delegation, a committee, a wedge.*
> *With four, you can start an organization.*
> *With six, you can hold a fund-raising party.*
> *A dozen make a demonstration.*
> *A hundred fill a hall.*
> *It goes on one at a time,*
> *It starts when you care to act*
> *It starts when you do it again after they said no,*
> *It starts when you say we and know who you mean, and each day you mean one more.*
>
> *(Margaret Piercy, 1980, p. 23)*

References

Batalden, P., & Stoltz, P. (1993). A framework for the continual improvement of healthcare: Building and applying professional improvement knowledge to test changes in daily work. *Joint Commission Journal on Quality Improvement, 19*(10), 424–452.

Bookman, A., & Morgan, S. (Eds). (1988). *Women in the politics of empowerment.* Philadelphia: Temple University Press.

Covey, S. (1991). *Principle-centered leadership.* New York: Summit Books.

Deming, W. E. (1993). *The new economics of industry, education, government.* Cambridge, MA: Massachusetts Institute of Technology, Center for Advanced Engineering Study.

Flexner, A. (1910). *Medical education in U.S. and Canada.* Birmingham, AL: Classics of Medicine Library.

Halloran, E., Sermens, R., & Barber, B. (1990). Decision support systems for nursing management and administration. In J. Osbolt, D. Vanderwok, & K. Hannah (Eds.), *Decision support systems in nursing* (pp. 29–40). St. Louis, MO: C.V. Mosby.

Madden, J. & Ponte, R. (1994). Advanced practice roles in the managed care environment. *Journal of Nursing Administration, 24*(1), 56–62.

Mason, D., Backer, B., & Georges, C. (1991). Toward the feminist model for the political empowerment of nurses. *Image: The Journal of Nursing Scholarship, 23*(2), 72–77.

Mason, D., Costello-Nickiatas, D., Scanlon, J., & Mangnuson, D. (1991). Empowering nurses for politically astute change in the work place. *Journal of Continuing Education in Nursing, 22*(1), 5–10.

Nazarey, P. (1993). The spirit of nurse empowerment: A leader's responsibility. *Emphasis: Nursing, 4*(2), 7–12.

Piercy, M. (1980). The low road. In *The moon is always female* (p. 23). New York: Alfred A. Knopf.

Reichelt, R., & Young, W. (1985). Professional nursing personnel: Data-based policy formulation. *Journal of Professional Nursing, 1*(3), 165–171.

Schmieding, N. (1993). Nursing empowerment through context, structure and process. *Journal of Professional Nursing, 9*(4), 239–245.

Stuart, G. W. (1986). An organizational strategy for empowering nursing. *Nursing Economic$, 4*(2), 69–73.

Watson, R., & Burkholder, J. (1990). Conflict resolution: Coping skills, empowerment and decision-making strategies for today's nurses. *Dermatology Nursing, 2*(1), 29–37.

15

Research Use in Advanced Practice Nursing

Mary T. Champagne ■ *Elizabeth M. Tornquist* ■
Sandra G. Funk

It is generally agreed that using research findings in practice is a good way to improve nursing care and outcomes for patients. Yet despite this widely held view and continuing increases in the quantity of clinical nursing research, the gap between nursing research and nursing practice remains. If we are to bring a scientific basis to practice, advanced practice nurses (APNs) must take a leadership role in research use. To paraphrase Donna Diers (1972), we must find the findings, select the good findings, and implement them in our practice (p.10).

Research use is usually thought of as the implementation and evaluation of a scientifically based innovation (Buckwalter, 1992). Some authors, however, have made a distinction between knowledge-driven and decision-driven models of research use (Cronenwett, 1992). According to the *knowledge-driven model*, research influences how we think without leading to any particular decision to change practice. From this perspective, we "use" research when we read a research article or attend a research conference to expose ourselves to new knowledge. The exposure helps us keep up with new thinking and information in a given field, and question the assumptions of existing policies or procedures. It stimulates a more reflective and questioning attitude. Weiss (1980) referred to this type of research use as "knowledge creep." The knowledge is there, on the "back burner," perhaps merging with other knowledge in forming a gestalt. The *decision-driven model* of research use, in which assessments and interventions are based on research findings, is what most of us think about when we think of research use. The implication is that nursing practice changes in a visible way because of the research we have reviewed or critiqued.

BENEFITS OF RESEARCH USE IN PRACTICE

Use of research has three main benefits for patients: it may help us understand the patient's situation more thoroughly, assess more accurately, or intervene more effectively (Funk, Tornquist, Champagne, & Wiese 1993). Qualitative studies that report the experiences of patients and their

Hickey JV: ADVANCED PRACTICE NURSING: Changing Roles
and Clinical Applications © 1996 Lippincott–Raven Publishers

families are powerful in that they make us more sensitive to patient situations and that understanding changes nursing practice. For example, the Eakes, Burke, Hainsworth, and Lindgren (1993) qualitative study of chronic sorrow in patients with infertility, cancer, Parkinson's disease, and multiple sclerosis helps us understand the periodic recurrence of intense grief associated with the losses these patients have experienced. This understanding changes the way we view the patient's situation, makes us more sensitive to needs, and thus changes the data we gather and even perhaps the way we intervene.

Other studies, including instrument development studies, help us assess more accurately to determine the need for an intervention or the effectiveness of an intervention. Beyer (1989), for example, noted that, although it was clear children were given far fewer doses of analgesics postoperatively than adults, it was difficult to determine whether the medication given was too little, enough, or too much because nurses had no way to accurately assess how much pain children were experiencing. She therefore developed and tested the *Oucher,* a pain intensity scale for the assessment and management of pediatric pain. Similarly, Holtzclaw and Geer (1995) identified a *mandibular hum*—the prodromal occurrence of palpable masseter contractions before visible shivering in hypothermic postoperative cardiac surgery patients—that may be a valuable predictive clinical sign for assessing shivering in such patients.

Still other studies have identified interventions that will decrease the cost of care or improve the quality of care and patient outcomes. A notable intervention study conducted by Brooten and her colleagues (1986) compared the cost and outcomes of two groups of low–birth weight infants who were treated with two different protocols. In the first group, preemies were discharged when they weighed 2200 g and met usual nursery criteria. They received standard care before and after discharge. In the second group, preemies were discharged early, even before they met the standard discharge weight, if they were physiologically stable. Families of infants in the early discharge group received education, home visits, counseling, and on-call availability of an APN for 18 months. The two groups of infants had similar outcomes; there was no difference in physical or mental development, number of hospitalizations, or acute-care episodes. There was however, a significant difference in the cost of care. The net savings for each infant in the early discharge group was $18,650. Brooten et al. estimated that if this intervention were implemented nationwide, $334 million might be saved annually without adverse effects on patient outcomes.

These uses of research in practice result in greater healthcare "value," which is a function of cost and quality (value = quality/cost). Value increases when higher quality care is provided at the same cost or the same quality of care is provided at lower cost. Whether we have national healthcare reform or reform through the marketplace in the form of managed competition, everyone in the coming years will be looking for greater value. As early as 1982, Fagin assessed the economic value of nursing research and concluded that research can lead to substantial savings of healthcare dollars and greatly enhance the quality of care. Better value is gained when practice is based on scientific evidence rather than on traditions, habits, or trial and error. In the changing healthcare marketplace, those providers who can show they bring greater value to patients will be in demand; those who do not will find themselves on the outside looking in.

BARRIERS TO RESEARCH USE IN PRACTICE

In addition to the healthcare value generated, when nurses engage in research-based practice, their view of themselves as professionals is enhanced and their work becomes more interesting and fulfilling (Cronenwett 1987; Goode & Bulechek, 1992; Titler et al., 1994). Yet nurses do not routinely use research findings in their practice (Brett, 1987; Coyle & Sokop, 1990; Ketefian, 1975; Kirchhoff, 1982). Miller and Messenger (1978) first reported on the barriers to using research that clinicians had identified. The most frequently mentioned problem was inability to obtain findings relevant to their practice. Other less frequently identified barriers included the time and cost involved in using research, resistance to change in the work setting, lack of rewards for using research in practice, and lack of understanding or uncertainty regarding the conclusions of research reports.

More recently, Funk, Champagne, Wiese, and Tornquist (1991) looked at barriers to using research identified by registered nurses. A stratified random sample of 5000 nurses drawn from the American Nurses' Association membership roster were mailed the BARRIERS questionnaire and asked to rate the extent to which each of 28 items was a barrier to using research to alter or enhance practice. The BARRIERS instrument has four subscales: (1) the characteristics of the nurse, that is, the nurse's research values, skills, and awareness (eight items); (2) characteristics of the setting, that is, barriers and limitations perceived in the work setting (eight items); (3) characteristics of the research such as its methodological soundness and the appropriateness of conclusions (six items); and (4) characteristics of the presentation of the research and its accessibility (six items).

Of the nurses who were sent the survey, 40% (n = 1989) responded, and 924 (46%) of these respondents reported that their primary job functions were clinical. These clinicians rated more than two thirds of the items on the BARRIERS Scale as great or moderate barriers. All eight items related to the characteristics of the setting were among the top 10 barriers. The two top barriers were the feeling that nurses did not have "enough authority to change patient care procedures" and had "insufficient time on the job to implement new ideas" (Funk et al., 1991, p. 91). When asked to list the top three barriers, clinicians identified insufficient time followed by lack of support from administration and lack of support from physicians. Thus, aspects of the setting were seen as the greatest barriers to use of research; these were followed by problems in the presentation and accessibility of the research. The nurse's research values and skills and the qualities of the research were seen as less problematic. When respondents were asked to list ways that the use of research findings in practice could be facilitated, the top three ways were increasing administrative support, improving the accessibility of research reports, and improving the nurse's research knowledge.

STRATEGIES FOR OVERCOMING BARRIERS

The responses of clinicians to the BARRIERS Scale give us some idea of why research is not used in practice and suggest how we might change that. First of all, it is clear that the work setting has a tremendous influence on the use of research in practice. Whether one works in a complex healthcare agency or a small office practice, administrative support and encouragement are critical. Studies that have looked at research use by hospital nursing staff (Champion & Leach, 1989; Linde 1990; Wilson, 1990) found that support from key nursing administrators—from the unit director to the director of nursing—was significantly and positively correlated with research use. Administrators' support for research use involves the creation of an organizational culture that values and uses research and in which questions are welcomed, critical thinking encouraged, and nursing care evaluated. In a setting with competing demands, no one is really going to believe research use is important unless the administration makes it seem important. In hospitals and clinics, nurse administrators and managers must not only speak of using research in practice, they must do so themselves and build this expectation into staff evaluations and rewards. Support for research use must be tangible. *Support* means the commitment of resources needed to accomplish the activity, including time for nurses to read research, pilot-test innovations, and develop new protocols, and funds for journals, library searches, copying, and perhaps consultation or conference attendance. APNs can spearhead efforts to use research by forming unit-level research committees to guide and organize the work or by forming quality improvement, total quality management, or policy or procedure committees that take a research-based approach to solving problems or revising protocols. APNs working in small group practices might link with a practice partner or join a research group in their professional specialty organization to look at new knowledge for practice.

Problems with the presentation and accessibility of research are also barriers to research use. Research reports are generally written by researchers for other researchers; at best they are dry and technical, and at worst they are filled with jargon understood only by other researchers. "They often emphasize the reliability and validity of instruments instead of discussing what was measured; they tend to focus on statistical tests rather than the magnitude and meaning of the findings; and they often fail to indicate what information may be applicable to practice" (Tornquist, Funk, Champagne, & Wiese, 1993, p. 177). Although some new journals and some specialty journals are presenting research in a clearer, more concise and user-friendly way, the old-fashioned approach modeled after the thesis and dissertation still predominates. APNs need to find ways to cut through the jargon to evaluate the significance of the problem being studied, the credibility of the evidence or methods used to answer the question or problem, the appropriateness of the conclusions, and the usefulness of the research for practice. Practical advice on how to read research is given by Tornquist and colleagues (1993). Other strategies for understanding difficult reports include consulting with research faculty in schools of nursing or within an agency.

It is also difficult to find a body of research on a particular topic in one place. For the most part, research conferences and research journals include studies on a wide variety of problems with insufficient focus on any one problem. As APNs, we can solve this problem, however, by obtaining library privileges at a health sciences library and conducting literature searches using computerized programs. If, in doing the literature review, questions arise about the sample, intervention, or other aspects of a study, the researcher can be contacted directly. Most researchers will be happy to talk about their work and will be interested in attempts to use their findings in practice.

In addition, the publications of the federal Agency for Health Care Policy and Research (AHCPR) can be useful. AHCPR was established to promote medical effectiveness research, develop databases for research, develop clinical guidelines, and disseminate research findings and clinical guidelines. It routinely publishes reviews of studies on clinical problems with summaries of treatment effectiveness; for example, a discussion of the effectiveness of intermittent positive pressure breathing was recently published (Duffey & Farley, 1994). AHCPR has also published research-based clinical practice guidelines on topics such as acute pain, depression, pressure sores, mammography, cataracts, and incontinence. AHCPR publications serve to bring together research on topics that may have relevance for your practice. The free publications of the AHCPR, including the *Research Activities*, *Provider Studies Research Note,* clinical practice guidelines, and the publication catalog can be obtained by contacting AHCPR Publications Clearinghouse, P.O. Box 8547, Silver Spring, MD, 20907 (800-358-9295).

RESEARCH USE MODELS

A number of models have been developed to improve the dissemination and use of research findings. In the late 1970s with funding from the U.S. Department of Health, Education, and Welfare, the Western Interstate Commission for Higher Education developed the Regional Program for Research Development with the goal of developing research use skills in clinicians. Clinicians who participated in the program first identified a practice problem and then looked for research to help solve it. Then, at an initial workshop, participants learned how to implement the research findings to make a change in their practice. Six months later, after the innovation had been implemented, they returned for a second workshop to discuss successful implementation strategies. Although the clinicians evaluated the program positively, many had difficulty finding appropriate research. Project staff noted, "Some participants came to Workshop I with research studies which exactly met their needs; others came with articles and frustration; and still others had not been able to find a single study that they could use" (Krueger, Nelson, & Wolanin, 1978, p. 287). The project staff concluded that the real problem with their approach was lack of access to good research and said no major use efforts should be undertaken until the products of research had been systematically identified, evaluated, and made ready for nurses to use in practice.

The next major research use effort attempted to do just that. The Conduct and Use of Research in Nursing (CURN) project aimed to promote clinical research activity and assist nurses to integrate research findings into their practice (Horsley, Crane, Crabtree, & Wood, 1983). Criteria for judging the applicability of research to practice were developed, and participants in the project helped develop 10 research-based protocols on problems such as the reduction of diarrhea in tube-fed patients and the prevention of pressure ulcers. The CURN model included identifying the clinical problem, summarizing the research, developing the innovation design and a protocol for implementing the intervention, and evaluating the outcomes. Unfortunately, the CURN approach assumed that implementation of research-based practice protocols is more static than is often the case. Clinical settings differ, patient situations differ, nurses differ, and the use of research requires practical assessment of the possibilities for change in a particular setting, ability to carry out the process of change, and ability to use clinical reasoning in applying and, often, adapting research findings to a particular situation.

The Nursing Child Assessment Satellite Training project, another major effort, used satellite communication technology to disseminate innovations to educators and practicing nurses and teach them how to use the innovations in practice (King, Barnard, & Hoehn, 1981). This project was successful in achieving its purpose. Despite the contributions made by each of these projects, however, use of research in practice has been infrequent.

More recently, The Dissemination Model developed by Funk and colleagues (1989b) was designed to overcome some of the problems with the accessibility and presentation of research. Based on this model, five national conferences were held to bring researchers and clinicians together to examine topic-focused research for practice. The model included improving the communication of the research so that it was understandable to clinicians and its relevance for practice was clear, and promoting ongoing dialogue between researchers and clinicians as innovations were tried in practice. Conference topics included pain, nausea, fatigue, mobility, rest, nutrition, and falls, as well as other issues in the care of the elderly, chronically ill, and acutely ill populations. Conference attendees—predominantly clinicians—felt that the implications of the research for practice were clear, the statistical analyses of the research were understandable, and the clinicians' perspective was presented. In addition, postconference evaluations at 6 months and 18 months revealed that conference participants had shared relevant innovations with their colleagues at home, nearly all had reevaluated their own practice in light of the new information, and more than 80% had tried using a research innovation in their practice (Funk, Tornquist, & Champagne, 1989a, 1989b).

Other approaches such as the regional research use conferences developed by Cronenwett at Dartmouth-Hitchcock Medical Center (Tornquist, Funk, & Champagne, 1995) have also been successful in increasing dissemination of research findings. Cronenwett's approach brings together clinicians and researchers who present research summaries related to clinical problems and suggest research-based solutions for practice.

The Stetler/Marram Model of research use (Stetler & Marram, 1976) has gained wide acceptance in practice and educational settings and has been used to facilitate research use at both individual and organizational levels. Stetler (1994) has recently refined and expanded the model (Fig. 15-1). The new Stetler Model for Research Utilization is based on four assumptions. The first is that individuals as well as organizations may be involved in the use of research, and planned change in a formal organization is not the only way research is used. The second, and most important, assumption challenges the rigid-specific, protocol-driven, or mechanistic notion of research use. Stetler notes that research usually provides us with probabilistic information, not absolutes. Thus, specific interventions should not be viewed as determining outcomes, but as affecting the probability of outcomes. Even with solid studies, examination of the means does not indicate whether each subject responded in the same fashion or to the same degree; variance is usually only partly accounted for; and patients, families, and

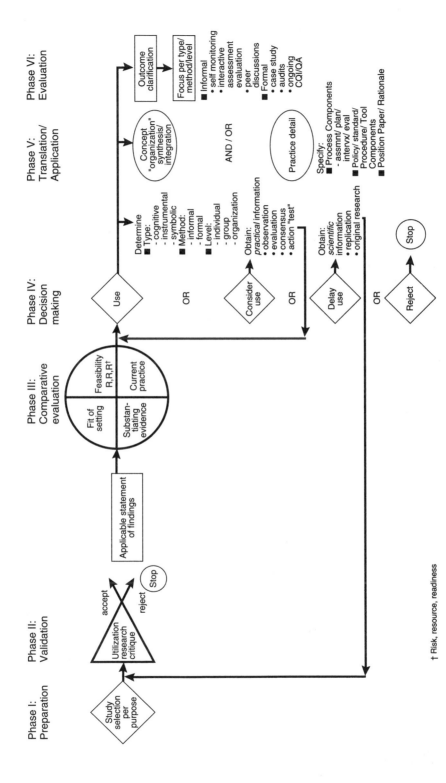

FIGURE 15-1 The Stetler model for research utilization. (*Note:* From Refinement of the Stetler/Marram model for application of research findings to practice by C.B. Stetler, *Nursing Outlook*, 1994).

situations are often unique and sometimes idiosyncratic. Thus, any research finding or innovation must be applied in the context of the clinical judgment of the skilled practitioner who is caring for the patient. The third and fourth assumptions suggest that in the real world (particularly when a deadline must be met), experiential and theoretical knowledge may be used along with research to make decisions; and lack of knowledge regarding research use may lead to inappropriate and ineffective use.

The model includes six phases in the use process: (1) preparation, or the purpose of the research review; (2) validation, in which a use critique of studies is done and studies are either accepted or rejected; (3) comparative evaluation, in which the fit and feasibility of the innovation are assessed and evidence of the benefit of the innovation and of current practice is reviewed; (4) decision making, which might be a decision to use, consider use, delay use until a later time, or reject; (5) translation/application, in which the exact nature of the practice implications are identified and the degree of adaptation is specified; and (6) evaluation, including clarification of formal and informal outcomes. Stetler's new prescriptive model, like most use models, is designed to facilitate use of research by the practitioner rather than to facilitate organizational adoption of research. Nevertheless, it can be used by both individuals and organizations to "mitigate some of the human frailties of decision making and thus to facilitate appropriate, effective, and pragmatic use; raise the consciousness of potential users; and increase the role of critical thinking in professional practice" (Stetler, 1994, p. 25).

The Iowa Model (Titler et al., 1994) is a heuristic, pragmatic approach to research use that evolved out of the Quality Assurance Model Using Research (Watson, Bulechek, & McCloskey, 1987) (Fig. 15-2). The model focuses on improving the quality of care. First triggers are identified that encourage nurses to think critically about current practice and identify problems that can be answered through the use or conduct of research. Triggers are powerful stimulants that cause nurses to question tradition and seek a scientific basis for their practice. Triggers may be problem focused, for example, clinical problems that arise frequently in practice or are discovered through total quality management or quality improvement programs; or they may be knowledge focused, arising from new knowledge or information including research literature, care philosophies, and standards and practice guidelines from federal agencies or professional organizations. Once a trigger is identified, the model suggests that the next step is to assemble, critique, and evaluate the relevant research for its applicability for practice. In Iowa, the critique and evaluation of the literature are usually done by those interested in the practice problems—either by a group of nurses including staff nurses, nurse managers, and APNs, or by a multidisciplinary team. Consultation with a nurse scientist is available during this phase.

Once the relevant literature has been evaluated, the group decides whether the research base is sufficient to warrant changing practice. When the research base is sufficient to guide practice, the group implements the steps necessary to bring practice in line with what is suggested by the research. In this stage, the baseline state and expected outcomes of the change are identified; the intervention is then designed by those who will be involved in implementing it, the practice change is piloted on one unit, and the change in practice is evaluated from both a process and outcome perspective. Based on this evaluation, methods of implementing the practice change may be modified, the innovation may be refined or adapted, or the outcome measures adjusted.

If the research base is insufficient for practice, the problem (trigger) is addressed in at least one of three ways: through the conduct of research when possible and appropriate, through a review of scientific principles that are related to practice and can help guide interventions, and through consultation with colleagues who are currently investigating the problem. Using any one of these three methods, practice may be changed. Although not specified by the model, it is likely that such practice changes would be developed, implemented, and evaluated on a pilot unit before use throughout the agency.

Following the development and pilot testing of the innovation, a second decision-making point in the model is reached: Should the practice change be made throughout the organiza-

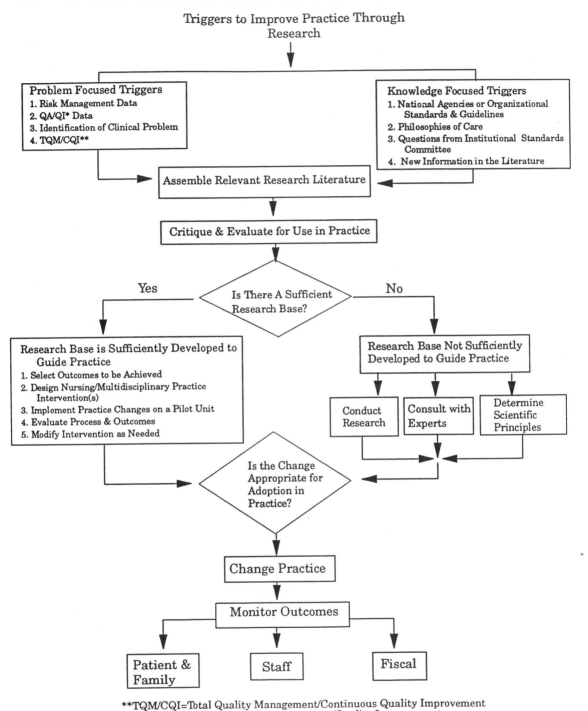

FIGURE 15-2 The Iowa Model: Research Based Practice to Promote Quality Care. (Adapted from Titler, M.G., Kleiber, C., Steelman, V., Goode, C., Rakel, B., Barry-Walker, J., Small, S., & Buckwalter, K. (1994). Infusing research into practice to promote quality care. *Nursing Research*, *43*, 307-313.)

tion? The authors of the model (Titler et al., 1994) have suggested that the following factors be considered in making this decision: costs and costs savings, effect on quality of care, increasing or decreasing patient risk of iatrogenic injury, competency of staff to carry out the innovation, and support of the administration in making the change. If the benefits of implementing the change are sufficient, using these criteria, the model recommends using a process of planned change in implementing the innovation. The model requires that patient and family, staff, and fiscal outcomes be monitored. The Iowa Model has successfully been used at the Iowa Hospitals and Clinics for the last few years. Its success is apparent in that more than 30 research use projects and 15 research studies have been initiated by nurses in practice at University of Iowa Hospitals and Clinics. Other nurses in practice have joined with faculty from the University of Iowa College of Nursing in Iowa City to participate in collaborative research studies. Through these projects and professional recognition of their achievements, the professional practice environment has been enriched for nurses.

HOW TO USE RESEARCH TO IMPROVE PRACTICE

Research findings can be used to change practice on at least two levels: the individual and organizational levels. On the individual level, the APN drives the change in his or her own practice or in the work setting. Most of the models previously described focus on research use on the individual level. Some focus primarily on changing one's own nursing practice; others focus on working within the organization to ensure that practice changes. In either case, the burden is on the nurse to "make things happen." On the organizational level, research use occurs because the organization facilitates and supports its use throughout the agency. Administrative support and organizational structures are in place to create an ethos and culture of research use to enhance the value brought to patients. At the organizational level of research use, the organization creates a climate in which the nurse is enabled to practice in a more scholarly and professional fashion, and in doing so, both the nurse and practice in the organization change.

Individual Use of Research

Regardless of the advanced practice role you hold, using research to validate or improve your individual practice is an essential part of your work. Begin reading research reports on a regular basis, especially if you are less than comfortable with research. Do not read them as you might have been taught in school—with a focus on technical jargon, statistical analyses, and the named design. Instead, focus on the clinical problem being studied, the credibility of the evidence presented, and the conclusions and their implications for practice (Tornquist et al., 1993). Subscribe to journals that routinely report clinical studies in your area of interest and get your name on the AHCPR mailing list. Discuss studies with colleagues and consult with experts or the author of the study if you have questions about the study or findings. Although it is true that only good research should be considered for use in practice, be wary of the "scholar" who finds every study fatally flawed. There is no perfect research design—the question is whether the methods used to produce the findings are sound enough to convince you that the findings are credible. The more you read research, the more comfortable you will become and the more confident you will be in evaluating the credibility of the work. Participate in other activities that expose you to research: join a journal club, attend research conferences, or become a member of your agency's research committee.

At the very least, you will begin to use research in the way described by Weiss (1980)—as "knowledge creep"—and this will increase your openness to new ideas and stimulate your thinking about your current practice. Some studies may help you better understand patient experiences or situations. Hawthorne's (1993) work on women with cardiac disease, for example, has described, in the women's own words, what this experience is like for them. After reading the study, your sensitivity to the experiences of women with cardiac disease will be heightened.

Your practice will change because you will do a better job of eliciting descriptions of what the experience is like for your own female cardiac patients and plan your care accordingly. As Cronenwett (1992) noted, "There is rarely a large body of replicated work about patients' experiences. But you will use what you read because the impact comes from reading the report" (p. 31). Use of research in this fashion carries few risks, and your increased sensitivity should benefit your patients.

If you intend to implement a research-based innovation that changes the way a patient is assessed or the interventions that are used in your practice, it will be easier to implement the change if there is a clearly identified need for change. For example, if a significant percentage of the patients on your unit are experiencing falls or elderly patients in your nursing home are developing pressure ulcers, the need for change will be clear. Also, when new knowledge, such as the use of closed-circuit suction for ventilated patients on positive end expiratory pressure, raises questions about current practice, the need for change may be clearer. Once a need for change has been identified, the relevant research literature needs to be reviewed and evaluated to determine if there is a sufficient research base. Integrated state-of-the-science papers, clinical practice guidelines, and meta-analyses are helpful in analyzing the research base. There is no magic rule as to "how many research studies" are sufficient to provide a sound research base. In general, though, the more risky or complex the intervention, the greater its cost, and the more questionable its efficacy, the greater the number of studies needed to support its use. If the risk to the patient is low, the cost small, and the potential benefit great, careful evaluation of a pilot implementation of the innovation may be warranted even if the number of supporting studies is small. When critiquing the research base, pay particular attention to whether the characteristics of the subjects and their environment are similar to those of your patients and their environment. Seek help from colleagues and experts, including study authors, during this phase of the process. Winning support from others and being clear about the evidence supporting the innovation and its potential benefits will help move the project forward (Cronenwett, 1989; Titler et al., 1994).

If the research base is strong and applicable to your setting, you will need to outline the innovation and how it will be implemented. Ask, What will it take to make this change? Whether you are in a small practice or a large healthcare agency, you must think through policies regarding change; ways to gain support from all who will be involved in or affected by the innovation; the time, costs, and other resources needed; and the legal and ethical implications of the change. The innovation may need to be adapted to fit your particular institution. If change is to be successfully implemented, both formal and informal leaders will need to give their support. Shared ownership by all involved provides the strongest guarantee of successful implementation (Clark & Hall, 1990; Goode & Bulechek, 1992).

You also will need to plan how to evaluate the effect of the innovation in your practice. In all studies, measuring value—that is, patient outcomes and costs—is important. Identify the patient outcomes you want to measure. Decide how information about your outcomes is currently recorded; whenever possible, use indicators and forms that are already being used to collect your outcome data. The greater the number of extraneous forms that you introduce for staff or others to fill out, the less likely you are to get the data you need. Before implementing the innovation, determine what level of change in your outcome measure you will consider clinically significant, warranting continued use of the innovation. Collect data on the outcome measures before and after the innovation to assess the change in outcomes. It may seem more daunting to determine the costs (time and resources used or saved) of the innovation, but this is a critical factor in every healthcare practice or agency. If necessary, seek out someone in your organization who can help you track cost data, both before and after the innovation. In addition, if you believe the innovation will affect the staff (and, in most instances, it will), you need to measure staff outcomes as well. After you evaluate the success of the innovation, be sure to share your data with colleagues involved in the practice change (Cronenwett, 1990; Lindquist, Brauer, Lekander, & Foster, 1990; Stetler, 1994; Titler et al., 1994).

Organizational Use of Research

We are just beginning to learn what factors or structures are critical to the development and success of organizational models for research use. The great success of the Iowa Model is related to two factors: first, it is a pragmatic heuristic model that is easy to use; second, the model is used in an organization that values and promotes the use of research in practice. For the organization, and for the nurses who work in that organization, critical thinking, risk taking, and databased decision making are a way of life.

Several key factors in creating a climate for research use involve removing the barriers to research use. In Iowa, administrative support for using research in practice and for conducting research is strong. The organizational structure includes research as a significant component. There is an overall department of nursing research committee and there are seven divisional research committees, one in each clinical division. Nurse executives in the organization are actively involved in research use and communicate the value of scholarly practice in tangible ways. Staff orientation and leadership development programs encourage staff to participate in nursing research and its use in practice. Clinical release time for doing research, tuition reimbursement for research coursework, and funding for attending research conferences convey clearly the value of research as a part of professional work. AHCPR guidelines are distributed to staff, as are research studies, integrative research reviews, and meta-analyses. At the unit level, staff are also provided time to carry out this part of their professional practice. They are encouraged to obtain research consultation and pilot research-based protocols, and release time from patient care is given for research activities such as attending journal clubs; collecting data; writing research-based practice protocols; preparing abstracts, talks, or papers; and participating in divisional committees. These structures not only remove barriers to research use but, more important, begin to bring together clinicians and researchers in a new way—as equal partners in the effort to use research to improve the quality of nursing care and reduce the costs of that care. Thus, the Iowa Model points the way. If we are to develop research-based nursing practice, all nurses must be involved in the work. There can be no class or caste divisions; the organizational culture and the individuals in the organization must value clinical scholarship and expect it from everyone.

References

Beyer, J. (1989). The Oucher: A pain intensity scale for children. In S. Funk, E. Tornquist, M. Champagne, L. Copp, & R. Wiese (Eds.), *Key aspects of comfort: Management of pain, fatigue and nausea* (pp. 65–71). New York: Springer.

Brett, J. L. (1987). Use of nursing practice research findings. *Nursing Research, 36,* 334–349.

Brooten, D., Kumar, S., Brown, L. P., Butts, P., Finkler, S., Bakewell-Sachs, S., Gibbons, A., & Delivoria-Papadopoulos, M. (1986). A randomized clinical trial of early hospital discharge and home follow-up of very low birthweight infants. *New England Journal of Medicine, 315*(15), 934–939.

Buckwalter, K. C. (1992). Research utilization awards: Utilization versus dissemination? *Reflections, 18*(3), 8.

Champion, V. L., & Leach, A. (1989). Variables related to research utilization for nursing: An empirical investigation. *Journal of Advanced Nursing, 14,* 705–710.

Clark, P. C., & Hall, H. S. (1990). Innovations probability chart: A valuable tool for change. *Nursing Management, 21*(8), 128V–128X.

Coyle, L. A., & Sokop, A. G. (1990). Innovation adoption behavior among nurses. *Nursing Research, 39,* 176–180.

Cronenwett, L. R. (1987). Research utilization in practice settings. *Journal of Nursing Administration, 17*(7–8), 9–10.

Cronenwett, L. R. (1989). Strategies for using research in practice. In S. Funk, E. Tornquist, M. Champagne, L. Copp, & R. Wiese (Eds.), *Key aspects of comfort: Management of pain fatigue and nausea* (pp. 321–332). New York: Springer.

Cronenwett, L. R. (1990). Improving practice through research utilization. In S. Funk, E. Tornquist, M. Champagne, & R. Wiese (Eds.), *Key aspects of recovery: Improving nutrition, rest and mobility.* (pp. 7–21). New York: Springer.

Cronenwett, L. R. (1992). Using research in practice. In S. Funk, E. Tornquist, M. Champagne, & R. Wiese (Eds.), *Key aspects of elder care: Managing falls, incontinence, and cognitive impairment* (pp. 28–38). New York: Springer.

Diers, D. (1972). Application of research to nursing practice. *Image: Journal of Nursing Scholarship, 5,* 2–11.

Duffey, S. Q., & Farley, D. E. (1994). *Intermittent positive pressure breathing: Old technologies rarely die* (AHCPR Publication No. 94-0001, Division of Provider Studies Research Note No. 18, Agency for Health Care Policy and Research). Rockville, MD: U.S. Public Health Service.

Eakes, G. G., Burke, M. L., Hainsworth, M. A., & Lindgren, C. L. (1993). Chronic sorrow: An examination of nursing roles. In S. Funk, E. Tornquist, M. Champagne, & R. Wiese (Eds.), *Key aspects of caring for the chronically ill: Hospital and home* (pp. 231–238). New York: Springer.

Fagin, C. M. (1982). The economic value of nursing research. *American Journal of Nursing, 82*(12), 1844–1849.

Funk, S. G., Champagne, M. T., Wiese, R. A., & Tornquist, E. M. (1991). Barriers to using research findings in practice: The clinician's perspective. *Applied Nursing Research, 4*, 90–95.

Funk, S. G., Tornquist, E. M., & Champagne, M. T. (1989a). Application and evaluation of the dissemination model. *Western Journal of Nursing Research, 11*, 486–491.

Funk, S. G., Tornquist, E. M., & Champagne, M. T. (1989b). A model for improving the dissemination of nursing research. *Western Journal of Nursing Research, 11*, 361–367.

Funk, S. G., Tornquist, E., Champagne, M., & Wiese, R. (1993). Caring for the chronically ill: From research to practice. In S. Funk, E. Tornquist, M. Champagne, & R. Wiese (Eds.), *Key aspects of caring for the chronically ill: Hospital and home* (pp. 3–7). New York: Springer.

Goode, C. J., & Bulechek, G. M. (1992). Research utilization: An organizational process [Special issue]. *Journal of Nursing Care Quarterly (Special Report)*, 27–35.

Hawthorne, M. H. (1993). Women recovering from coronary artery bypass surgery. *Scholarly Inquiry for Nursing Practice, 7*, 223–244.

Holtzclaw, B. J., & Geer, R. T. (1995). Clinical predictors and metabolic consequences of postoperative shivering after cardiac surgery. In S. Funk, E. Tornquist, M. Champagne, & R. Wiese (Eds.), *Key aspects of caring for the acutely ill: Technological aspects, patient education, and quality of life* (pp. 226–233). Springer: New York.

Horsley, J. A., Crane, J., Crabtree, M., & Wood, D. (1983). *Using research to improve nursing practice: A guide.* New York: Grune & Stratton.

Ketefian, S. (1975). Application of selected nursing research findings into nursing practice: A pilot study. *Nursing Research, 24*, 89–92.

King, D., Barnard, K. E., & Hoehn, R. (1981). Disseminating the results of nursing research. *Nursing Outlook, 29*, 164–169.

Kirchoff, K. T. (1982). A diffusion survey of coronary precautions. *Nursing Research, 31*, 196–201.

Krueger, J. C., Nelson, A. H., & Wolanin, M. O. (1978). *Nursing research: Development, collaboration, utilization.* Germantown, MD: Aspen Publishers.

Linde, B. J. (1990). The effectiveness of three interventions to increase research utilizations among practicing nurses. *Dissertation Abstracts International, 51*, 1195B (University Microfilms No. 9013960).

Lindquist, J. R., Brauer, D. J., Lekander, B. J., & Foster, K. (1990). Research utilization: Practical considerations for applying research to nursing practice. *Focus on Critical Care, 17*(4), 342–347.

Miller, J. R., & Messenger, S. R. (1978). Obstacles to applying research findings. *American Journal of Nursing, 78*, 632–634.

Stetler, C. B., & Marram, G. (1976). Evaluating research findings for applicability in practice. *Nursing Outlook, 24*, 559–563.

Stetler, C. B. (1994). Refinement of the Stetler/Marram Model for application of research findings to practice. *Nursing Outlook, 42*(1), 15–25.

Titler, M. G., Kleiber, C., Steelman, V., Goode, C., Rakel, B., Barry-Walker, J., Small, S., & Buckwalter, K. (1994). Infusing research into practice to promote quality care. *Nursing Research, 43*, 307–313.

Tornquist, E. M., Funk, S. G., & Champagne, M. T. (1995). Research utilization: Reconnecting research and practice. *AACN Clinical Issues, 6*(1), 105–109.

Tornquist, E. M., Funk, S. G., Champagne, M. T., & Wiese, R. A. (1993). Advice on reading research: Overcoming the barriers. *Applied Nursing Research, 6*, 177–183.

Watson, C. A., Bulechek, G. M., & McCloskey, J. C. (1987). QAMUR: A quality assurance model using research. *Journal of Nursing Quality Assurance, 2*(1), 21–27.

Weiss, C. H. (1980) Knowledge creep and decision accretion. *Knowledge: Creation, Diffusion, Utilization, 1*, 381–404.

Wilson, L. E. (1990). An analysis of selected variables influencing the acceptance of an innovation (autonomous nursing units) by nurses in an acute care setting. *Dissertation Abstracts International, 50*, 3927B. (University Microfilms No. 9004842)

C H A P T E R

16

Cost-Containment Initiatives: Analysis of Clinical Resource Use

Valinda R. Rutledge ■ *Cynthia A. Bennett*

POSITIONED FOR THE FUTURE

Healthcare today is undergoing radical change not experienced since the mid-1980s, when diagnosis-related groups (DRGs) were introduced for Medicare reimbursement. In the past, an attempt to shift costs from the Medicare and Medicaid population to the commercial population did not result in a decrease in general healthcare costs. However, the change underway is the result of the demand for market competition (see Chap. 13), which has led to cost reductions, with the emphasis on reducing overall healthcare costs.

The key goal of the leadership of any organization is to develop a vision that will ensure the continued viability of the organization. The leadership's articulation of this organizational vision allows employees to set targets and see the "finish line." Without a shared organizational vision, the staff will struggle to understand the end point. Without the staff's understanding of their leadership's vision, the internal environment is filled with chaos and uncertainty as external societal changes continue to erupt. Staff may experience the same feelings as sailors in a tiny rowboat without oars on a windswept sea. Once leaders develop the vision, skills can be taught to allow the staff to navigate the turbulent sea.

The leadership should articulate a vision of how the organization will be defined in the future as it interacts with external market forces. Senior management must look beyond next year and anticipate major shifts in healthcare. Waiting for the market to affect the organization before making any changes leaves the organization in a reactive mode and decreases its future options.

Currently, the payer's primary focus is on price, with little emphasis on quality measures. Questions about quality are arising, including whether it has been sacrificed for lower costs. Has the primary goal become to use the minimal amount of resources on each patient rather than to align healthcare resources with consumer needs (Patton & Katterhagen, 1994)?

Hickey JV: ADVANCED PRACTICE NURSING: Changing Roles
and Clinical Applications © 1996 Lippincott–Raven Publishers

Number slashing as a substitute for a detailed analysis of value (cost/quality ratio) can cause erosion in quality. However, visionary leaders will realize that, with consumer pressure, the pendulum will inevitably swing back to value measurement; hence, these leaders will position their organizations to be poised for success.

Because a healthcare organization represents a collection of subsystems that interconnect in multiple ways, the strategies of the leadership are extremely complex. Each subsystem (eg, medical practice, nursing practice, marketing, finance, and hospital ancillary departments) has its own set of goals based partly on departmental, professional, and personal considerations. Some subsystems such as medical practice have fragmented into smaller microcosms of specialists and generalists. The concept of fragmentation among departments is common as the changing environment threatens previous roles and responsibilities. Departments in the fee-for-service environment, which once were viewed as revenue producers, are suddenly generating costs in a capitated system. This fragmentation can lead to unhealthy competition among departments, which results in duplicative efforts and forces costs to rise (Patton & Katterhagen, 1994). Departmental energies are often focused on maintaining personnel and tasks rather than appropriately aligning departmental resources with the vision of the organization.

As the entire healthcare system undergoes rapid change, the effects on individual healthcare organizations will radiate inward to each of their subsystems. Initially, subsystems will attempt to maintain equilibrium by resisting change, which will cause tension. This attempt will continue until new directions are accepted and accommodated by each subsystem. An understanding of systems theory is essential for the leadership, who must steer their organizations through this difficult transitional time.

Organizational leadership must develop effective strategies with an understanding of external and internal causal factors. Sophisticated information systems are integral to defining these causal factors and for allowing organizations to position themselves for success. A detailed understanding of current cost standards and patterns will enable staff to modify or change their behavior within the context of the parameters of the vision.

Identification of "champions" in each subsystem will help integrate the process within the organizational mainstream. Champions should have the following characteristics:

- be highly respected among professional colleagues
- be viewed as clinically competent within their department
- have knowledge about cost structures
- have the energy to move change through the system
- have consistency of purpose

Working with these champions will facilitate the change internal to the group and foster organizational integration of the process. Consultants and administrators, without the help of such champions, will experience greater resistance, increased chances of sabotage, and the withholding of critical information.

This chapter identifies and discusses trends related to external causal factors. The infrastructure of healthcare costs is defined and explained as are definitions associated with quality management and outcomes assessment. The authors outline a framework for analyzing costs and value and demonstrate practical applications to illustrate the concepts in the context of outcomes assessment projects.

EXTERNAL FACTORS

The three external factors that affect the profit margin of each organization are payer mix, market share profiles, and the extent to which the components of the healthcare system are integrated. Understanding the trends related to each of these factors, the interconnections among them, and their linkage to the bottom line is crucial to the success of an organization. Choosing a strategy that focuses on one of the three causal factors will ultimately affect the other two in unanticipated ways. As the market becomes increasingly competitive, the need to forecast the effect of a strategic direction, such as collaborating with another hospital or healthcare system on a specific program, and its bearing on the bottom line, will become crucial. Forecasting models are becoming a commonplace tool for the hospital administrator and clinician as they jointly make strategic decisions.

Nongovernmental health plans can be divided into three broad categories: fee-for-service, managed care, and capitated. The traditional health plan has been fee-for-service (also referred to as indemnity insurance); in 1981, 95% of all Americans younger than age 65 years were covered by this type of plan (Touse, 1993). However, by 1990, the number had declined to 19%, with a corresponding high growth in the number of managed care plans. Indemnity plans have allowed patients the freedom to choose physicians and hospitals. In the past, there was no incentive to reduce costs because each hospital ancillary department, such as a pharmacy, could bill their services separately. Hospital ancillary departments were viewed as revenue producing, whereas other areas such as nursing units were viewed as cost centers. In a current fee-for-service payer system, care providers continue to have no incentive to conserve resources because they are able bill for services such as reading x-rays or interpreting laboratory tests. However, in an attempt to reduce costs, some indemnity plan strategies have been put in place: surgical second opinions, admission precertification, and case management above a specific dollar amount (Alkire & Stolz, 1993). From a healthcare organizational viewpoint, patients with fee-for-service health plans will generate the highest net margin (because the reimbursement is based on straight charges) and are usually actively recruited to use services within the organization. (*Net margin* can be calculated by subtracting total cost from net revenue.)

As healthcare costs soared, employers began to purchase more managed care health plans, and the number of indemnity plans decreased. In managed care plans, access to services is controlled to reduce costs by directing patients to specific physicians and hospitals contracted to provide discounted services. Contracts can be bundled to include both hospital and professional fees to avoid cost shifting. Examples of managed care plans are health maintenance organizations, preferred provider organizations, and point-of-service contracts. With heavy market penetration by managed care plans, hospital net margins have decreased dramatically. In southern California, patient days fell 50% as the market moved from a predominantly fee-for-service to a capitated environment (Cerne, 1994). Providers are now selected primarily on price; thus, reducing costs within an organization quickly becomes paramount to survival. Contracts may have to be signed that are at or below the variable cost level in an attempt to maintain a break-even patient volume.

Capitated health plans, another type of commercial plan, are a payer system in which healthcare organizations assume part of the risk by providing total healthcare to a designated population at a set price per month per member (Kongstvedt, 1993). The payment is based on number of enrollees and not on number of services provided. If the population is stable, yearly budgets can be developed in advance based on the surveyed population's health needs. The focus shifts from the acute care hospital to the outpatient setting, and other alternative approaches, such as home care and subacute facilities, are used to decrease costs. In response to the high organizational risk, care providers develop innovative methods to treat patients. Preventive programs are also developed to maintain the health of the population. Unfortunately, in fee-for-service systems, preventive health programs are seldom funded because of the lack of financial incentives.

In a capitated system, the integration of different alternatives to hospitalization must be seamless. If a healthcare organization lacks a vital component and acquires the services from outside its network, its costs will dramatically increase. The commonly used alternatives to the acute-care hospital are skilled nursing facilities, subacute facilities, home healthcare, and rehabilitation services. Experience has shown that as the number of capitated payers increases, the organization's bottom line will erode quickly if costs are not significantly decreased and alternatives to hospitalization are not encouraged. Thus, integration of hospitals and care providers is the key to success in both managed care and capitated environments. In systems in which integration has not occurred, cost shifting will occur without any resulting reduction in total costs.

Additionally, one possible consequence of a capitated environment is underuse of resources (Kongstvedt, 1993). In an effort to decrease resource consumption, patients could possibly not receive adequate care, and quality of care could decline. However, well-coordinated outcomes assessment teams can alleviate this concern. As we confront the difficult decisions that may result from the rationing of care, clinicians are in a position to ensure quality yet cost-effective care.

An analysis of organizational market share and referring physicians' payer mixes will identify areas of risk with changes in the market. The geographic service area of an organization can be subdivided into four divisions: local, immediate, remote, and beyond remote. The *local* service area is within 30 minutes driving distance, whereas the *immediate* service area is within 60 minutes. Both of these areas would be at minimal risk if referring physicians' contracts were converted to managed care. However, *remote* (between 1 hour and 3 hours driving distance) and *beyond remote* (greater than 3 hours) would be at a greater risk if the referring organization were to have a large number of managed care contracts. The reason for this is that frequently a managed care contract will inhibit the authorization of referrals from a remote or beyond remote area unless no provider nearby has the necessary expertise, or unless the tertiary hospital to which patients are to be referred has a "carved-out" area of expertise, such as transplants, recognized by the specific payer (see Chap. 9 for a more detailed discussion of "carve-outs").

INFRASTRUCTURE OF COSTS

Before changes in reimbursement, in a predominantly fee-for-service environment, total hospital charges would be representative of the revenue. However, with commercial payers' negotiating a discount, an increasing number of managed care contracts, and changes in government reimbursement, the key number to review is net revenue. *Net revenue,* or *adjusted revenue,* is calculated by subtracting discounts from the total reimbursement. In some areas of the United States, discounts could be as high as 50% of total charges.

Costs can be classified using several different methodologies depending on a manager's perspective and needs. Service businesses such as hospitals have defined and categorized costs differently than manufacturing companies. Terms such as *cost of goods* and *conversion costs* found in manufacturing budgets are foreign to hospital balance sheets. Total costs can be divided into two categories: direct and indirect. *Direct costs* are traced to a specific test/exam or service provided to patients. Examples of direct costs are those associated with nursing hours, lab tests, and radiologic exams. Direct costs are considered to be controllable at the department manager level.

Conversely, *indirect costs* cannot be attributed to specific patient services. Indirect costs include administrative salaries and material management facilities. A specific type of indirect cost, classified as "allocated," is assigned using a type of base. The base used could be square footage, number of full-time equivalents, or hours of service. Costs such as payroll and electricity are assigned using one of these criteria. The indirect/direct cost ratio can be as high as 50%. Indirect costs are frequently viewed as uncontrollable costs at the department manager level.

At a higher level of management, all costs are controllable; the amount of control will vary based on the type of costs. Direct costs typically decrease at a steady rate. Indirect costs often decrease at a slower rate than direct costs; however, decreases in indirect costs are incrementally larger than decreases in direct costs. For example, if the entire payroll system were automated, allocated payroll costs would decrease in one large, single amount.

The next level of cost classification involves the behavior of costs in relationship to changes in workload level. *Variable costs,* the first classification of cost behavior, change proportionately as the number of patients increases or decreases. These costs include patient supplies such as linen. Figure 16-1 represents the linear relationship between variable costs and the volume of patients: as the number of patients increases, linen costs increase. *Fixed costs,* the second classification of cost behavior, remain constant as the number of patients increases or decreases. An example of fixed costs are administrative salaries. Figure 16-2 represents fixed costs in relation to volume of patients. *Mixed costs* are products of a combination of variable and fixed costs, such as labor costs associated with a nursing unit. Variable costs would be registered nurses' salaries, whereas a fixed cost would be the head nurse's salary. Most cost-accounting systems avoid the term *mixed costs* and attempt to differentiate between *fixed* and *variable.*

Overall, the majority of costs in a hospital can be divided into the following four categories for cost analysis:

1. variable direct labor (eg, nursing hours)
2. variable direct supplies (eg, pharmaceutical costs)
3. fixed direct labor (eg, head nurse salaries)
4. allocated (eg, administrative salaries)

Questions to ask when costs are submitted for analysis include

- Are the numbers inclusive of direct variable costs?
- What indirect costs are attached?
- What amount of allocated costs are included and what is the base assignment used?

Investigating the answers to these questions and examining trends of fixed, variable, and allocated costs will allow for major opportunities to quickly identify cost-containment initiatives. For example, practitioners may find that variable direct costs associated with cases grouped by a certain DRG have been steadily declining, whereas indirect costs have increased proportionately. The practitioners are able to demonstrate the effect on total cost of changes in practice and clinical resource use. In turn, the initial analysis indicates that administrative and other overhead costs have not been reduced in proportion to variable costs.

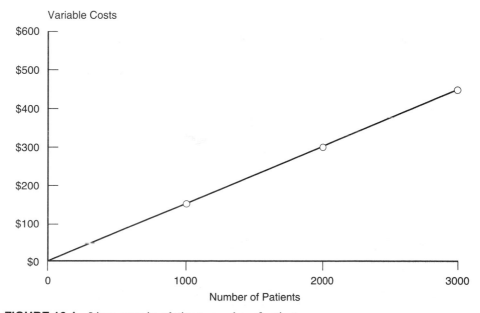

FIGURE 16-1 Linen costs in relation to number of patients.

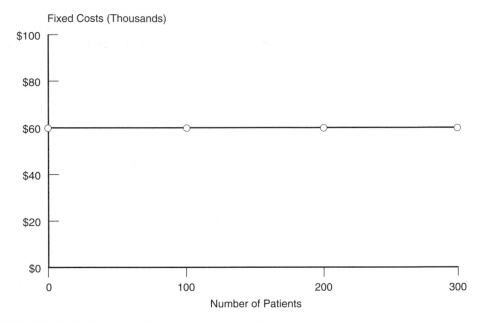

FIGURE 16-2   Fixed costs in relation to number of patients.

After net or adjusted revenue and total costs are determined, net margin can be calculated as follows:

Gross revenue	$ 1,000,000
Discount (25%)	− 250,00
Net revenue	$ 750,000
Net revenue	$ 750,000
Total costs	− 500,00
Net margin	$ 250,000

If a program is unable to generate a profit (ie, has a positive net margin) or is not, at minimum, at breakeven (ie, net revenue equals total cost), then the program is at future risk. If the program is central to the mission of the organization, then the revenue of the program may need to cover only the direct costs and not the indirect costs. The following example demonstrates a situation in which the revenue from the program covered the direct costs but was unable to cover the indirect costs without additional patient volume:

Net revenue	$ 750,000
Direct costs	− 500,00
	$ 250,000
Indirect costs	− 300,000
Loss	(50,000)

The *break-even point* is the number of services provided to patients at which adjusted revenue equals total costs (including direct, indirect, and allocated costs). Calculation of the break-even point allows the manager to determine the appropriate volume needed to support program costs. Additionally, it allows for forecasting the effect of changes in either volume or adjusted revenue on the net margin. The calculation is demonstrated as follows with regard to a radiology program with high fixed costs:

The net revenue of each radiologic exam is $400.
The variable cost of each exam is $100, but the fixed cost (machine cost) is $2,000,000.
The break-even point is 6666 exams.

$$400x = 100x + 2,000,000$$
$$300x = 2,000,000$$
$$x = 6666$$

Standard unit costs—predetermined expectations of costs (including labor and material) based on targets set by management—are developed to "benchmark"(ie, compare organization's costs against market norms). For example, if the standard unit cost of a urine test at Hospital A were $12.50 (including labor and materials), whereas it was only $10.00 at Hospital B, decreasing use of the test at Hospital A in cases grouped under a specific DRG would not necessarily affect the variable direct cost of the laboratory department for that DRG.

The budget for the following year can be forecast using the standard costs multiplied by the projected number of tests/exams and services to be provided. This budget allows the manager to track departmental productivity in relation to the targeted costs. For example, when indirect costs are eliminated in large increments, the standard costs will correspondingly decrease. Controlling costs in relation to the standard costs should be done at the department manager level, whereas clinical resource use analysis should be accomplished at the care provider level.

APPLICATION OF A COLLABORATIVE MODEL OF PRACTICE IN COST-CONTAINMENT INITIATIVES

As described in Chapter 10, "the purpose of collaboration among healthcare professionals is to enhance quality of care and improve patient outcomes that 'could not be offered in practices organized differently'" (Kitzman, 1986, p. 141). With the emergence of the joint-practice model of collaborative practice, the acute-care nurse practitioner (ACNP) and the physician "provide care to patients as a team" (Chap. 10, p. 154) and "the concept of interdependency is emphasized . . . with the complementary application of roles . . ." (Chap. 10, p. 155). Under this model, the ACNP's reporting relationship is "matrixed"—the ACNP is responsible to a physician director for patient outcomes relative to medical management of patients and responsible to a nursing director for issues relating to professional practice, program development, and system improvement.

Because the ACNP role in a joint-practice model at the University of Rochester/Strong Memorial Hospital has evolved into a nationally recognized prototype of advanced nursing practice, it is referenced in this chapter. The scope of practice and professional standards for the ACNP at that hospital are outlined in Table 10-1 as statements of practice responsibilities; performance criteria for the ACNP, presented in Table 10-2, reflect the standards of practice. The following sections consider five performance criteria (Table 16-1) and explore applications in operationalizing performance relative to cost-containment initiatives.

KEY DEFINITIONS ASSOCIATED WITH QUALITY MANAGEMENT AND OUTCOMES ASSESSMENT

Before beginning a discussion of cost-containment initiatives, the following terms should be defined. These definitions, which evolved in the 1980s and 1990s, have been published by The Joint Commission on Accreditation of Healthcare Organizations (JCAHO)(Davies, Thomas, Lansky, Rutt, Stevic, & Doyle, 1994; JCAHO, 1990) for consistency in interpretation. The JCAHO is a nationally recognized not-for-profit organization that surveys healthcare organizations on a 3-year cycle to determine voluntary adherence to preestablished standards.

TABLE 16-1 **Five Performance Criteria**

Professional Role	Performance Goal	Performance Criteria
Care delivery	Direct/indirect care	1. Delivers direct care and coordinates interdisciplinary care plan for patients, requires the expertise of an advanced practitioner.
	Consultation	2. Serves as consultant in improving patient care and nursing practice based on expertise in area of specialization.
Clinical Coordination	Quality improvement/ critical analysis	3. Identifies system-specific problems requiring evaluation or change.
		4. Provides direction for and participates in unit or service quality improvement programs.
		5. Evaluates the effect of changes in clinical practice and formulates recommendations regarding appropriateness and cost-effectiveness.

Source: see Chapter 10, Table 2.

- *Outcome:* the result of the performance (or nonperformance) of a process; a good outcome is a result that achieves the goal of the process (Davies et al., 1994, p. 7)

    A number of goals exist for the healthcare process. Many are directly related to a patient's health, for example, to avoid adverse effects of care such as return hospitalizations and secondary infections.

    Other goals for the healthcare process are not directly health related, for example, to minimize the cost of care by avoiding unnecessary diagnostic tests and treatments (Davies et al., 1994, pp. 7-8).
- *Outcome indicator:* an indicator that measures what happens (or does not happen) to a patient after a process is (or is not) performed (JCAHO, 1990, p. 112)
- *Outcomes measurement:* the systematic, quantitative observation of outcome indicators at a certain point in time (Davies et al., 1994, p. 9)
- *Outcomes monitoring:* the repeating measurement of outcome indicators over time in a manner that permits inferences about what produced the observed patient outcomes (eg, patient characteristics, care processes, or resources)(Davies et al., 1994, p. 9)
- *Outcomes management:* the use of information and knowledge gained from outcomes monitoring to achieve optimal patient outcomes through improved clinical decision making and service delivery (Davies et al., 1994, p. 9)
- *Outcomes assessment:* measurement, monitoring, and feedback of outcomes (Davies et al., 1994, p. 9)

    Managing outcomes is accomplished by managing the care process that generates the outcomes, which is primarily the domain of clinicians and the organizations in which they work. The job of an outcomes assessment team in outcomes management is to provide clinicians with useful, meaningful, accurate data and to help them interpret the data as they analyze and modify the care process (Davies et al., 1994, p. 9).
- *Continuous quality improvement (CQI):* an approach to quality management that builds on traditional quality assurance methods by emphasizing the organization and systems (rather than individuals), the need for objective data with which to analyze and improve processes, and the ideal that systems and performance can always improve even when high standards appear to have been met (JCAHO, 1990, p. 110)

- *Practice guideline:* descriptive tool or standardized specifications for care of the "typical" patient in the "typical" situation; developed by a formal process that incorporates the best scientific evidence of effectiveness with expert opinion; synonyms or near synonyms include *practice parameter, preferred practice pattern, algorithm, protocol,* and *clinical standard* (JCAHO, 1990, p. 113)
- *Comorbidity:* disease or condition present at the same time as the principal disease or condition of a patient (JCAHO, 1990, p. 109)
- *High-volume function:* a key function that is performed frequently or affects large numbers of patients (eg, diagnostic testing)(JCAHO, 1990, p. 111)
- *High-risk function:* a key function that exposes individual patients to a greater chance of adverse occurrences if not carried out effectively or appropriately; also applies to services that are inherently risky, even when effective and appropriate, because of certain patient attributes or newness of the services (JCAHO, 1990, p. 111)
- *Appropriateness of care:* the degree to which the correct care is provided, given current state-of-the-art knowledge (JCAHO, 1990, p. 109)
- *Timeliness of care:* the degree to which care is provided to patients when it is needed (JCAHO, 1990, p. 115)
- *Efficiency of care:* the degree to which the care received has the desired effect for which it is used (JCAHO, 1990, p. 110)
- *Effectiveness of care:* the degree to which care is provided in the correct manner, that is, without error, given current state-of-the-art knowledge (JCAHO, 1990, p. 110)
- *Efficacy of care:* the degree to which a service has the potential to meet the need for which it is used (JCAHO, 1990, p. 110)

    Clinical research historically has relied on the randomized controlled trial. This methodology can demonstrate the efficacy of treatment under ideal circumstances, but it cannot demonstrate effectiveness in routinely delivered care. Multisite observational studies have shown large variations in outcome between and within sites (Davies et al., 1994, p. 8).
- *Continuity of care:* the degree to which the care needed by the patient is coordinated among practitioners and across organizations and time (JCAHO, 1990, p. 109)

COST ACCOUNTING/DECISION SUPPORT SYSTEM AS A PRIMARY DATA SOURCE

This section familiarizes readers with the level of data sophistication available in many hospitals. Cost-accounting/decision support systems receive data from the hospital medical record system, the admission/discharge/transfer (ADT) patient tracking system, and patient accounting system. Patient demographic data, data elements required by payers on the UB-92 form, ICD-9-CM and procedure codes and CPT-4 procedure codes assigned after the patient is discharged, and any other data elements regularly abstracted by the medical record department staff are transferred to the cost accounting/decision support system. The *UB-92 form* is a uniform billing form that was updated in 1992 by the Health Care Financing Adminstration for billing 11 payers. *ICD-9-CM* refers to the *International Classification of Diseases, 9th Revision, Clinical Modification* (World Health Organization, 1979) and is a coding schematic required by the Medicare Catastrophic Coverage Act of 1988 for reporting inpatient/outpatient diagnoses and surgical procedures when billing government or private insurance carriers for reimbursement. *CPT-4* refers to Current Procedural Terminology, 4th Edition (American Medical Association, 1977) and is the most widely accepted nomenclature for the reporting of professional procedures and diagnostic services performed by physicians under government and private health insurance programs.

    In addition, volumes, costs, and charges associated with the hospital tests/exams and services for which the patient was billed during a hospital stay are also transferred. The data are usually available in the cost accounting/decision support system for report generation the month following the discharge date. Most systems have the capability to summarize the patient's billable hospital tests/exams and services by the day of stay, that is, hospital day 1, hospital day 2, and so forth, or by a portion of the stay (eg, preoperative period).

If the hospital has a patient severity system, a severity-of-illness score for each patient's hospitalization is also transferred to the cost accounting/decision support system. A severity score is assigned to a patient's hospital stay based on factors such as age, principal diagnoses, comorbidities, complications, and surgical procedures. Severity scores can explain differences in the use of ancillary hospital services in cases in which there are similar diagnoses and procedures.

Data Quality Control

The integrity of the data in the cost accounting/decision support system is the same as its integrity in the system from which it originated. As part of a hospital's continuous quality improvement program, there are data quality control checks incorporated in daily tasks to ensure levels of data completeness and accuracy. For example, in one hospital, peer cross-checking is done by the admissions department staff on a sample of data entries on each shift. The medical record department coding supervisor regularly assesses the accuracy of ICD-9-CM and CPT-4 coding on a representative sample of cases and provides feedback to staff as needed. Likewise, supervisory staff on nursing units and in hospital departments monitor the completeness and accuracy of charges entered on the computer; staff compare computer data entry with entries made in medical records and in department logs.

Resources for Data Access, Analysis, and Interpretation

The data dictionary of the cost accounting/decision support system serves as a guide to the data elements, their definitions, and the source of data entry. Likewise, the cost structure for each patient billable test/exam or service, that is, indirect, direct fixed, and direct variable, can be readily referenced by the cost center (or hospital ancillary department).

In many hospitals, the finance department is the owner of the cost accounting/decision support system and the outcomes assessment staff are active users of the system; in other hospitals, the system is co-owned by the finance department and the outcomes assessment department. In either scenario, the respective departments become the focal resources for data access, analysis, and interpretation. Their participation on teams that undertake outcomes assessment projects is important.

IMPLEMENTATION OF A COST-CONTAINMENT INITIATIVE AS AN OUTCOMES ASSESSMENT PROJECT

An outcomes assessment project can be characterized in terms of a series of seven steps to be accomplished:
1. Identify a DRG or a group of diagnoses or procedures to investigate.
2. Assemble a team.
3. Refine the field of interpretation, transform the data into information, and interpret the information.
4. Statistically manipulate the data.
5. Provide feedback.
6. Develop cost-effective algorithms.
7. Apply the algorithms.

Because the intent of this chapter is to provide a framework for analysis, templates for a logical progression of analysis are provided in a detailed discussion of step 3, refine the field of interpretation, transform the data into information, and interpret the information. The templates offer a consistent methodology for analysis in cost-containment initiatives; the template subjects are as follows:

- review of average lengths of stay and cost trends over time
- payers
- geographic service areas
- medical staff services and departments
- nursing unit locations during the hospital stay
- principal diagnoses and associated secondary diagnoses
- principal diagnoses and associated principal and secondary procedures
- continuity of care (eg, admission sources and discharge dispositions)
- costs associated with hospital department resources received by patients
- costs associated with specific clinical resources received by patients (eg, tests, exams, or drugs).

Identify a Diagnosis-Related Group or a Group of Diagnoses or Procedures to Investigate

The first step in a new outcomes assessment project is to decide which DRG or groups of diagnoses or procedures to study. One academic hospital (we will refer to it as University Medical Center) took a top-down strategic approach by identifying DRGs that had the most negative net margins during the previous 12-month period. Diagnosis-related groups with negative net margins were further subdivided by the organizational structure of the hospital, that is, vertically by the departments of medicine and surgery, respectively, and horizontally by service lines such as cardiovascular, oncology, neurology/orthopedics/rehabilitation, digestive, children's services, and women's services. The hospital then benchmarked the average lengths of stay of cases by DRG with those of other hospitals of the same type (academic versus community) and of the same size in terms of the number of discharges per fiscal period. Opportunities for reduction in patient days were next calculated by DRG; in turn, the hospital projected dollar savings associated with the reduction in patient days. Selection of DRGs to study were made based on opportunities for patient day reduction, associated savings, and the number of cases per annum expected to be affected. The analysis was segmented in line with the organizational structure; therefore, the data could be readily reviewed with administrative and medical staff leadership responsible for each area.

Benchmark data can be obtained from other hospitals, acquired from state agencies, and purchased through membership in organizations such as University Hospitals Consortium. Typically, benchmark data are available at the DRG level. Whereas charge data are in the public domain, cost data are less frequently shared because of the sensitivity of internal cost accounting methodologies. Data that are dated within 1 year of the current year are the most relevant for comparison purposes and the most challenging to acquire.

Assemble a Team

The earliest course of development of a project is usually cooperatively set by a physician project champion, a hospital administration representative, a member of the outcomes/decision support staff, and members of the involved clinical department. The clinicians "own" the project, and hospital administration and the director of the outcomes/decision support staff provide necessary management services for the project.

A critical role is that of project coordinator. The person who serves in this role is typically a member of the outcomes/decision support staff or can be a member of the clinical department. An ACNP can fill this role after having gained experience as a participant in several teams. The project coordinator brings together all the skills and resources needed to carry out a project. Working with the physician project champion, a project coordinator should possess the characteristics of a change agent who communicates, solves problems, innovates, and champions the larger agenda. Of particular importance are interpersonal skills; contact with individuals throughout the institution often requires considerable sensitivity to competing professional and personal agendas as well as the ability to avert possible conflicts in a nonadversarial manner (Davies et al., 1994). The comprehensive role of project coordinator offers a challenging application of the three ACNP performance criteria for the professional role of clinical coordination and the performance goal of quality improvement/critical analysis (see Table 16-1).

Refine the Field of Interpretation, Transform the Data into Information, and Interpret the Information

After DRGs or a group of diagnoses or procedures is selected, several templates of analysis can be applied to expedite the assessment process. As is demonstrated with the following applications, areas for more in-depth investigation can be readily identified.

Comparison of Average Length-of-Stay and Cost Trends

Comparison of average length-of-stay and cost trends involves a comparison of the previous 3 years with the current year, depending on data availability. Subject to comparison are the annual number of cases; the annual average lengths of stay; the annual total, indirect, direct fixed, and direct variable costs on a per case and per day basis; and the annual net revenue and net margin on a per case and per day basis.

Relative changes in total days of stay need to be considered in carrying out this analysis. (*Total days of stay* is the sum of the lengths of stay of the cases in a population in a given period.) Increases in cost per day become apparent from year to year when there appears to be a decrease in cost per case. Likewise, the percentage of change in cost per day can be greater or less incrementally from year to year compared with cost per case.

As indicated in the length-of-stay and cost trend summary for a DRG in the digestive service line, there was an 11.05% decrease in total cost per case, whereas there was a 6.02% increase in total cost per day from fiscal year 1993 to 1994. The difference in the percentage of change between total cost per case and total cost per day can be attributed, in part, to the drop in average length of stay of 1 full day (Table 16-2). The percentage of decrease in total cost per day is larger than the percentage of decrease in total cost per case from fiscal year 1991 to 1992. This can be explained by the 87.96% increase in total patient days from 1991 to 1992; both an increase in total cases and lengths of stay (ie, total days of stay) are to be recognized.

Note that costs are concentrated or spread across lengths of the hospitalizations in calculating cost per day. When there is a high frequency of either extremely short or long lengths of stay, increases or decreases in cost per day from year to year should be interpreted in terms of the corresponding decreases or increases in total days of stay.

TABLE 16-2   **Comparison of Average Lengths-of-Stay and Total Cost Trends for a DRG in the Digestive Service Line, 1991–1994**

Fiscal Year	Total Cases	Total Days	Average Length of Stay	Total Cost per Case ($)	% Change Preceding Year	Total Cost per Day ($)	% Change Preceding Year
1991	89	565	6.3	6846		1078	
1992	154	1062	6.9	6576	– 3.94	954	– 11.50
1993	181	1101	6.1	7377	12.18	1213	27.15
1994	195	995	5.1	6562	– 11.05	1286	6.02

Increases or decreases in total costs can be proportionately related to increases or decreases in either indirect or direct costs; however, there is often a combination of changes in both indirect and direct costs that affect the total cost figure. As can be seen in Table 16-3, the 11.05% decrease in total cost per case from 1993 to 1994 for the DRG was primarily related to the 19.78% decrease in direct variable cost per case, although the 2.74% decrease in indirect cost per case also had an effect. There were increases in all cost categories on both a per case and a per day basis from 1992 to 1993, most significantly with respect to direct fixed costs. Although direct variable costs decreased from 1993 to 1994, direct fixed costs continued to rise (Table 16-4).

Changes in direct variable costs are under the control of clinicians with respect to the volumes of tests/exams and services ordered. Changes in indirect costs and direct fixed costs, in terms of labor, supplies, and other resources needed to deliver the tests/exams and services, are under the control of hospital administrative and managerial staff. Therefore, the outcomes assessment team submitted the findings to the administrative director of the digestive service line and senior management.

To assist the outcomes assessment team in carrying out the analysis, bar charts of the length-of-stay and cost parameters were drawn to visually depict the changes over time. Figure 16-3 is a bar chart of the changes in average lengths of stay from fiscal year 1991 through 1994 for University Medical Center. The figure also illustrates target average lengths of stay using benchmark average lengths of stay for the DRG for 1993 and 1994, respectively, from a midwestern hospital and from a west coast hospital.

Payer Analysis of the Current Year

A payer analysis of the current year compares the number of cases, average lengths of stay, total cost, net revenue, and net margin per case and per day for each major payer. A pie chart of the percentage of cases by major payers in conjunction with bar charts of net margin (per case and per day, respectively) for each payer provide for a quick analysis of the payer mix by the outcomes assessment team. Figure 16-4 is a pie chart of the percentage of cases by payer; Figure 16-5 is a bar chart of net margin per case for each payer. The selected cases were grouped by a DRG and were only those patients admitted or discharged by physicians in the department of medicine at University Medical Center.

Many of the patients (48.9%) were covered by Medicare; moreover, net margin per case, –$2961, and net margin per day, –$1,733, were lowest for patients covered by Medicare (see Figs. 16-4, and Table 16-5). Although net margins were also negative for patients under managed care plans and who paid their own bills, these patients represented less than 1% of the total cases, respectively. However, with the percentage of cases under managed care plans expected to increase dramatically in the near term, the overall net margin per case is expected to

TABLE 16-3 **Comparison of Cost Trends Per Case for a DRG in the Digestive Service Line, 1991–1994**

Fiscal Year	Total Cost per Case ($)	% Change from Preceding Year	Indirect Cost per Case ($)	% Change from Preceding Year	Direct Fixed Cost per Case ($)	% Change from Preceding Year	Direct Variable Cost per Case ($)	% Change from Preceding Year
1991	6846		2473		391		3982	
1992	6576	– 3.94	2345	– 5.18	438	12.02	3793	– 4.75
1993	7377	12.18	2592	10.53	756	72.60	4029	6.22
1994	6562	– 11.05	2521	– 2.74	810	7.14	3232	– 19.78

TABLE 16-4 **Comparison of Cost Trends Per Day for a DRG in the Digestive Service Line, 1991–1994**

Fiscal Year	Total Cost per Day ($)	% Change from Preceding Year	Indirect Cost per Day ($)	% Change from Preceding Year	Direct Fixed Cost per Day ($)	% Change from Preceding Year	Direct Variable Cost per Day ($)	% Change from Preceding Year
1991	1078		390		62		627	
1992	954	– 11.50	340	– 12.82	64	3.23	550	– 12.28
1993	1213	27.15	426	25.29	124	93.75	662	20.36
1994	1286	6.02	494	15.96	159	28.23	633	– 4.38

drop below the current figure of -$734. Changes in net margin for the DRG can be forecast based on differences in the net margin for cases currently under managed care plans and in net margins for commercial Blue Cross/Blue Shield and other commercial payers.

Net margin per day by major payer should also be considered because the number of cases or average length of stay of cases covered by specific payers may be extremely low or high. Moreover, when evaluating the effect of the shift in care setting from inpatient to outpatient, net margin per day by payer is used. For example, for a certain DRG, there is a shift in se-

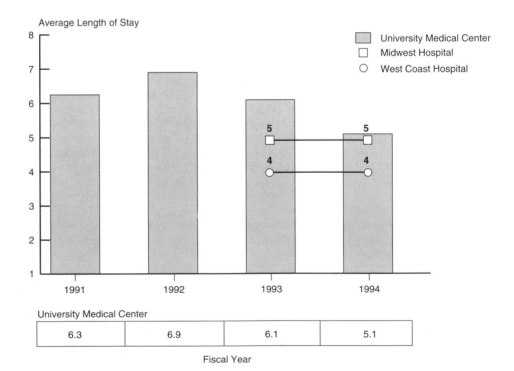

FIGURE 16-3 DRG XXX: DRG description, fiscal years 1991-1994, University Medical Center, Digestive Services: Average length of stay.

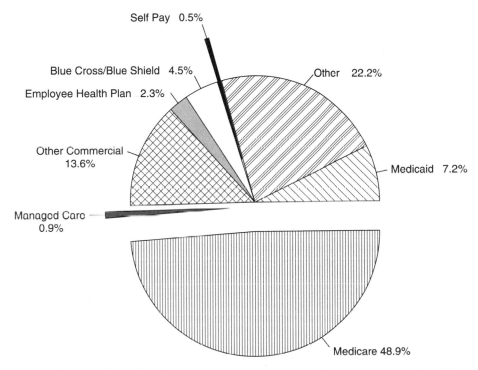

FIGURE 16-4 DRG XXX: DRG description, fiscal year 1994, University Medical Center, Department of Medicine: Percentage of cases by payer.

quencing when comparing the ranking of payers from lowest to highest net margin per case to the ranking of payers from lowest to highest net margin per day. The overall net margin per day is $308 and that net margin per day for patients covered by Medicaid is $235 (Table 16-5).

With the knowledge of changes in reimbursement for a certain DRG (or a group of diagnoses or procedures) based on recently signed managed care contracts or forthcoming changes in reimbursement structures set by the federal government or state agencies, the payer mix analysis provides information for forecasting the cumulative effect on the net margin before the changes in reimbursement are instituted. For example, when the Medicaid reimbursement structure for psychiatric cases changed from a per diem rate to a per case rate, changes in net margin could be predicted for high-volume diagnoses (eg, patients with depressive disorders) for patients who do or do not undergo specific high-risk procedures (eg, such as electroconvulsive therapy). Further analysis was conducted to determine changes in net margin by age ranges. In addition, the continued economic viability of inpatient as opposed to outpatient management was evaluated.

Geographic Service Area Analysis

A geographic service area analysis of the current year involves a comparison of the number of cases, total cost, net revenue, and net margin per case and per day for each defined geographic service area. Patient source locations with respect to market analysis, new program feasibility analysis, and established program continued viability analysis were addressed earlier. There are

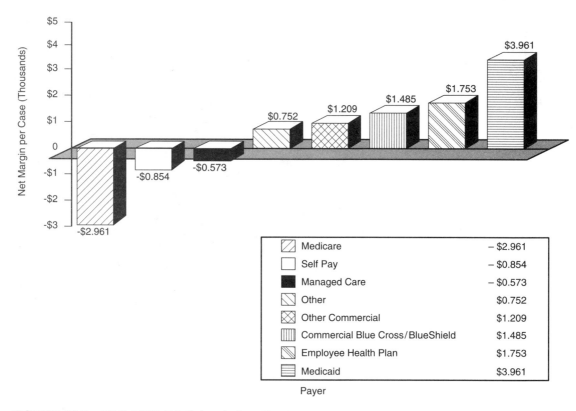

FIGURE 16-5 DRG XXX: DRG description, fiscal year 1994, University Medical Center, Department of Medicine: Net margin per case for each payer.

generic steps in evaluating the profitability of managing cases from different geographic service areas. Similar to the payer analysis, a pie chart of the percentage of cases by geographic service area in conjunction with bar charts of net margin (per case and per day, respectively) for each geographic service area can assist an outcomes assessment team in carrying out their evaluation.

In assessing the economic effect on transferring a major portion of business associated with a DRG of the oncology service line from inpatient to outpatient, University Medical Center determined the percentage of patients who traveled a driving distance of more than 3 hours. Figure 16-6 demonstrates that 18% of the patients either commuted from more than 3 hours away in the state (14%) or from outside of the state (4%). In addition, net margin per case and per day were ascertained for each geographic service area. Figure 16-7 indicates that it was not profitable for the hospital to manage these patients. It can be surmised that overall net margin for the DRG may increase should business patient be converted to the outpatient arena.

Net margin per day by geographic service area is used when forecasting the effect of the shift in care setting from inpatient to outpatient because patients will be managed on this basis. Table 16-6 shows shifts in sequencing when comparing the ranking of geographic service areas from lowest to highest net margin per case with lowest to highest net margin per day.

TABLE 16-5 Comparison of Net Margin Per Case and Net Margin Per Day for a DRG

Rank	Payers	Net Margin per Case	Rank	Payers	Net Margin per Day
Lowest net margin per case			*Lowest net margin per day*		
	Medicare	–$2.961		Medicare	–$175
	Self pay	–$824		Managed care	–$57
	Managed care	–$573		Self pay	–$52
	Other	$752		Other	$48
	Other commercial	$1209		Other commercial	$73
	Commercial Blue Cross/Blue Shield	$1485		Commercial Blue Cross/Blue Shield	$103
	Employee health plan	$1753		Employee health plan	$133
Highest net margin per case	Medicaid	$3961	*Highest net margin per day*	Medicaid	$235

Medical Staff Services and Departments of Physicians Admitting or Discharging Cases

To determine differences in practice patterns, it becomes necessary to focus assessment of a DRG on patient management by certain medical staff services or departments of physicians who admitted or discharged the cases under study. Such an assessment examines the number of cases, average lengths of stay, and total cost per case and per day by medical staff service or department. For example, at University Medical Center, the majority of cases in a DRG in the digestive service line were admitted or discharged by physicians in the department of med-

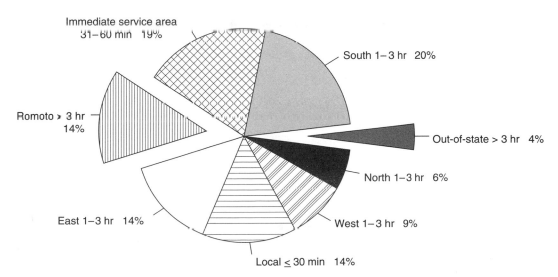

FIGURE 16-6 DRG XXX: DRG description, fiscal year 1994, University Medical Center, Department of Medicine: Percentage of cases by geographic service area.

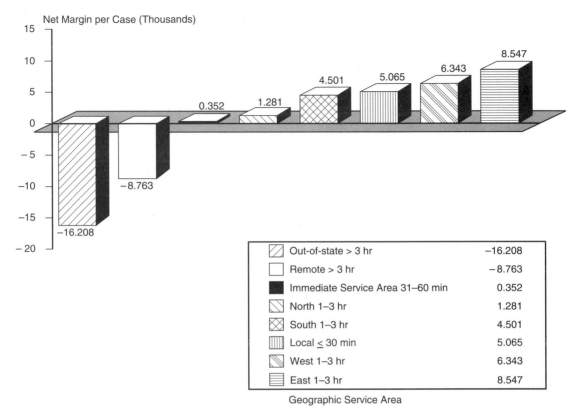

FIGURE 16-7 DRG XXX: DRG description, fiscal year 1994, University Medical Center, Department of Medicine: Net margin per case by geographic service area.

icine. As expected, the medicine and gastroenterology services managed the majority of patients admitted or discharged by the department of medicine (Fig. 16-8).

The length-of-stay and cost parameters can be further evaluated with respect to individual physicians who admitted, discharged, or were the attending physicians on the cases under study. The other parameters and variables described in the remaining sections can also be analyzed in terms of individual physicians who managed the cases.

Nursing Unit Locations

In an analysis of nursing unit locations during hospital stay, case selection is based on any one of the nursing units a patient was on during a hospitalization. In addition, data are summarized for the entire hospital stay.

At University Medical Center, the medical director of the pediatric intensive care unit was the physician champion of an outcomes assessment team whose objective was to understand the reasons for negative net margins associated with pediatric cases grouped under certain DRGs. Of particular interest was a subset of DRGs in which the majority of patients spent a significant portion of their hospital stay on the pediatric intensive care unit.

The two DRGs selected for evaluation had relatively higher volumes of cases compared with other DRGs grouping pediatric cases with negative net margins. It was decided to study the DRGs in tandem because patients grouped under the respective DRGs are managed on ventilators during their stays—a high-cost and high-risk mode of treatment.

TABLE 16-6   **Net Margin Per Case and Per Day by Geographic Service Area for a DRG in the Oncology Service Line**

Rank	Geographic Service Area	Net Margin per Case	Rank	Geographic Service Area	Net Margin per Day
Lowest net margin per case			*Lowest net margin per day*		
	Out-of-state	−$16,208		Out-of-state	−$715
	Remote > 3 h	−$8,763		Remote > 3 h	−$458
	Immediate service area 31–60 min	$352		Immediate service area 31 60 min	$19
	North, 1–3 h	$1281		North, 1–3 h	$70
	South, 1 3 h	$4501		South, 1–3 h	$198
	Local, ≤ 30 min	$5065		Local, ≤ 30 min	$268
	West, 1–3 h	$6343		West, 1–3 h	$326
Highest net margin per case	East, 1–3 h	$8547	*Highest net margin per day*	East, 1–3 h	$629

As part of the assessment process, benchmark average lengths of stay of the respective DRGs were referenced. Although the average length of stay for one of the DRGs was in line with the benchmarks, the average length of stay for the second DRG was almost twice that of one of the benchmarked institutions. Because there was a clear opportunity to investigate extended lengths of stay in cases grouped under the second DRG, the outcomes assessment team also analyzed hospital ancillary department utilization patterns. Practice patterns in terms of clinical resource utilization should always be evaluated in concert with length-of-stay patterns because even if there are reductions in length of stay, the same utilization practices and related costs may be condensed into a shorter time period.

Hospital ancillary department utilization per day as percentages of total cost per day is shown in a pie chart for each DRG, respectively, in Figure 16-9. Per day utilization was chosen for comparison because of the significant difference in average lengths of stay for the DRGs. Interestingly, the percentages of consumption were found to be within 5 percentage points for each hospital ancillary department. Commensurately, as can be seen in Figure 16-10, there was at most a $38 per day difference when reviewing the dollar amounts related to use of services, except when comparing costs associated with emergency room and transportation to the medical center.

Next steps include identification of any differences in use of specific clinical resources (eg, tests/exams or drugs). If the hospital had a patient severity system, cases could be selected with respect to severity-of-illness scores to relate clinical resource use type and frequency to comorbidities and complications. An analysis would first be conducted at the aggregate level. Attending physician practice patterns would then be compared. A final analysis could be carried out at the individual case level. Examples of more in-depth analyses follow.

Principal Diagnoses and Associated Secondary Diagnoses That Make Up a Diagnosis-Related Group

Carrying out a detailed analysis of a DRG often requires breaking down the DRG and identifying the high-volume principal diagnoses managed at the institution that compose the DRG.

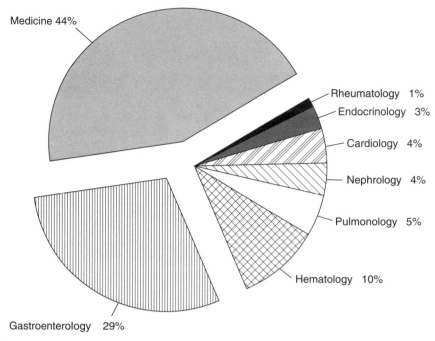

Medicine 44%

Rheumatology 1%

Endocrinology 3%

Cardiology 4%

Nephrology 4%

Pulmonology 5%

Hematology 10%

Gastroenterology 29%

FIGURE 16-8 DRG XXX: DRG description, fiscal year 1994, University Medical Center, Department of Medicine: Percentage of cases by discharge service.

There are other times when the analysis of clinical resource use can only be meaningful if it is done at the diagnosis level.

This analysis considers the number of cases, average lengths of stay, and total cost per case and per day for cases discharged with each secondary diagnosis. Parameters are summarized at the principal diagnosis level. For example, the principal diagnoses rolled up into the DRG in the digestive service line were too broad in scope for evaluation at the DRG level to be meaningful. Therefore, analysis of use of drugs, lab tests, and radiologic exams was focused by capturing the hospital ancillary service data by the groups of diagnoses in Table 16-7.

On the other hand, a DRG may not capture the entire patient population that should be considered in assessing the continuity of care provided to a group of patients. For example, on review of the return hospitalizations of patients in DRG 473: Acute Leukemia Without Major OR Procedure, Age Greater Than 17, patients were found to return with a secondary diagnosis of acute leukemia. (A principal diagnosis of acute leukemia directs cases into DRG 473.) The outcomes assessment team concurred that patients with either a principal or secondary diagnosis of acute leukemia defined the population more completely. At the particular medical center, these cases rolled up into 21 different DRGs, but primarily into DRGs 492, 473, and 398; the cases represented only percentages of total cases grouped under the respective DRGs.

Principal and Secondary Procedures Associated With Each Principal Diagnosis That Make Up a Diagnosis-Related Group

This analysis examines principal and secondary procedures associated with each principal diagnosis that compose a DRG. The analysis considers the number of cases, average lengths of stay,

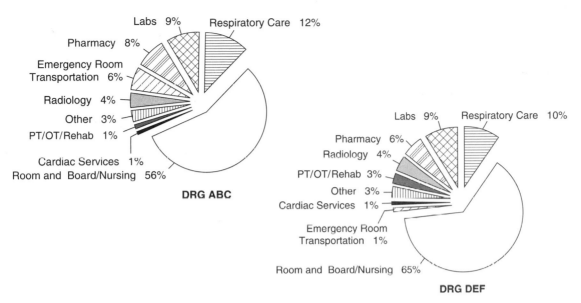

FIGURE 16-9 Hospital ancillary department utilization, University Medical Center: Percentage of total cost per day of hospital ancillary service department utilization for patients who spent part of their hospital stay in the pediatric intensive care unit in fiscal year 1994.

and total cost per case and per day for cases discharged with each secondary procedure. Parameters are summarized at principal procedure level and then at the principal diagnosis level.

For example, psychiatric patients aged 65 years or older who had a depressive disorder were found to have longer lengths of stay when they underwent electroshock therapy or had certain secondary diagnoses, namely, non–insulin dependent diabetes (type II diabetes), atrial fibrillation, and urinary tract infections. To learn if length of stay could be predicted in terms of variables such as age, admission source, discharge disposition, specific "medical" or "psychiatric" secondary diagnoses, or the number of hospital days between the date of admission and the date of the first electroshock therapy treatment, the outcomes assessment team asked that a multiple regression (ie, a multifactorial analysis with two or more predictors) be performed. The data obtained for the analysis were on an individual case basis. (Interpretation of a regression analysis is discussed in the section Statistically Manipulate the Data: Test of Prediction.)

A different approach was undertaken by another outcomes assessment team. The team identified cases of patients discharged with a principal diagnosis of either gastric ulcer or duodenal ulcer with hemorrhage who had comorbidities or underwent procedures unrelated to the principal reason for the hospitalization. This subset of patients was likely to have interventions that could extend their lengths of stay. Differences in procedures performed and differences in the use of clinical resources in the remaining cases were then reviewed as being specific to the diagnosis and management of a gastric or duodenal ulcer with hemorrhage. Algorithms of "best practices" could be developed based on an analysis of this more homogenous sample of cases.

Continuity of Care Analysis

Continuity of care analysis is conducted in terms of admission sources and discharge dispositions. This analysis considers the locations from which patients were admitted or to which patients were discharged (eg, home without home healthcare, home with home healthcare, a nursing home, or a skilled nursing facility).

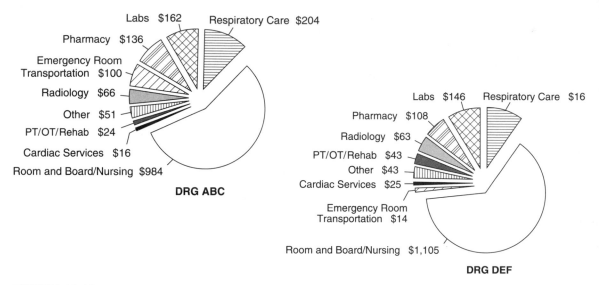

FIGURE 16-10 Hospital ancillary department utilization, University Medical Center: Hospital ancillary service departmental total cost per day for patients who spent part of their hospital stay in the pediatric intensive care unit in fiscal year 1994.

Sources of admission and discharge dispositions of psychiatric patients aged 65 years and older who had a mood disorder, for example, were determined. Lengths of stay for cases discharged to nursing homes, skilled nursing facilities, and other acute-care facilities were only somewhat longer than for patients discharged to their homes. Admission source and discharge disposition were variables that were included in the multiple regression run to predict influence on length of stay.

Issues concerning continuity of care were readily apparent to another outcomes assessment team on review of readmitted cases grouped under DRG 127: Congestive Heart Failure. The number of patients returning through the emergency room was higher than expected. On the other hand, the number of patients admitted without prior use of home healthcare services was lower than expected. The outcomes assessment team recognized the need for:

- enhanced patient/family education for postdischarge, including a patient education video and specific information on congestive heart failure in a take-home handbook
- development of clinical guidelines for discharge and referral to a subacute-care facility versus a nursing home or a skilled nursing facility
- intensified case management guidelines for the timely identification of patient candidates for discharge home with home health services.

As the project coordinator or as a member of an outcomes assessment team, the ACNP can play a critical role in identifying concerns and recommending remedial action plans.

Costs Associated With Hospital Ancillary Department Services

The costs associated with hospital ancillary department services received by patients are summarized by medical staff services of physicians who admitted or discharged the patients. The analysis considers total cost per case and per day of patient consumption of the named hospital ancillary department services. Use of the named hospital ancillary departments is attributed to management by medical staff services who admitted or discharged the patients and is totaled for all medical staff services.

TABLE 16-7 **Breakdown of Cases and Total Cost for a DRG in the Digestive Service Line Into Meaningful Groups of Principal Diagnoses**

ICD-9-CM Codes: Principal Diagnoses	ICD-9-CM Descriptions: Principal Diagnoses	% of Total Cases	% of Total Cost
531.40	Chronic stomach ulcer with hemorrhage		
531.41	Chronic stomach ulcer with hemorrhage & obstruction	27	17
532.40	Chronic duodenal ulcer with hemorrhage, w/o obstruction		
578.0	Hematemesis		
578.1	Blood in stool	27	14
578.9	GI hemorrhage, unspecified		
537.83	Angiodysplasia of stomach & duodenum with hemorrhage	12	11
569.85	Bowel angiodysplasia & hemorrhage		
562.12	Diverticulosis of colon with hemorrhage	11	12
562.13	Diverticulitis of colon with hemorrhage		
535.01	Acute gastritis with hemorrhage		
535.31	Alcoholic gastritis with hemorrhage		
535.41	Other specific gastritis with hemorrhage	8	17
535.51	Unspecified gastritis or duodenitis with hemorrhage		
535.61	Duodenitis with hemorrhage		
456.0	Esophageal varices with bleeding		
530.7	Gastroesophageal laceration hemorrhage syndrome	5	15
530.82	Esophageal hemorrhage		
531.00	Acute gastric ulcer with hemorrhage, w/o obstruction	3	9
532.00	Acute duodenal ulcer with hemorrhage, w/o obstruction		
531.60	Chronic gastric ulcer with hemorrhage & perforation	1	5
532.60	Chronic duodenal ulcer with hemorrhage & perforation		

GI, gastrointestinal; w/o, without.

For a DRG or a group of diagnoses or procedures under study, pie charts displaying percentages of the overall total cost per case and percentages of the overall total cost per day, respectively, that use of each hospital ancillary department represents, assist an outcomes assessment team in readily seeing the relative differences in clinical resource consumption across departments. In Figure 16-9, pie charts of cases in two different DRGs were displayed for comparison of hospital ancillary department consumption per day as percentages of the overall total cost per day for each DRG. The selected cases were admitted or discharged by all medical staff services of the pediatrics department. Per day use was chosen for comparison due to the significant difference in average lengths of stay for the DRGs.

Similarly, pie charts of hospital ancillary department consumption per day as percentages of the overall total cost per day can be compared in cases grouped by the previously listed diagnostic categories that compose a DRG in the digestive service line. Hospital ancillary department use could be attributed to each of the medical staff services of the department of medicine that admitted or discharged the patients. Percentages of the overall cost per case (and per day) are frequently the highest for services consumed from the laboratory, pharmacy, and radiology departments after those for room and board and nursing services.

Costs Associated With Specific Clinical Resources

This analysis addresses the costs associated with specific clinical resources received by patients (eg, tests/exams or drugs). A detailed listing of hospital ancillary services billable to the patient by charge code is summarized by hospital department. The number and percentage of cases that consumed the test/exam or service, the quantity of the test/exam or service consumed per case and per day, and the direct variable cost of the test/exam or service per case and per day are denoted.

The 80:20 rule, often referenced in cost accounting applications, implies that usage of 20% of tests/exams and services results in 80% of direct variable costs. With this rule in mind, a statistical process control (SPC) framework can be considered in initiating an analysis of patterns of the use of specific clinical resources received by patients. One test for detecting special causes in variation with statistical process control identifies a pattern of "behavior" that is greater than three standard deviations above or below the average or mean "behavior." The occurrence of this pattern suggests a special cause—one that should be investigated. With regard to clinical resource use, when the percentage of cases that consume a specific test/exam or service is more than three standard deviations above or below the average percentage of use of hospital ancillary department services by the cases under study, the utilization pattern should be investigated. Likewise, when the quantity of the specific test/exam or service consumed per case or per day is three standard deviations above or below the average consumption per case or per day of services of that hospital ancillary department, the utilization pattern should be investigated. Investigation can be prioritized in terms of the direct variable cost of the test/exam or service.

Overuse can result from standing orders. When outcomes assessment teams continue to identify such causes, centralized monitoring programs established as part of the hospital's continuous quality improvement program can collectively summarize the findings and offer recommendations for hospital-wide implementation. Centralized monitoring programs include medical staff committees such as a pharmacy and therapeutics committee that oversees drug use evaluation and infection surveillance and control.

Obviously, use patterns of specific tests/exams or services that are between two and three standard deviations above the mean usage of services of a hospital ancillary department may warrant investigation. Identifying overuse patterns within these parameters requires clinician input. Outcomes assessment teams have sought the expertise of medical directors of laboratory services and radiology services, respectively, in assessing use patterns and in algorithm development.

Isolated instances of inappropriate use can be identified on evaluation of the aggregate data. For example, on review of respiratory therapy use for cases in DRG 014: Specific Cerebrovascular Disorders Except Transient Ischemic Attack admitted or discharged by the neurology service of the department of medicine, supplemental oxygen therapy was found to have been administered in approximately one third of the cases. In some cases, oxygen therapy was started in the emergency room. The outcomes assessment team led by a physician champion of the neurology service recommended that oxygen therapy not be routinely used in an acute stroke patient unless the patient had evidence of hypoxia or another medical condition that requires supplemental oxygen. A memorandum was sent to the neurology staff and emergency department staff. In addition, the team's findings and recommendation were presented, discussed, and accepted in bimonthly meetings attended by the neurology and emergency staff and residents. Follow-up monitoring will be conducted on a quarterly basis to ascertain any changes in practice.

Redundancy in the use of radiologic exams was suspected by the same outcomes assessment team on review of the aggregate data delineating consumption of radiology department services by cases in DRG 014: Specific Cerebrovascular Disorders Except Transient Ischemic Attack. An analysis of billable charge codes, which indicate consumption of radiologic exams by individual patients, revealed that 30% of the patients underwent both magnetic resonance imaging of the head and computerized tomography of the brain. The outcomes assessment team led by a physician champion of the neurology service reviewed cases with emergency department physicians. They concurred that some patients will require an emergent head computerized tomography scan when admitted during the night to rule out cerebral hemorrhage, subdural hematoma, and other entities. However, they agreed that a stable patient with either a stroke or transient ischemic attack could be admitted and undergo magnetic resonance imaging the next morning. The team requested assistance from the medical and administrative directors of radiology services to prioritize scheduling for brain magnetic resonance imaging for these patients.

Likewise, use of specific drugs in cases in DRG 127: Congestive Heart Failure, in which physician 1 was the attending physician, was compared with use by other physicians of the same medical staff service Use was compared in terms of percentages of total patients managed who received the specific drug and the average quantities of the drug received. The severity-of-illness scores of patients managed by physician 1 were almost identical to the severity-of-illness scores of patients managed by the peer group. (Table 16-8).

After reviewing detailed charge-level data, outcomes assessment teams are in a position to recommend action plans. Physician-specific data are referred to chairpeople of medical staff departments for discretionary follow through. In this case, continuing education for physician 1 may be recommended. Another recommendation may involve revision of standing orders. Follow-up monitoring of individual practice patterns can also be done on a regular basis, as requested by medical staff department chairpeople.

Statistically Manipulate the Data

A common-language outline of frequently used statistical manipulations is presented to facilitate an understanding of how data are transformed into information.

Test of Relationship

The *chi-square test* can detect differences in absolute counts of events. The test compares the frequency of an observed occurrence with the frequency of an expected occurrence (based on previous as well as concurrent experience) and assesses whether the observed and expected occurrences are or are not different (Kazandjian, 1991). However, it compares counts and not

TABLE 16-8   **Use of Drugs for Patients Diagnosed With Congestive Heart Failure**

| Pharmaceutical | % of Cases in Which Patients Received Pharmaceutical | | Quantity per Case | | |
	Physician 1	Average for Comparison Group	Physician 1	Average for Comparison Group	Difference
Cefotaxime, 1 gram injection	7	7	29	15	+14
Heparin, 10,000 units/ml	7	3	19	4	+15
Meperidine, 25 mg injection	7	3	39	6	+33
Albuterol inhalant, 3 ml unit dose	47	17	32	23	19
Alprazolam, 0.25 mg tablet	7	12	26	9	+17

Source: Whitmore, B.C. (1994). Using refined DRGS in resource management initiatives. The Quality Resource: The Newsletter of the Quality Assurance Section of the American Health Management Association, 12(5), p. 4.

rates, proportions, or percentages. The chi-square test can be performed on small numbers in both the observed and the expected; often, statistical tests require larger sample sizes (eg, 30 or more observations).

Test of Prediction

Regression analysis is a statistical procedure that results in information on the relative influence of a variety of independent or predictor variables on an outcome (dependent) variable. Length of stay is an outcome variable that has been discussed frequently in this chapter.

After defining a sample universe (eg, cases grouped under a certain DRG), a series of regression analyses are conducted to arrive at the shortest list of factors, that is, those with the greatest probability of making a difference, in predicting certain lengths of stay. For example, the final regression model for cases with depressive disorders was able to show which of the previously listed variables influenced the length of stay, how large the influence was, and whether the influence increased or decreased the likelihood of the length of stay. *Beta weights* are the values that the regression analysis assigns to the variables assumed to have influence on the outcome variable; the more a beta differs from 0, the greater the influence of a predictor variable. If the beta of a predictor variable is positive, its presence increases the likelihood of the outcome variable; if the beta of a predictor variable is negative, its presence decreases the likelihood of the outcome variable (Bogue, 1991).

Although, regression analysis cannot determine causality, it can partially describe the independent and collective relationship of a number of variables hypothesized for association with an outcome variable. Regression helps to predict what would happen if the value of an independent variable were changed; that is why regression analysis is used in predictive model generation (Kazandjian, 1991).

Test of Difference

The *two-sample* t *test* compares the means or averages of two samples (ie, testing whether there is a statistically significant difference in the means, or whether one mean is larger or smaller than the other). The test is based on several mathematical assumptions that are not exactly satisfied in practice.

The most crucial assumption is that of *independence* of the two samples; if the samples are taken from different populations and if there is no connection between the elements of one sample and those of the other, the independence assumptions should be valid. The assumption that both populations are normally distributed is less crucial. Based on the Central Limit Theorem, normal distribution is determined largely by the combined size of both samples ($n_1 + n_2$), and the assumption should be valid when $n_1 + n_2$ is at least 30. Although sample variances differ because of random variation, there is an assumption of equal variance. However, if the sample sizes are equal, the universal conclusion is that even a substantial difference in variance has remarkably little effect. Test results may be in serious error when the larger variance is associated with the smaller sample size. In such a situation, an alternative to the two-sample t test is the Wilcoxon rank sum test (Hildebrand & Ott, 1983).

The result of a statistical test is often summarized by stating that the result is statistically significant at the specified *p*-value. The *p*-value is called the attained-significance level of a statistical test. A sample result with an associated *p*-value > 0.05 is considered to be "not statistically significant." To say that a difference is "statistically significant" or "statistically detectable" is to say that the observed result cannot easily be attributed to random variation alone (Hildebrand & Ott, 1983).

Provide Feedback

Data analysis requires statistical expertise and interpretation of findings requires clinical expertise. However, most clinicians and hospital administrators are not adept at interpreting statistical information (Davies et al., 1994). Therefore, analyses should be presented in ways that project participants can understand and use. The project coordinator or the outcomes/decision support staff are required to have a basic understanding of the statistics involved and skills to communicate and explain the analysis. In these early evolutionary stages of outcomes methodology, the transformation of raw data to useful information demands a considerable degree of exploratory statistical work and frequent data interpretation sessions with clinicians (Davies et al., 1994). To achieve true efficiency and integration with the care process, it is important that most statistical analyses become routine and standardized.

Develop Cost-Effective Algorithms

It is increasingly recognized that physicians' behavior is heavily influenced by their perceptions of what is "accepted" or "standard practice." Thus, practices espoused by peer leaders and accepted by peers can be more influential than scientific knowledge about pathophysiology or clinical outcomes. Mere distribution of published guidelines has been shown in a number of studies to be ineffective as a single intervention in changing physician behavior. Effective implementation requires that providers accept, adopt, and use the guidelines.

Guideline development needs to be facilitated by the clinician champion with attention paid to the professional and educational needs of physicians, residents, nurses, and hospital ancillary department staff. Preconceived objections that algorithms represent a challenge to autonomy and are a form of "cookbook medicine" also need to be addressed.

Throughout the process of guideline development, the project team should be sensitive to practitioners' concerns. The team should:
- include practitioners in the process of initial algorithm development
- be receptive to suggestions for algorithm review and modification
- acknowledge that some patients may be treated more appropriately in a manner different from what the algorithm states and respect the role each provider plays in the management of individual patients.

Apply the Algorithms

In reflecting on the five performance criteria for the ACNP mentioned earlier, consider the criteria that relate to care delivery: direct/indirect care, which involves delivery of direct care and coordination of an interdisciplinary care plan for patients and requires the expertise of an advanced practitioner, and consultation, in which the ACNP serves as a consultant in improving patient care and nursing practice based on expertise in an area of specialization. These criteria denote the integral role the ACNP can have in applying algorithms in a collaborative model of practice as the ACNP and the physician as a team provide care to patients.

During interdisciplinary patient rounds in which the patient's care plan is established, evaluated, and continuously updated, algorithms can offer a common language for the team in clinical decision making and can facilitate communication between practitioners. As stated in Chapter 10, "In the healthcare environment of today with its many complexities and potential for fragmentation, it is imperative to establish organizational structures [consistent with the joint-practice model of collaborative practice] that reflect . . . professional interdependence" (p. 155). Only with such structures in place can healthcare services be delivered in a high-quality, yet cost-effective, manner.

References

American Medical Association. (1977). *Current procedural terminology* (4th Edition, updated annually). Chicago, IL: Author.

Alkire, A., & Stoltz, S. (1993). Employer's view of managed health care: From a passive to an aggressive role. In P. R. Kongstvedt (Ed.), *The managed health care handbook* (2nd ed., pp. 255–264). Gaithersburg, MD: Aspen Publishers.

Bogue, R. J. (1991). Transforming data into information: A case study. In D. R. Longo & D. Bohr (Eds.), *Quantitive methods in quality management: A guide for practitioners* (pp. 127–136). Chicago, IL: American Hospital Publishing.

Cerne, F. (1994). Dollars & sense: Creating incentives to effectively manage change. *Hospitals & Health Networks, 67*(7), 28–30.

Davies, A. R., Thomas, M. A., Lansky, D., Rutt, W., Stevic, M. O., & Doyle, J. B. (1994). Outcomes assessment in clinical settings: A consensus statement on principles and best practices in project management. *Joint Commission Journal on Quality Improvement, 30*(1), 6–16.

Hildebrand, D. K., & Ott, L. (1983). *Statistical thinking for managers.* Boston: PWS Publishers.

Joint Commission on Accreditation of Healthcare Organizations. (1990). *Primer on indicator development and application: Measuring quality in healthcare.* Oakbrook Terrace, IL: Author.

Kazandjian, V. (1991). Statistical testing: Is what you see really there? In D. R. Longo & D. Bohr (Eds.), *Quantitative methods in quality management: A guide for practitioners* (pp. 15–25). Chicago, IL: American Hospital Publishing.

Kitzman, H. (1986). Education in nursing. In J. E. Steel (Ed.), *Issues in collaborative practice* (pp. 139–159). Orlando, FL: Grune & Stratton.

Kongstvedt, P. R. (Ed.). (1993). *The managed health care handbook* (2nd ed.). Gaithersburg, MD: Aspen Publishers.

Patton, M. D., & Katterhagen, J. G. (1994). Critical pathways in oncology: Aligning resource expenditures with clinical outcomes. *Journal of Oncology Management, 3*(4), 16–20.

Touse, J. (1993). Medical management and legal obligations to members. In P. R. Kongstvedt (Ed.), *The managed health care handbook* (2nd ed., pp. 481–493). Gaithersburg, MD: Aspen Publishers.

Whitmore, B. C. (1994, September/October). Using refined DRGs in resource management initiatives. *The Quality Resource: The Newsletter of the Quality Assurance Section of the American Health Information Management Association, 12*(5), 1-4.

World Health Organization. (1979). *International classification of diseases, 9th revision, clinical modification* (updated annually): Reston, VA: St. Anthony Publishing.

The Advanced Practice Nurse: Innovative Models for Caring

17

Primary Care: Improving Health Promotion and Disease Prevention

Introduction: Sandra L. Venegoni

Primary care, a healthcare term commonplace during the last quarter of this century, has been used in a variety of ways to describe different practice models (see Chap. 5 for a detailed historical perspective of primary care). As we approach the new millennium, the National Academy of Sciences Institute of Medicine (IOM) has charged its Committee on the Future of Primary Care to revisit and redefine its original 1978 definition of primary care. After 2 years of work, this new, provisional definition takes into account the changes that have occurred in healthcare since 1970 and the changes projected to occur during the next 5 to 10 years. This new definition considers major concerns of the healthcare reform era: issues about the healthcare costs; the advanced and specialized knowledge and techniques available to healthcare providers; the trend toward large, integrated delivery systems with enrolled populations; and the use of teams to provide healthcare.

Primary care, as defined in the Institute of Medicine interim report (Donaldson, Yordy, & Vanselow, 1994) is "the provision of integrated, accessible healthcare services by clinicians who are accountable for addressing a large majority of personal healthcare needs, developing a sustained partnership with patients, and practicing in the context of family and community" (p. 15). Central to the definition of primary care is the patient–clinician partnership that is formed and the specific description of each person in this relationship. The individual who seeks care is considered in the context of the family and community in which he or she lives. This context may include living conditions, dynamics of the family unit, work situation, and cultural background of the family and community. The individual may or may not be ill at the time he or she seeks care. The predominant need may be for advice, information, or preventive care. The committee work was guided by several critical assumptions, one of which stated that "primary care will be an important instrument for achieving stronger emphasis on health promotion and disease prevention" (p. 6)

Hickey JV: ADVANCED PRACTICE NURSING: Changing Roles and Clinical Applications © 1996 Lippincott–Raven Publishers

The clinician enters into a relationship with a patient under two conditions. There is the expectation that the relationship will continue over time and because the clinician has the authority to direct patient care. The clinician uses a recognized scientific knowledge base as the foundation for the primary care delivered. However, primary care teams, rather than a single individual, deliver much of the care as part of an integrated delivery system that serves a defined population.

The three exemplars in this chapter portray advanced practice nurses (APNs) who are active in the delivery of primary care and personify the Institute of Medicine's definition of primary care. The exemplars describe the APNs' relationships with a distinct clientele who have unique family and community situations. The APNs deliver both illness care and healthcare with an emphasis on ways to improve health promotion and disease prevention for their patients. These practitioners function as team members who serve a specifically defined patient population.

In Exemplar A, Dunn and Graves describe the faculty practice model of the Community Nursing Organization (CNO) at a university school of nursing. The model is but one example of the 250 community nursing centers throughout the United States. The unique patient–clinician relationship meets the needs of some of society's most vulnerable and underserved populations: homeless people and other at-risk individuals. The CNO provides primary healthcare to these groups and simultaneously fulfills the major characteristics of a nursing center and expressed integrated mission of academia: education, scholarship, and service. Two long-range goals for the CNO are to offer collaborative education of students from multiple disciplines and to carry out research (hence, strengthening the Institute of Medicine's definition of *teams*). It is hoped that additional research will demonstrate that the CNO is an effective model of health service delivery that can provide affordable healthcare. Both of these goals are highly desirable and needed as APNs move into the 21st century.

If primary care by definition needs to be accessible and focused on preventive care, then Butts in Exemplar B met this requirement by providing healthcare where a large number of Americans spend a great portion of their day—in the workplace. Long before it was in vogue to have health promotion and wellness programs in the workplace, the practitioner in this exemplar seized an innovative opportunity to demonstrate that the relatively young and healthy members of this industrial setting could be assisted to not only remain healthy, but even become healthier. More than 10 years of successful practice and collaboration with community practitioners have proven that the APN can make a significant difference and provide cost-effective care to members of the workforce. Indeed, primary care in this exemplar is truly "health where the people are located."

In Exemplar C on school health programs, Gulbrandsen demonstrates that primary healthcare can be provided to youngsters who spend their days in their "workplace": the school system. Given the correlation between a student's health status and success in their schoolwork, this exemplar illustrates the type of primary healthcare and preventive care that can be carried out in this environment and the contributions APNs can make to the team. Over a 10-year growth period, full-time equivalents in the health department in the school district described have increased from 10.00 to 21.75, with 16.00 of these full-time equivalents being nurse practitioners prepared at the master's level. These individuals collaborate closely with local health departments and private healthcare providers to provide individualized care needed by each child. Other than the home setting, the APNs are, indeed, closest to the child's world and, therefore, able to provide the needed continuity of care.

The healthcare providers in each of the exemplars stand out for their innovative and creative beginnings in their respective roles. They all took risks in beginning the type of service and primary care they deliver, and yet all have had demonstrable success in their endeavors. It is an ongoing challenge for APNs to accept these types of risks and to capitalize on the opportunities, wherever they are, to meet their patients' health needs.

Community Outreach Model of Faculty Practice

Barbara H. Dunn ■ *Sandra L. Graves*

This exemplar describes the development of a faculty practice in an academic nursing center at the Virginia Commonwealth University (VCU), Medical College of Virginia (MCV), School of Nursing, in Richmond. The nursing center, called the Community Nursing Organization (CNO), provides primary healthcare services to several vulnerable and under-served populations in the Richmond area. It also provides practice opportunities for faculty members, community-based clinical experiences for students, and a rich source of data for research and ultimately policy development.

Following an overview of academic nursing centers in general, the evolution of the VCU/MCV CNO is described, including how needs were identified, consistent community relationships were developed, services were established, and faculty and students were involved. Also addressed are the focus of care, scope of services, types of populations served, and specific considerations with these populations. The exemplar concludes with a discussion of costs, outcomes, and issues related to the challenges of providing community-based health services.

ACADEMIC NURSING CENTERS

Nurse-managed centers and clinics developed in the 1970s in response to several trends, including increasing numbers of nurses interested in alternative models and systems of care, recognition that some populations had unmet health-related needs, and concern about a growing gap between nursing education and service. Academic nursing centers are that subset of nurse-managed centers affiliated with schools of nursing. Although it is difficult to obtain accurate numbers, more than 70 schools of nursing probably have nursing centers (Barger, Nugent, & Bridges, 1993).

According to an American Nurses' Association task force formed in 1987 to develop guidelines (Aydelotte et al., 1987), nursing centers are characterized by direct patient access to professional nursing services, patient-centered services that focus on health and optimal functioning, and services that respond to the health needs of the target populations and communities. The nurse provider is responsible and accountable for patient care and professional practice, and is reimbursed at a reasonable rate (Aydelotte et al., 1987, p. 1).

There are generally at least four purposes for academic nursing centers: to provide community service, student education, clinical research, and faculty practice (Barger & Bridges, 1989, 1990; Barger et al., 1993). As Walker (1991) has stated, these centers allow nursing conceptual models to be applied to practice and administration. In addition, they provide a demonstration site for the intradisciplinary practice of nursing and for interdisciplinary and interagency collaborative efforts.

Centers may operate from one clinical site and target a single population, but more often provide a variety of services for different patient groups at several locations. Typically, nurse practitioner and community health faculty members are involved in providing services. In a few well-established centers, faculty must undergo a formal application process to be granted practice privileges. Consultation and referral to physicians or other disciplines may be arranged contractually, or on some other agreed-on basis within a particular agency or setting. There may be a formal quality assurance program that includes evaluation of services and personnel, including faculty who participate (Aydelotte et al., 1987; Higgs, 1988).

A 1990 survey of nursing schools (Barger et al., 1993) has provided a typical profile of schools with nursing centers. The schools are large (with an average of 34 full-time equivalent faculty), have graduate programs, and are located in public institutions without health science centers. They usually do not require practice of faculty, use it as a criterion for promotion or tenure, or have a formal faculty practice plan. A significant portion of the funding for the nursing center comes from the affiliated school. One report (Higgs, 1989) has suggested that, in some centers, faculty volunteer efforts provide what is largely uncompensated care.

Financial viability is a major concern for nursing centers, particularly among those in state institutions for which budgets are declining. Fragile funding may account for the transient nature of a number of academic nursing centers. According to Barger et al. (1993), some centers in operation when schools were surveyed in 1985 were no longer operational by early 1990. Besides institutional funding, centers are also supported by fee-for-service payment, third-party reimbursement, contracts, grants, in-kind support, and use of free space (American Association of Colleges of Nursing, 1991, 1992; Elsberry & Nelson, 1993).

At the federal level, grant support for nursing centers is available through the U.S. Department of Health and Human Services (DHHS), Division of Nursing. These 5-year grants, which are intended to demonstrate methods of improving access to primary healthcare in medically underserved communities, are funded under Title VIII, Section 820(b), of the Public Health Service Act of 1944 (Nursing Special Projects Grants). To establish stable long-term funding, however, some nursing centers have sought status as federally certified Rural Health Clinics (RHCs) or Federally Qualified Health Centers (FQHCs), which are eligible for reimbursement under Medicare and Medicaid.

In addition, several CNO demonstration projects have been funded by the DHHS Health Care Financing Administration. These 5-year projects, which ended in 1994, provided care to Medicare recipients for a particular reimbursement rate. The Health Care Financing Administration evaluation of these demonstration projects will determine whether this financing model will be extended to other nursing centers.

With continuing debate about healthcare reform, major changes in the organization and financing of services are forecast. The future for nursing centers and other alternative models of service delivery is not yet clear, particularly in a managed care or managed competition environment. In this environment, nonphysician providers or providers not affiliated with large service networks may have little opportunity to be designated preferred providers, therefore increasing costs to consumers who choose to use their services. For example, the Virginia Medicaid program has a federal waiver (waiving the requirement that gives patients freedom of choice in selecting providers) to provide services to pregnant women and children under a managed care plan called Medallion. Currently, Medallion designates only physicians as primary care providers, seriously limiting access to the populations by nurse practitioners, certified nurse-midwives, and physician's assistants.

COMMUNITY NURSING ORGANIZATION

In the spring of 1992, the authors and other faculty members conducted a feasibility study to establish a nursing center at the VCU/MCV School of Nursing. As part of that study, a community needs assessment was completed. The assessment involved a review of available data from Richmond and surrounding areas and interviews with a variety of health and social services providers. Among other things, it identified unmet health needs among homeless and at-risk populations in Richmond that nurse-managed services, in part, could meet.

The school CNO was formally established in fall 1992. It is a distinct organizational entity within the school that reports directly to the dean (Fig. 17-1). It was conceptualized as a *center without walls* under whose umbrella multiple faculty-led projects would eventually develop. Consistent with the missions of the university and the School of Nursing, the CNO chose as its initial focus high-risk populations in inner-city Richmond. The Homeless and At-Risk Populations (HARP) project was the first developed because of identified needs as well as the interests of faculty involved. For HARP, an *at risk population* is defined as low income families with young children (primarily female headed) and elderly people, particularly those residing in high-poverty and medically underserved areas of the city.

During the pilot phase of HARP (the 1992–1993 academic year), additional data were collected from homeless and at-risk people and other service providers for use in designing CNO services (Virginia Commonwealth University, 1993). Furthermore, relationships with community-based providers became more formalized, and project staff sought consultation from several nationally known individuals with expertise related to nursing centers and home-

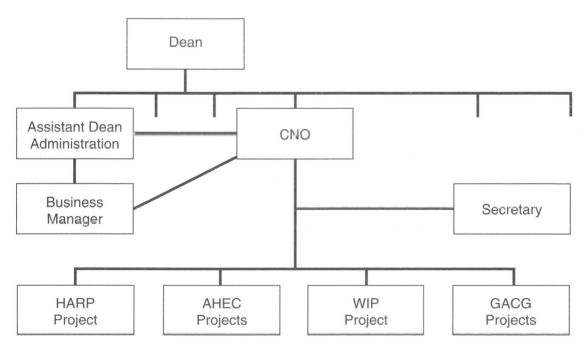

FIGURE 17-1 Organizational chart: Community Nursing Organization, School of Nursing, Virginia Commonwealth University, Medical College of Virginia. CNO, community nursing organization; HARP, homeless and at-risk population; AHEC, area health education center; WIP, women in prison; GACG, governmental agency contracts and grants.

less healthcare. Additionally, project staff were members of a Faculty Practice Task Force that explored the development of a formal faculty practice plan and relationships between the CNO and any plan that might be established.

Funding for the CNO during its first year of operation came from the nursing school budget, two grants, and two contracts. The grants included one from the MCV Foundation, which partially paid the CNO director's salary, and another through the Virginia Department of Health. The Virginia Department of Health grant was part of the federal Cooperative Agreement Educational Linkage program (of DHHS, Health Resources and Services Administration) that sought to increase student primary healthcare experiences in community-based sites that targeted underserved populations. In addition, there were two time-limited contracts for nurse practitioner services: one with a rural health district for weekly pediatric clinics and another with a county mental health and mental retardation agency for monthly developmental screening clinics (referred to as Governmental Agency Contracts and Grants in Fig. 17-1).

The school continued its financial support a second year (1993–1994) while project staff pursued external funding sources for HARP and other projects. The county mental health and mental retardation agency contract continued a second year, and a new contract was signed with the Virginia Department of Corrections. This new contract provided nurse practitioner services for a weekly women's health clinic at a regional prison facility (referred to as the Women in Prison project in Fig. 17-1).

During its third year of operation (1994–1995), the dean again committed funds for general CNO support. The CNO also received grant funding from the Greater Richmond Area Health Education Center Program (referred to as AHEC projects in Fig. 17-1) as a subcontractor on two proposals submitted by cooperating community-based agencies. These proposals were both for nurse practitioner services. One of the proposals was for the Richmond Area High Blood Pressure Center to provide clinical evaluation services 16 hours per month for center patients; the other proposal was for Fan Free Clinic to provide clinical services 8 hours per week at its Street Center location (serving primarily homeless men) and 8 hours per month at its Hanover Avenue location (serving homeless and high-risk women and children).

In addition, the authors received Medicaid provider numbers, enabling reimbursement for services provided to children under the Early and Periodic Screening, Diagnosis and Treatment program. Further discussion of costs and financing can be found in the section Issues and Outcomes.

TARGET POPULATIONS

Richmond is a city of 200,000 (1990 census) with a population that is 43.4% African-American. One in five Richmond residents has an income below 100% of the federal poverty level and two in five are 200% below poverty level. Despite these statistics, fewer than half of Medicaid-eligible residents are actually enrolled (Richmond City Health Department, 1991; Richmond Community Action Program, 1993).

The City of Richmond is a federally designated Medically Underserved Area (MUA) and Health Professional Shortage Area (HPSA). There are 11 census tracts with medically underserved area designations and eight with health professional shortage area designations, most in the downtown, east end, or near southside areas of the city; another four census tracts have dual designations (all east end). These are also the areas with the highest percentage of poverty-level residents and, therefore, the largest at-risk populations.

The typical Richmond resident is an African-American woman younger than age 45 years with children. People aged 65 years and older compose 15% of the population and are predominantly white women (Richmond City Health Department, 1991). Many of these women and children are low income, live in female-headed households (38.9% are poverty-level), and have marginal housing (Richmond Community Action Program, 1993). The serious drug and violence problems in the city increase the vulnerability of these women and children and put them at-risk for a variety of health and other social problems, including homelessness. Other groups at high risk for homelessness include those doubling up with family or friends, those with unstable employment, victims of domestic violence, substance abusers, and the chronically mentally ill.

The average homeless person in Richmond is an African-American male younger than age 40 years. One third of these individuals are veterans and more than 35% have serious mental health or substance abuse problems. Although many homeless people are employed, most homeless families (90% headed by single women) are supported by social services payments (Richmond Department of Mental Health, Mental Retardation, and Substance Abuse Services, 1993). In 1991, Richmond had 10,986 requests for temporary shelter and denied almost 5000 requests primarily because beds were full. Consistent with state and national trends, an increasing proportion of these requests come from families with children (Children's Defense Fund, 1994; Virginia Coalition for the Homeless, 1993). An unknown number of additional people never made requests and remained on the streets.

Health Status

The effects of poverty on health status are well known. The combination of poverty and loss of housing and other social supports can have devastating and long-term effects on health. What follows in regard to homeless people is also true for those at high risk of homelessness, only to a lesser degree.

Homelessness is the result of a complex set of social, psychological, and health-related problems. The homeless population has more difficulty with access to the traditional medical care system than any other group. Access problems are related to lack of insurance, service hours and organization, staff attitudes, lack of transportation, psychological distress, and frequent inability to comply with recommendations.

Homeless people are less likely to use outpatient services, although they suffer more illness than the general population. Rates of physical morbidity are higher (30% to 40%, with at least one chronic condition), and they have twice the incidence of mental illness. Health problems may be related to adverse health habits such as smoking, alcohol, and drug use. When combined with the adverse effects of street life, particularly sleep deprivation and poor nutrition, these problems may be exacerbated (Wood, 1992).

Homeless individuals are more likely to be products of seriously dysfunctional families (e.g., in which there is parental drug or alcohol abuse or child physical or sexual abuse). Often, they continue the cycle of poverty and dysfunction. Their perceptions of their own and their children's health status is poorer than that of the general population. For many women and children, homelessness is related to domestic violence. Once on the street, women are likely to be victims of repeated rape and other trauma. If they become pregnant, they may receive inadequate prenatal care and deliver low–birth weight infants. Their children have developmental, nutritional, and emotional problems that are more severe than those of other poor children, and their children are sick twice as often as children with homes. Homeless children also frequently miss school and repeat grades (Children's Defense Fund, 1994; Wood, 1992).

Health Services

In general, the availability of various services for homeless and at-risk individuals is inversely related to the proportion of people needing those services (Fig. 17-2). Therefore, the smallest subgroup—those in long-term shelters or transitional housing—receive the most intense services, whereas the largest subgroup—those on the street or at high risk—are mostly invisible and unserved.

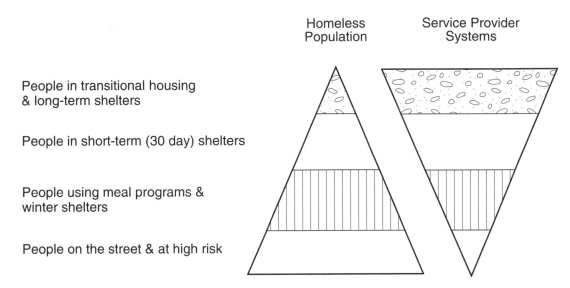

People in transitional housing
& long-term shelters

People in short-term (30 day) shelters

People using meal programs &
winter shelters

People on the street & at high risk

Homeless
Population

Service Provider
Systems

FIGURE 17-2 Relationship between homeless and at-risk populations and service provider systems.

Health services received by homeless and high-risk people are usually episodic and focus on acute problems. When these individuals do obtain services, often late in the course of an illness, they frequently use the emergency room or are hospitalized. Convalescence after hospital discharge may occur on the street or in marginal housing, where it is difficult to comply with medical recommendations or obtain follow-up care. It may also be difficult or impossible to get prescriptions filled, usually because of cost. Because patients may give the address of a shelter, or a fictitious address, health providers may not know the individuals are homeless. Consequently, it becomes difficult to adapt treatment recommendations to special needs or to determine service use by this population (Weinreb, 1992; Wood, 1992).

The five major sources of care for homeless and high-risk people in Richmond are (1) the VCU/MCV Hospital emergency room, outpatient clinics, and inpatient units; (2) the Department of Veterans' Affairs Medical Center; (3) Richmond City Health Department; (4) Cross-Over Health Center; and (5) Fan Free Clinic at the Street Center. Services from these sources of care are provided on-site during usual business hours or at the 24-hour emergency room. They typically are organized according to the traditional medical model of service delivery, are physician directed and provided, and are not necessarily targeted or modified for the special needs of homeless people.

Fan Free Clinic at the Street Center, as a subcontractor to the Daily Planet, a mental health provider, receives federal funding under the Stewart B. McKinney Homeless Assistance Act of 1987 (section 340 of the Public Health Service Act of 1944) to provide health services for the homeless population. These funds are administered by the DHHS, Bureau of Primary Health Care, Division of Special Populations. The bureau also funds Community and Migrant Health Centers. However, the Street Center environment is inhospitable for women and children, so the primary population served is men. None of these providers has services designed to meet the particular needs of homeless women and children.

Furthermore, there is minimal integration of services among health and other providers and limited coordination of care. There is little orientation toward health promotion and prevention, particularly health education, health maintenance, and age-appropriate screening, testing, immunization, and counseling. Shelter and meal program staff have limited access to education on health-related topics, and usually do not have a health professional with whom they can consult.

The CNO faculty believed that more effective nontraditional health services were needed, particularly for women and children, to increase access, promote health, and reduce inappropriate use of costly hospital-based care. Homelessness is most often a temporary condition, so that long-term health status should be a consideration in the design of services for this population. Improvements in health status may prevent long-term homelessness. Likewise, the most important preventive health strategy for these individuals is the resolution of their homelessness (Weinreb, 1992).

HARP PROJECT

The HARP Project is a cooperative effort of the CNO and 16 community-based public and private organizations. This nurse-managed community outreach model provides primary healthcare services that emphasize health promotion and prevention. Its purpose is to increase access and improve the comprehensiveness of primary healthcare services for a medically underserved and largely uninsured population: individuals and families who are homeless or at-risk of homelessness in Richmond. Access is improved by taking care to sites where homeless and at-risk people congregate, making services available at times convenient for patient populations, and offering a variety of services unavailable from other sources. The project complements and extends rather than duplicates existing services.

It is also consistent with the goals and objectives of *Healthy People 2000* (DHHS, 1992), and specifically addresses three broad public health goals. Those goals are (1) increasing the span of healthy life for Americans (by improving health status, early detection and treatment of disease, and better management of chronic conditions); (2) reducing health disparities among Americans (by increasing access to health services for homeless and other at-risk populations and improving long-term health status); and (3) achieving access to prevention services for all Americans (by emphasizing health promotion and prevention services for this underserved population).

Primary project staff during the first 2 years (1992–1994) were five advanced practice nurses, all of whom have faculty appointments in the School of Nursing. These nurses included three clinical specialists—in community health, mental health, and women's health, respectively—and two nurse practitioners—one family and one pediatric (the authors). The percentage of time dedicated to the project for these faculty members ranged from 20% to 50% of effort. Other faculty were involved, placing students in project sites for community-based clinical experiences. Students to date have included undergraduates in community health and pediatric clinical courses and graduate nurse practitioner students in women's health and child health courses. Undergraduate nursing students and second-year medical students, as well as faculty and alumni, have also been involved as volunteers in tuberculosis and blood pressure screening programs for homeless people.

Community Collaboration

During its first 2 years of operation, CNO staff expended significant effort developing relationships with staff in community-based agencies serving homeless and at-risk populations. Most of these organizations are social services agencies that provide shelter, meal programs, and other support services to homeless people or have programs targeted at particular at-risk groups, such as victims of domestic violence and children and elderly residents of high-poverty areas. Sixteen organizations provide direct or in-kind resources to HARP, including access to their patient groups, space, and staff support (Table 17-1).

TABLE 17-1   **Cooperating Community-Based Agencies by Type of Service**

Housing Providers	*Health Service Providers*
CARITAS	Cross-Over Health Center
Emergency Shelter, Inc.	Fan Free Clinic
Freedom House	Richmond City Health Department
SRO of Richmond: Clay House	Richmond High BP Center
St. Joseph's Villa	
YWCA Battered Women's Shelter	*Mental Health Providers*
	Daily Planet, Street Center
Meal Program	Richmond Street Team
St. Paul's Episcopal Church	
	Child Care Providers
Neighborhood Center	RCAP: Head Start
Peter–Paul Development Center	YWCA Childcare Program

BP, blood pressure; CARITAS, Congregations Around Richmond Involved to Assure Shelter; RCAP, Richmond Community Action Program; SRO, single room occupancy.

These community organizations support CNO efforts to provide health services, but not financially. These typically small, nonprofit agencies are underfunded and often overextended in terms of staff workload. Homeless and at-risk individuals have the most complex social, psychological, and health problems imaginable. On the other hand, agency staff are often young, inexperienced, and trying to survive in organizations that frequently are in crisis. It should not be surprising, then, to find high rates of burnout and turnover in these agencies. Given this environment, it has been a particular challenge to attempt to coordinate schedules and services with these community-based providers. It has required much reconsideration and reorientation of priorities and roles, with HARP project staff essentially being guests in the space of other agencies.

Data were collected from agency leadership and staff during the first year of CNO operation, and needs have been assessed on an ongoing basis since. Needs identified by service providers included staff education on health-related issues; availability of a health professional for staff consultation, patient evaluation, or referral; and coordination of care with other health service providers. HARP project services for community providers were designed based on their self-identified needs and with the knowledge that these supportive services to staff could indirectly benefit the patients they serve.

Services and Sites

Data collected from homeless people during the first year of operation guided the design of services. Needs identified included comprehensive physical assessment, health education and counseling, health promotion and prevention services, age-appropriate screening, testing, and immunization; and improved availability of services after working hours and at locations where homeless people congregate. Information continues to be gathered from patient populations as the project evolves.

Services are provided at a variety of sites, including meal programs, homeless shelters (winter, short term, and long term), a battered women's shelter, a transitional housing unit, childcare centers, a neighborhood center, and a clinic site (Table 17-2). The three categories of patient services are (1) individual, family, or group counseling sessions; (2) outreach screening and health promotion clinics; and (3) health maintenance clinics. In addition, services provided to or with other providers include staff education, consultation, patient evalua-

TABLE 17-2 HARP Project Services, Sites, and Personnel

Health Services	Sites	Personnel
Health Maintenance Clinics	Fan Free Clinic	NPs, WHS,* students
Screening/Health Promotion Clinics	Meal Program:	
	St. Paul's Episcopal Church	FNP*, students
	Shelters:	
	CARITAS*	Staff, students
	YWCA Battered Women's Shelter	NPs on call
	Freedom House	MHS*, NPs on call
		NPs on call
	Child Care:	
	YWCA child care program	PNP*, students
	RCAP*: HeadStart	All staff, students
	Neighborhood Center:	
	Peter-Paul Development Center	FNP, CHS*, students
Counseling	SRO of Richmond*:	
	Clay House	MHS, students
	Emergency Shelter, Inc.	MHS, others
	Agency Requests	Staff as indicated
Staff Education	All Agencies	All staff, students

KEY: CARITAS, Congregations Around Richmond Involved to Assure Shelter; CHS, community health specialist; FNP, family nurse practitioner; MHS, mental health specialist; PNP, pediatric nurse practitioner; RCAP, Richmond Community Action Program; SRO, single room occupancy; WHS, women's health specialist.

tion, care coordination and referral, and mass screening. Project staff have also regularly attended monthly meetings of the Greater Richmond Coalition for the Homeless.

Counseling Sessions

These sessions were provided by the project staff's mental health specialist to individuals and women's groups at a transitional housing unit and a homeless shelter. Referrals for individual or family counseling developed as a result of the group sessions and regular presence of the project staff member; referrals came from agency staff and patients themselves.

Screening/Health Promotion Clinics

These outreach clinics provide health screening, health education and counseling, physical assessment, minor acute problem assessment and management, monitoring and follow-up of chronic conditions, evaluation of mental health status or crisis intervention, age-appropriate immunizations, and referral and coordination with other providers. Other screening includes annual citywide tuberculosis screening in cooperation with the city health department and targeted blood pressure screening in cooperation with the high blood pressure center. Clinics are held in four types of locations: (1) meal programs, held weekly in cooperation with a downtown church-sponsored lunch program; (2) shelters, held at least monthly at a family shelter for homeless women and children and at a winter cots program at rotating church sites (from November to March), and available on an on-call basis to another long-term homeless shelter and a domestic violence shelter for women and children; (3) child care centers, held weekly at a homeless child care program and scheduled during a 3- to 5-week period in the fall and spring at a Head Start program; and (4) neighborhood center, held weekly at a church-affiliated center with programs for elderly people and school-aged children.

Health Maintenance Clinics

These clinics are held weekly in space provided by Fan Free Clinic at its Hanover Avenue location. A children's clinic (staffed by the pediatric nurse practitioner) and a women's clinic (staffed by the family nurse practitioner and a women's health specialist) are held Monday afternoons. Appointments for these clinics are made by telephone or on a walk-in basis through the Fan Free Clinic manager. Transportation from shelter sites can be arranged by agency staff.

Services in these clinics include history-taking, risk appraisal, and physical examination; assessment of mental health status and coping strategies; age- and gender-appropriate health screening, testing, and immunization or vaccination; health education and counseling; assessment and management of minor acute problems; monitoring and follow-up of chronic conditions; completion of medical forms for school, work, and entitlement programs; and referral to and coordination with other providers and settings. Screening, testing, and counseling are consistent with the recommendations of the U.S. Preventive Health Services Task Force (1989). In addition, materials from the *Put Prevention Into Practice* project (DHHS, 1994) were incorporated when they became available in mid-1994.

Administration

Records for the health maintenance clinics and outreach screening are maintained at the Fan Free Clinic Hanover Avenue location, using clinic forms. In addition, HARP project staff use staff-developed permission forms and another form summarizing findings and recommendations because many children are seen without parents or a guardian present. Standard health department information forms are provided to the parent or guardian before children receive immunizations. The Fan Free Clinic provides the project with supplies and vaccines for outreach screening sites, as well as consultation and referral from its medical director.

In Virginia, nurse practitioners are licensed by the state and required to have an identified supervising physician with whom they collaborate. The nurse practitioner project staff also have prescriptive authority (limited by state law to Schedule VI drugs), which also requires a collaborating physician and a signed practice agreement. Pediatric consultation and referral are available from the Fan Free medical director as well as through a collaborative agreement with a pediatrician on the VCU/MCV Department of Pediatrics faculty. These physicians are available on an on-call basis, and conduct a monthly chart review of patients who needed prescriptions or referrals.

Project staff use staff-developed clinical privileges documents to describe and delineate each clinician's scope of practice. Staff also regularly use standard references and staff-developed clinical protocols for common problems of women and children, which enable them to provide standards across sites and providers.

ISSUES AND OUTCOMES

A variety of issues related to development and institutionalization of the CNO and HARP project include those related to faculty roles, community agency characteristics, short- and long-term financing, population considerations, and project evaluation.

Faculty Roles

In regard to faculty roles, the mission statements of the university and School of Nursing relate to teaching, research, and service by faculty members. However, as in many other universities, the reward structure does not place equal emphasis on community service and faculty practice. In the School of Nursing, a Faculty Practice Task Force (1992–1993) made recommendations regarding the development of a formal practice plan. Those recommendations could not be implemented, in part, because the university placed a moratorium on the establishment of separately incorporated faculty practice plans. Establishing a reward structure for practice remains essential to the full implementation of the CNO.

With the national shift toward community-based primary healthcare and a renewed emphasis on underserved populations, health professions schools are beginning to revise their curricula and clinical experiences. Change is difficult, particularly when it means new ways of thinking about faculty roles, models of service delivery, clinical sites, and patient groups. To fully operationalize this model of health professions training, priorities will need to focus on community-based faculty practice and student learning.

In the HARP project, staff also place a high value on the development of personal relationships with agency staff. Good interpersonal skills and a cooperative attitude are critical to the organizational and political success of the CNO.

Agency Characteristics

Additionally, major differences exist between the way the university system approaches tasks and that of the cooperating community-based agencies. For instance, faculty are accustomed to planning activities as much as a year or at least a semester in advance (e.g., course planning). On the other hand, the community agencies, because of small overextended staffs, often do not have the luxury of planning, and may be coping day to day. In terms of clinical services and student experiences, the needs of the community agencies (in regard to time and skills) do not always easily match the students' schedules, experiences, or skill levels. Consequently, a great deal of time must be spent coordinating schedules so that students, other faculty members, patients, and community agency staff have positive experiences.

Another issue related to community agency characteristics is the compensation level of staff in these agencies vis-à-vis faculty members. These are primarily social services agencies whose staff make less than $35,000 per year (even the executive directors, in some cases). Faculty compensation (considering salary and a healthy state benefits package) is significantly more than $35,000. Thus, discussion of the value of clinical services and the negotiation of contracts is a delicate subject. To minimize the tension, an attempt is made to avoid breakdown into hourly rates. This is done by bundling services, that is, giving a total annual value or cost that includes clinical and counseling services, staff consultation, staff education, supplies, laboratory and equipment resources, and a quality assurance mechanism.

Because of high stress and low salaries, the nonprofit community agencies typically have high staff turnover rates. As a result, coordination is more difficult, as is the establishment of personal relationships with agency staff, an element that is crucial to the cooperative effort.

Financing Issues

Academic nursing centers are expensive programs for schools of nursing to operate. Even with part-time involvement of faculty, costs in faculty salaries alone may be in the range of $100,000 to $200,000 annually. This creates tremendous pressure to secure external sources of funding, either through grants, contracts, or third-party payment.

In the short-term, grants and time-limited contracts may provide the necessary start-up and initial development funds. However, time spent searching for funding sources, writing grants, and negotiating contracts seriously limits direct service efforts. For the long term, a stable source of funding must be identified. The CNO and HARP project staff are in the process of seeking both short- and long-term funding.

Although all of the patients served by the project are medically indigent, many of them are either ineligible or have not applied for Medicaid. For those eligible, assisting with enrollment in the entitlement programs for which they qualify is a priority. However, until the goal of universal health insurance coverage is accomplished, the costs for many of these individuals will continue to be covered by specifically targeted state and federal grants.

Population Considerations

Special considerations in providing health services to homeless and other high-risk individuals include the following. Cultural competence and sensitivity is a major issue. The typical homeless person in Richmond is a young, African-American male, and the overwhelming majority (more than 90%) of individuals receiving HARP project services are African-American and very low income. To date, four of the five project staff are Caucasian, and all are middle-class women.

Major differences also exist in orientation to time, place, and priorities between the population served and the care providers. Life on the street requires a short-term survival orientation, with the activities for a day defined by day of the month, location and time of meal programs, shelter hours, and the weather. Priorities revolve around personal safety and meeting basic physiologic requirements rather than higher-order needs. In this instance, any health-related concern that is not emergent could be considered a higher-order need. Likewise, primary prevention or health promotion may be a foreign or remote consideration.

Especially in the homeless population, alienation is a core issue. Individuals frequently have a history of abusive, violent relationships, often including sexual abuse. For these individuals, development of any trusting relationship is a challenge. These difficulties are exacerbated by issues related to substance use and mental illness. Because of these psychological issues, relationships with these patients develop slowly over a long time or they do not develop at all. Consistent staffing at clinical sites is therefore important.

Another issue relates to the motivations of service providers in relation to this population. Not infrequently in healthcare as well as other social services, professionals work out or act out their own psychological issues in their relationships with patients. This is dangerous as well as nontherapeutic, particularly with this most vulnerable of populations. Much has been written in the past few years about codependency and caretaking behavior. Project staff have given thoughtful consideration to their motives and behavior to ensure that clinical providers are caregivers rather than caretakers.

Project Evaluation

Special issues are involved in the evaluation of services for homeless people. Many homeless people survive by remaining invisible (or at least inconspicuous) and are reluctant to be tracked or studied for evaluation purposes. The transient nature of this population, and their multidimensional problems, must be considered in choosing appropriate effectiveness indicators. A national survey of healthcare providers to the homeless (Hunter, Crosby, Ventura, & Warkentin, 1992) demonstrated limited development of outcomes-based evaluation methods.

Outcome evaluation may also be affected by community agency characteristics. That is, the nature and extent of record-keeping in many of these organizations is limited. Computerization may be entirely dependent on donation of equipment or acquisition through grant funding. Furthermore, actual data entry may depend on the adequacy of staffing and the urgency of other priorities.

Moreover, the literature has indicated little outcomes-based evaluation of either academic or freestanding nursing centers (Barger et al., 1993). However, design of meaningful outcome measures is a goal of the HARP project. Development of an outcomes-based evaluation program is included in the 5-year plan, with consultation anticipated.

In terms of process indicators, the HARP project is increasing access to primary health-care services, particularly for homeless and high-risk women and children. During the 1993–1994 academic year, with essentially one full-time equivalent provider, there were approximately 1100 patient contacts and more than 250 contacts with agency staff and volunteers. The project is also improving early detection of preventable and treatable problems and enhancing the monitoring and follow-up of chronic conditions. These activities are accomplished through referrals made from health maintenance clinics and outreach sites, through ongoing tuberculosis screening of patients and agency staff, and through blood pressure monitoring and referral coordination.

In the long-term, and with a computerized portable database for the project, other indicators will be assessed. These include the following six objectives, which are also evaluation criteria: (1) to increase knowledge of preventive self-care strategies, (2) to improve health status, (3) to reduce inappropriate use of emergency rooms and other hospital-based care, (4) to expand the capacity of agency staff to handle health-related concerns, (5) to improve coordination of care and integration of services among providers, and (6) to document qualitative differences in care provided and qualitative and quantitative differences in outcomes of nurse-managed care.

Ultimately, the CNO hopes to develop a model community-based nursing practice for the collaborative education of nursing, medical, and other health professions students in community-oriented primary care. In such a model, the faculty member uses the community as classroom and brings the community to the classroom, which enriches the student experience and provides a perspective otherwise lacking. Finally, nursing centers such as the CNO at the VCU/MCV School of Nursing hope to demonstrate a cost-effective alternative model of health services delivery for underserved as well as other populations.

Acknowledgment: The authors of this exemplar would like to recognize other faculty members involved in the development of the Virginia Commonwealth University/Medical College of Virginia Community Nursing Organization. They are Nancy Langston, PhD, RN (Dean); JoAnne K. Henry, EdD, RN (Director); Marcia Davis, MS, MsEd, RNC, WHCNP, ANP; Terry Phillips, MSN, RN; and Carolease Wallace, MPH, RN.

Note: References are cited at end of chapter.

Industry-Sponsored Comprehensive Healthcare in the Workplace

Jimmie K. Butts

Ideas color our world with possibility.
They are everywhere and take all guises...
Be ever alert, ever watchful,
to seize opportunity, to recognize possibilities
and assess potential.
Grasp firmly
an idea whose time has come.
Put aside your fears
and reach for what might be.
(From a poster by Great Performances, Inc., 1990)

HEALTHCARE IN THE WORKPLACE

Until I became personally involved in healthcare in the industrial setting, or workplace, I never thought of applying my nursing skills in a setting that seemed so routine, with so little hands-on nursing unless there was a crisis—an emergency. Then opportunity knocked. The opportunity to establish a nurse-managed healthcare facility in a corporate setting that became a trendsetter for other companies came to me in 1984.

That year, the director of human resources at SAS Institute Incorporated (SAS Institute), a small (about 300 employees) software development firm in Piedmont Region, North Carolina, recognized that healthcare costs were spiraling and adversely affecting company profits. The company was using a commercial insurance plan and the expenses were exorbitant for its population of young and healthy employees. A search was begun for an alternative to the typical commercial health insurance available.

One of the alternatives considered was to hire a nurse practitioner to develop on-site primary healthcare and a wellness program that would assist employees in choosing healthy lifestyles. This is where I came in.

In 1976, I completed the certification program to become a family nurse practitioner at the University of North Carolina at Chapel Hill School of Nursing. This program enabled me to acquire advanced practice skills. The convenience, nurturing, health education—all of which contributed to the documented success of the primary care program at SAS Institute— would have been impossible for a registered nurse in an industrial setting who did not have advanced practice skills. Without such training and skills, I could not have taken an appropriate medical history, requested (and many times performed) the appropriate diagnostic tests, made a medical diagnosis, and treated with medical judgment, prescribing the correct procedures or medications that a nurse in advanced practice is privileged to perform.

SEIZING THE OPPORTUNITY

In January 1984, David Russo, director of human resources at SAS Institute, and I discussed several concerns regarding a nurse-managed on-site primary healthcare and wellness program. He wanted to know what a nurse with advanced practice skills could do for the company, whether the company needed a company doctor, how a company medical department could benefit the company, and what could be done to improve the quality of care and lower costs. Here was an opportunity to design a program that included health education, preventive medicine, quality nursing, and early identification of risk factors and an opportunity to document the value of those services using an SAS Institute-developed software system. In April 1984, I accepted the challenge of developing a nurse-managed program that most nurses only dream about. Without education and experience in advanced practice, I would not have qualified for this new and exciting job.

I spent the first months making an informal needs assessment, doing blood pressure screenings, and educating employees (e.g., about managing high blood pressure, about caring for a sick child). In addition, I spent many hours designing the physical facility, ordering supplies and equipment, planning for future staffing, and surveying vendors. Contracting for laboratory services was a major cost-control factor. Also, a physician was hired to serve as a consultant to comply with the North Carolina laws stipulating that a nurse practitioner could perform medical acts only with physician backup.

The SAS Institute Health Care Center opened on July 23, 1984, soon thereafter, the company information systems department designed and installed a computer software system that simplified documentation of medical records. The system can compare the cost of company-provided services to the cost of the same services provided in the community at large. Using the software, the medical office manager tracks the figures and is able to report immediately figures that support this innovative program.

From the day the center opened until the present, there has never been a dull moment. Initially, I may have seen only eight patients a day; however, scheduling, doing lab work, taking vital signs, and transcribing notes kept me busy.

SERVICES PROVIDED

By mid-1985, about 1 year after the Health Care Center opened, the director of Human Resources and I determined a second nurse practitioner was needed. I then became the manager of the Health Care Center and continued to see patients in addition to my new responsibilities. As the company grew and added facilities out of state, the Health Care Center grew. The population enlarged and a remote development site was added. As the new manager of Corporate Health Services, my management and administrative duties expanded, thus requiring that I broaden my skills in those areas.

By March 31, 1994, when I retired, the center was seeing 60 patients a day. The staff consisted of 17 full-time people and a consulting physician who spent 4 hours a week at the center reviewing medical records, offering advice, and "keeping us out of trouble"—a phrase he used to describe his role as our consultant.

HEALTH CARE CENTER MISSION STATEMENT AND GOALS

From its inception, the Health Care Center has followed established goals and objectives, with measurable outcomes. The mission statement for the Health Care Center contains four aims:

1. to provide comprehensive assistance to employees and their families to meet their healthcare needs
2. to contribute to the establishment of a healthy working environment for employees
3. to provide the most reliable and current health information for all age groups
4. to empower employees to become wise consumers of healthcare.

Patient care is the first priority. The most efficient way to see patients, do lab work, document findings, attend meetings, and so forth is to schedule appointments rather than see them on a walk-in basis, except in emergencies. This policy permits a routine that allows adequate time with the patient and time to document findings accurately. Administrative time is built in for planning and implementing health education events, follow-up with patients, and research regarding epidemiology, needs assessment, and cost-effectiveness.

After 10 years of experience, the system continues to work; providers include full-time nurse practitioners, contract nurse practitioners, a licensed practical nurse, nursing assistants, medical technologists, a nutritionist, and a work-family administrator. A strong support staff includes medical transcriptionists, medical receptionists, and a medical office manager who manages the administrative staff and handles cost studies. In addition, the following three contract employees offer special services: a geriatric counselor who has a master's degree in social work, a geriatric nurse practitioner, and a certified psychological counselor.

The consulting physician worked 4 hours a week, teaching, counseling, reviewing the medical notes, and occasionally seeing a patient at the nurse practitioner's request. Two additional on-site physicians have been hired to expand center services to 24-hour call and hospital admission, if needed. The new physicians report to the manager of Corporate Health Services, a nurse practitioner.

Types of Care Provided

The Health Care Center provides various types of care, including acute care, physical examinations, emergency care, allergy injections and immunizations, counseling, and information to help employees choose a private healthcare provider.

Acute Care

Acute care at the center is provided at the following visits:
- brief visits for first aid or blood pressure checks
- routine visits, which are usually 15-minute exams for complaints of cold symptoms, infections, or other symptoms
- health checks, which are usually 15-minute exams in which the healthcare provider takes the patient's medical history; checks vital signs; examines the musculoskeletal system and heart and lungs; looks for hernia; and makes other pertinent considerations before clearing employees to participate in activities in the on-site recreation and fitness center.

Physical Examinations

During comprehensive physical examinations, the healthcare provider performs laboratory tests, makes health risk appraisals, records a complete health history, administers electrocardiograms and spirometries that are age and risk related, and performs a complete head-to-toe examination. Physicals are not mandatory; rather, anyone who requests an examination may have one and will be reminded to return at appropriate intervals for checkups.

Emergency Care

Employees, dependents, and visitors with injuries, those who faint or are in diabetic crisis, and so forth, are treated by the nurses in the Health Care Center or referred to either a physician on site or in the community. The nurse practitioners also are available to go to the site of the emergency and treat or assist even when community rescue services are involved.

Allergy Injections and Immunizations

Staff at the center administer immunizations after confirming the wishes or protocols of the person's private physician or the local health department. The licensed practical nurse can give the injections when the nurse practitioner is present and prepared to treat any reactions.

Counseling

Counseling is available for identification and management of stress or anxiety. Through the Generation to Generation program at the center, employees who seek guidance in working with elder family members and, at times, needy young family members, or in dealing with grief, for example, may receive counseling about available community resources. Also, the staff nutritionist offers counseling on obesity and other health problems, including problems related to diet (e.g., elevated cholesterol or anemia). The staff nurse practitioners or staff nutritionist, or the social workers or professional counselors with whom the Health Care Center contracts, may provide behavior modification for problems such as smoking and alcohol use. The exercise physiologist from the on-site recreation and fitness center works closely with the nutritionist and the Health Care Center staff on many of these programs.

Support To Choose a Private Healthcare Provider

The company does not subscribe to a preferred provider organization or a health maintenance organization. Instead, it gives the employees information to help them choose their own providers. It is more cost-effective if the provider has a collegial relationship with the Health Care Center staff and allows patients to use center services, such as laboratory examinations, electrocardiograms, immunizations, and so forth at company cost rather than the employee's cost.

BENEFITS OF THE HEALTH CARE CENTER

Convenience

The convenience of the Health Care Center is a major benefit for the employees and the company. Employee patients seen by appointment can be back at their workplace in 30 to 60 minutes. In contrast, if they had to leave the premises for appointments, they might not return for several hours. For instance, surveys taken in fall 1991 showed that community providers rarely saw patients at the appointed time. Obviously, this results in lost time, which costs the company and can affect both employee and company schedules.

Early Identification of Risk Factors

It is well known that early examination often reveals risk factors that can be reduced through early treatment. The Health Care Center continues the practice of health promotion, risk reduction, and disease prevention through screening and early treatment. Long before healthcare received so much press, SAS Institute and its self-funded insurance plan paid for physical examinations, mammograms, and well-baby care.

Wellness Programs

From its inception, the Health Care Center has offered programs to employees and their families to teach them about their health and how to become wise healthcare consumers. In 1985, the Wellness Committee of providers was formed and the wellness coordinator became the chairperson. This working committee now provides approximately 50 programs a year; as many as 10,000 people have participated in programs in 1 year.

Quality Care

Quality care is foremost. The nurse practitioners and the consulting physicians have a review system that enables them to identify health risks, helps the center to lower overall costs, and results in a healthier, wiser population. Services vary. One of the nurse practitioners is certified in Brazelton examinations of newborns. Another practitioner has a strong background and experience in treatment of substance abuse and the emotional components of illness; she serves as liaison to the employee assistance program, which assists employees to obtain early treatment for emotional illness before more costly treatments are needed. Another practitioner has considerable experience with adolescents as well as the unique problems faced by the minority community. In addition to working in their areas of interest, each practitioner has served in an administrative role as team leader or supervisor.

Quality care is also provided through the Generation to Generation program, which offers resources, education, and support to patients who are dealing with issues involving elderly family members. Furthermore, the Health Care Center administrator offers information and referrals for families all across the United States. She created the newsletter *Elderline,* a quarterly publication written and produced at SAS Institute at a reasonable cost; *Elderline* is available to all employees.

The Health Care Center makes creative use of the staff's special talents and skills. For example, a staff nurse practitioner implemented the federally mandated Blood-borne Pathogen and Infectious Disease Program for Workplace Safety, saving the company the $7000 to $10,000, an amount an outside consultant would have charged for that service. The medical laboratory technologist designed the laboratory procedures to be certified to comply with CLIA 88 laws, thus saving another several thousand dollars in consulting fees. The nutritionist provides services to diabetics and other patients with nutritional problems. She and the wellness coordinator from the on-site recreation and fitness center have had better than average success with weight loss and fitness programs.

The administrative staff and medical support staff also contribute in meaningful ways to this team of caregivers. All are valued for their individual and collective contributions. The medical receptionists work just as they would in a private office: they schedule appointments, which involves triage skills; handle innumerable phone calls; and remain ever pleasant. The consulting physicians are competent and caring, carefully review the medical records, and advise the staff in collegial ways. Respect begets respect. The team approach to healthcare works well at SAS Institute. Because retention of qualified staff is vital, SAS Institute developed a cost-effective program of quarterly continuing education events that provide current information for and support the professional growth of staff members. All staff members are encouraged to seek affiliation with their professional organizations and to reach constantly for the next level of performance and expertise. An audit team approach is currently being implemented to support a system of peer review and quality assurance.

COMPANY SUPPORT OF THE HEALTH CARE CENTER

SAS Institute paid third-party reimbursement to nurse practitioners, midwives, clinical nurse specialists in psychiatry, and master's-prepared social workers long before other companies or insurers did. Furthermore, the company implemented family leave policies before the law was passed. In addition, the president of SAS Institute, Jim Goodnight, executive vice president, John Sall, and director of human resources, David Russo, have given their support philosophically and financially so that healthcare can consist of quality, cost-effective services.

These are exciting times—those of us in advanced practice have so many opportunities that our dilemma is what to choose! Never before has there been such a high level of acceptance of nurse-midwives, nurse anesthetists, nurses who provide psychological services, and others in advanced practice.

Clinical skills, education, experience, courage, devotion to the profession of nursing, a vision, and faith in leaders, colleagues, and patients have all contributed to the success of the center. However, the nurse practitioners who provide primary care are the key element in its success. Patients who see a nurse in advanced practice and have their problem accurately diagnosed and appropriately treated will come back for future treatment, and word of mouth will bring others in. The Health Care Center has "satisfied customers" who have received quality care.

Another key factor in the success of this innovative model of healthcare has been the cooperation of community providers and their support of the nurse practitioners. Community physicians continue to seek referrals and offer to help us in many ways. The workplace is an appropriate and fitting site for healthcare centers. Using advanced practice nurses, an interdisciplinary team approach offers a cost-effective way to keep employed Americans healthy, useful, and productive members of society.

Note: References are cited at end of chapter.

C

School Health Services: A Case Study of the Madison Metropolitan School District

Mary Wachter Gulbrandsen

The goals of helping young people participate fully in their learning, feel safe in securing the healthcare they need, and reducing or eliminating those health problems that interfere with achievement are reasons that health services continue to be an integral part of the school environment. A pediatric nurse practitioner who chooses to practice pediatric nursing in the school setting will face a host of challenges and opportunities unique to that environment and population.

SETTING

School is where children spend the majority of their waking hours, and it is the "workplace" for nearly one fifth of the U.S. population, if both children and adults are counted (Green & Kreuter, 1991). Schools offer the opportunity for preventive health teaching as well as the management of primary healthcare needs. It has been known for years that education affects health. But only recently has it been made clear that academic achievement will require attending to health in the broadest sense because a child's health status directly affects his or her academic success (National Health/Education Consortium, 1990).

School health services support the educational mission of a school district by providing professional support to students to help them progress through their education by removing, limiting, or attenuating barriers to that end. School nursing is thus an integral part of the educational mission. "In today's world, schools can only accomplish their education mission if they attend to students' emotional, social, and physical problems" (National Commission on the Role of the School and the Community in Improving Adolescent Health, 1990, p. 38).

Nursing care in the school setting is important for all children but especially for children with chronic health problems who have specific needs for technical nursing procedures during the school day and for children with untreated acute health problems that are interfering with their ability to learn. This has been true in the Madison Metropolitan School District in Wisconsin where health services in the schools have undergone major changes. These changes have come about because of the increased social needs of the children in the city as well as the numbers of children attending school who require some form of healthcare. In today's America, the school may represent the only stable environment a youngster experiences and may be the most logical place to provide some of the necessary healthcare to children.

SIGNIFICANCE OF THE SCHOOL AS A HEALTHCARE SETTING

Schools gather together children who are economically and ethnically diverse, who live in many different family structures, who have different abilities and disabilities, and who have a variety of health problems and concerns. Schools have changed; thus, school nursing must also change. School districts face concomitant challenges and are expected and sometimes mandated to provide increasing levels of care within the school setting. School nurses in Madison have developed a strong practice framework to face these challenges and capitalize on the opportunities inherent in school nursing in the 1990s by embracing the need for preventive teaching and assuring that primary healthcare is available for all children. Advanced practice nurses in the school setting are a key part of this team of school care providers.

School nurses, particularly nurse practitioners, are governed by federal, state, and local laws guiding their practice. Many of the federal regulations pertaining to public services for people with disabilities affect the services schools (and school nurses) are required to provide. Pertinent state regulations range from the description of requirements for school nurse certification to the laws that govern child abuse reporting. Prescriptive authority for advanced practice nurses has been written into law in the state of Wisconsin. This law offers the nurse practitioner working in a school setting the potential ability to at least diagnose and treat those illnesses for which a child should not miss school or a parent miss work.

The Nurse Practice Act gives guidelines for the responsibilities and obligations of nurses in each state; the act is particularly important for the more autonomous nurse practitioner. The local board of education determines school district operations and policies. School nurses must stay abreast of legislation and policy at all levels and integrate changes in their practice.

The practice of a pediatric nurse practitioner, within the context of school health services, encompasses a wide range of services:

- providing traditional nursing services, such as direct care, counseling, screening programs, health education, advocacy, and participation in services to students with exceptional educational needs
- diagnosing and treating minor acute illnesses (under established protocol)
- becoming involved in districtwide decision-making committees regarding educational issues and other current concerns schools are being asked to address.

FRAMEWORK FOR NURSING CARE

The preceding services, and many others, are provided under a nursing practice framework that guides the Madison health services program. This framework states that

- nurses bring unique skills and knowledge to the school setting
- health services must be a part of the support services to the school population and system and must work in collaboration with families and community agencies outside the school
- health services must be staffed by highly qualified nurse practitioners, nurses, and nurse's assistants, who are organized in a differentiated staffing pattern to serve students, their families, and sometimes staff
- health services must provide both traditional and some nontraditional health services in every school building, although the population in each building may shape the exact nature of services provided
- health services must be provided to increase students' knowledge and ability to make decisions about their own health and healthcare and to help them act on those decisions.

This last goal is critical to the educational mission of the school district; by assisting students to increase their knowledge to make decisions about their own health and healthcare and to help them act on those decisions, they can become more active learners. The nurse and nurse's assistant in each health office strive to provide a child-oriented, safe, open environment in which all children feel they can access healthcare by a trusted adult. Children return to class more than 90% of the time after receiving the care they need so they can continue to participate in their school day.

HISTORICAL OVERVIEW

Historically, the Madison Metropolitan School District received health services from the Madison Health Department; however, in the 1983–1984 school year, the district, for a variety of reasons, decided to employ its own health services staff. The allocation for nurses has increased from 10 full-time equivalents during that year to a total of 21.75 full-time equivalents in 1993. This is a direct reflection of the board of education's belief that health services are an important part of the educational mission of the Madison schools.

Of the 30 nurses who currently fill the school nurse full-time equivalents, 19 are master's-prepared nurse practitioners and one is working on her master's degree. When health services were first brought under the employment of the Madison Metropolitan School District in 1983, only five of the then 15 nurses were master's-prepared in nursing. It has become almost an essential part of the broad range of nursing services provided in the district that a majority of the school nurses on staff have this advanced education. Having expertise in technical procedures in a nonhealthcare institution, diagnosing a broad range of health problems in children and families, coordinating healthcare within a variety of settings, and having physical examination skills and broad knowledge in the diagnosis and treatment of pediatric healthcare problems enhance the school nurse's ability to help young people be successful in school by removing unnecessary health barriers to learning.

POPULATION

The combined 43 schools in the Madison district have an enrollment of 24,800 students. The nurse/student ratio is approximately 1:1100. The health services staff is differentiated by both education and job description. Staff members include an administrator who is master's-prepared in pediatric nursing and certified as a pediatric nurse practitioner; master's-prepared nurse practitioners in program support roles; school nurses, most of whom are also master's-prepared nurse practitioners, but all of whom are minimally prepared at the baccalaureate level; and technically trained nurse's assistants. A pediatrician from the University of Wisconsin–Madison medical school serves as the medical adviser. The administrator and some of the nurse practitioners also hold joint appointments with the School of Nursing, University of Wisconsin–Madison.

Nurses and nurse's assistants are assigned to each school in the district based on a formula that factors total enrollment, the number of low-income students, the numbers of students who move in and out during the course of the school year, the number of students with exceptional educational needs, and the number of students with special healthcare needs. A nurse may be assigned to between one and three schools, depending on the factors listed; in addition a nurse's assistant is assigned to each school for part of every day. The nurse and assistant make up the health services team assigned to each building. A program support nurse is assigned to each team to provide support, assistance with difficult situations, and guidance to nursing practice.

Because schools have a mandate to provide free public education to all children grades 1 through 12 and for all children with disabilities aged 3 years to 21 years, the school nurse must have a strong developmental framework in his or her practice. This is particularly true because so many of today's young people face a number of threats to their well-being. Poverty, lack of insurance, limited understanding of and access to healthcare systems, untreated acute and severe chronic health problems, chemical abuse, assaults, and violence all challenge youths and their caregivers. The problems become particularly severe and intractable when multiple risks occur simultaneously for the same child at a time of great change and development in his or her life.

The Madison Metropolitan School District has a tradition of high student achievement and educational excellence. Seven of the 43 schools have received presidential awards as National Schools of Excellence. The median scores on standardized achievement tests in reading and mathematics have been at approximately the 70th percentile for many years. American College Test (ACT) and Scholastic Aptitude Test (SAT) scores are consistently above the national average. In 1993, almost 75% of the graduating seniors planned to attend postsecondary schools. The students are always well represented among state champions in interscholastic athletics and many receive statewide honors in performing and expressive arts.

Madison has experienced a dramatic change in demographics over the past 25 years. The city has changed from a relatively homogeneous, predominantly white-collar community to a city of increasing ethnic and socioeconomic diversity. In 1968, when the school population was approximately 34,000, 2% ($n = 680$) of the students were ethnic minorities. In 1993, with a school population of 24,452, 25.4% ($n = 6200$) of the students were from minority groups.

These demographic changes have been particularly significant during the past decade. Since 1983, the school population has increased by 9%, whereas the proportion of minority students has more than doubled, from 11% to 24%. According to a community assessment completed in 1993 (United Way of Dane County, 1993) the child poverty rate (the percentage of persons under age 18 living in households below the poverty level) in Madison/Dane County at the time of the 1980 census was 7.3%. In the 1990 census (Kaplan, 1993), the child poverty rate in the Madison Metropolitan School District had risen to 13.9%. On another measure of economic need, more than 25% of elementary school students are eligible for free or reduced lunch. In addition, one out of every five Madison students lives in a female-headed household, a family configuration highly correlated with poverty and poorer educational outcomes. Moreover, homeless children, almost unknown in the Madison community in 1988 numbered 1400 during the 1992–1993 school year. The majority (800) of the children were preschoolers, with most of the remainder of elementary school age.

The geographic mobility of children in the Madison schools, another major impediment to successful learning, has been growing steadily. During the 1992–1993 school year, 24 students moved into or out of an elementary school for every 100 students present on the date of the official enrollment count. High rates of mobility are strongly correlated with low achievement.

The change in demographics has increased the diversity in the Madison Metropolitan School District, enriching the educational experiences of all children and helping to prepare students for life in an increasingly multicultural society. However, the changes have also brought challenges to a community and school district frustrated that the educational environment that has successfully nurtured past populations has been less successful with the new student body. However, the Madison district has maintained its tradition of academic excellence. The school district is now at a critical juncture. The district and community continue to scrutinize how public education is being provided so that all of the young people of the district can succeed. All of these factors continue to challenge the health services staff in providing necessary health services for educational success. The overall absence rate of the district has continued to remain stable, with an average daily absence rate of 8% over the course of the school year. This low rate is partially due to the diligence of the health services staff in monitoring attendance patterns of students from very young ages and by having staff who can evaluate a child's condition and carry out an intervention without necessarily sending a child home.

One of the most striking changes in the student demographics (which provide the base of knowledge for determining how health services will be provided) is the number of young people coming to school without their basic needs having been met. A steady increase of students who come to school tired, hungry, inadequately clothed, or living in unsafe conditions has been documented.

Even in 1978, when school health programs were being reexamined, the healthcare issues under discussion centered around changing families, changing expectations of healthcare, alcohol and drug use, and accidents. Today's problems are even more severe (e.g., violence, mental illness, and new communicable diseases) and have become markedly so in a short time. School systems are recognizing the need for change again as they respond to these changes in the childhood experience.

INTERVENTIONS

Direct nursing services continue to account for the majority of health services activities. These services are generally provided to students referred directly to the health office or to those who come in on their own. In Madison, approximately 70 students are seen each day in each high school health office. Districtwide, more than 12,000 student contacts occur each month, not including administration of medications or performance of procedures.

Overall, males and females are somewhat evenly represented in the number of visits to the school health office. Students with exceptional education needs are seen by health services staff in greater numbers than their nondisabled peers. Although students with disabilities represent only 12% of the district population, they account for 27% of the health office visits. Children who live in poverty represent approximately 23% of the population, yet make 38% of the visits to the health office. Unquestionably, poverty affects a child's health status and ability to easily access healthcare.

Children in elementary school are seen more frequently for unmet basic needs and medication administration than older students. Students across all levels seek assistance for first aid and basic healthcare needs, but numbers rise somewhat as students mature and make healthcare decisions on their own. High school students seek counseling services much more frequently than younger students.

Although the incidence of chronic illness has not increased tremendously since the mid-1980s, there have been changes that have influenced both the survival and longevity rates of children with chronic health problems. These changes have resulted in increased mobility and school attendance. Certain chronic illnesses (e.g., asthma, attention deficit disorder, and neurologic conditions) have increased among the district population since 1986. Some of these increases may be due to improved recognition and diagnosis of conditions. Others, such as neurologic disorders, are most likely related to increased survival of very premature infants, prenatal exposure to drugs and alcohol, and exposure to lead in the early years of life. National trends support an increase in chronic, severe asthma in children. Two nurse practitioners on staff in collaboration with a private healthcare clinic are training specific community members in certain neighborhoods in how to manage asthma incidents without having to necessarily resort to emergency room care.

Nursing procedures such as catheterization, suctioning, blood glucose monitoring, tracheostomy care, medication administration, and coordination of care are all provided to students with chronic healthcare problems. Currently, about 50 students in the district must have specific nursing procedures provided daily. More than 600 medications are given daily; additionally, there are many orders for medication and procedures as needed. Nurses may delegate nursing procedures to less skilled staff, whom the nurses train and supervise.

In addition to nursing care for children with chronic illnesses, screening programs such as hearing, vision, depression, blood pressure, and scoliosis, and the monitoring of immunization status are all provided to students. Home visits, phone calls, or any other necessary follow-up are completed, because the district believes that no screening program should be initiated unless appropriate follow-up services can be guaranteed.

Students with exceptional educational needs make up about 10% of the school population. Their needs may range from speech and language therapy services to the many related services of occupational and physical therapy or nursing services to deal with severe and profound cognitive and physical disabilities. Nurses in these instances will sit on the multidisciplinary team to determine the need for exceptional educational programming. They may assist in defining student goals or they may provide necessary related health services to maximize the benefit of the educational program for the student.

Counseling and crisis management account for the second area of greatest need among students in Madison schools. Counseling services may range from helping a student who is struggling with a math class to crisis management with a young woman who has just found out she is pregnant.

Health education, another major priority area, can occur in many ways. Both through individual health contacts and in group discussions, children can acquire knowledge and make sound decisions. Nurses are actively involved in student health curriculum development, consultation to classroom teachers, direct teaching in the classroom, and the conduct and development of staff inservices.

School nurses also act as liaisons with community organizations and in advocacy roles for children. They may coordinate care for one child among several community healthcare agencies, or they may speak on behalf of the district to a legislative panel examining, for instance, the drinking age for minors.

Innovative health services programs have also contributed to making the Madison school district better able to serve all children's needs. In many ways, these programs have also helped keep the nurse's role challenging and exciting. Programs such as providing complete health assessments for homeless students have been developed. The parents of homeless children have been particularly receptive to these services and have managed to follow through with care under difficult circumstances. Instead of implementing school-based health clinics, the district chose to operate under the Robert Wood Johnson model of the late 1970s, in which nurses and nurse practitioners provide expanded healthcare services at all grade levels and are part of the school system staff instead of being part of an outside agency that comes into the school system. This successful model does not have to deal with enrollment issues or confidentiality issues, and it ensures that all children in the school setting have access to basic healthcare services.

In Wisconsin, Early Periodic Screening and Diagnosis is provided to children through a program called Healthcheck. Nurse practitioners in the Madison schools, in collaboration with the local public health departments and private healthcare providers, are involved in providing all of the components of the Healthcheck screen in clinics located at neighborhood schools. In the future, these clinics will be provided regularly and will be available not only to children who are eligible for medical assistance but to children who do not have insurance or means to pay for private healthcare. Early observations from these clinics have indicated that the children receive the healthcare, immunizations, and follow-up that they need, that families are more comfortable coming to the school setting for educational reasons, and that the children's attendance improves.

These clinics in Madison do not intend to compete with private healthcare providers, but rather to act as a means by which all children can gain entry into the healthcare setting and, in so doing, receive necessary examinations and immunizations. Goals are to provide clinics in a setting with which families are comfortable—the school—and to help children locate and access primary healthcare through the private healthcare providers in the city.

Many of the nurse practitioners on staff also hold joint appointments with the University of Wisconsin–Madison School of Nursing. As a result of these joint appointments and the strong staff commitment to providing learning opportunities for healthcare professionals, the Madison school district is also used as a pediatric setting for undergraduate and graduate nursing students, and medical students, and residents from the School of Medicine, University of Wisconsin–Madison. The district has become a popular clinical site because this is where children are during the day; it is rare that a child would leave a secondary or tertiary care setting and return to school in a short time.

Continued increases in the numbers of students with special healthcare needs will mean that nurse practitioners will provide more and more care coordination among several agencies and families. For example, one of the school nurse practitioners sat on a state committee that studied early childhood initiatives to define how the relevant public laws would be implemented in Wisconsin. The Madison schools continue to respond to the increasing ethnic diversity of the district, making expanded health services a priority in this area. Additionally, nurses continue to be involved in implementing a strong alcohol and drug program including prevention, intervention, and aftercare services.

OUTCOMES

Measuring the effectiveness of health services is critical in determining whether educational dollars should continue to be spent for the provision of healthcare. The Madison district health services staff submits an annual report to illustrate not what the staff have done but what the results of those activities have meant for the success of students in school and for their personal well-being. School nursing must focus on the outcomes for children and families and must do so through strong evaluative processes. Continuing to document nursing activities, document children's success both before and after nursing interventions, and develop new interventions to meet the changing needs of the population within the overall social context are essential if children are going to benefit overall.

REIMBURSEMENT ISSUES

Funding health services in schools will continue to be a challenge as educational dollars become increasingly scarce. Accessing the federal medical assistance dollars for school health services for eligible children is an option that many school districts, including the Madison school district, are exercising. Writing maternal and child healthcare grants is another avenue used to secure money for these necessary services. However, neither the health nor the educational success of young people will be achieved until communities as a whole decide that the health of children is a priority and set common goals by which to measure the success of their programs.

Today, as always, families are—or should be—the center of all children's lives. The mission of public schools is educating young people to be productive members of society. That mission can only be accomplished by bringing children, their families, and services—including public and private healthcare—together in coordination and collaboration. Schools should be a center for this collaboration.

Debate will always arise about the proper role of the school. Critics protest that schools are not social services agencies and should not be expected to remedy all of the nation's social ills. But, as the Carnegie Council on Adolescent Development (1989) has pointed out, "Where the need directly affects learning, the school must meet the challenge. So it is with health" (p. 61). School health services are part of this education mission and should be a part of the school organization, but also a part of the broader structure of the community.

Currently, the school nurse staff of the Madison district is reviewing how best the health needs of students can and should be met in this community. Several specific criteria will help determine the direction the deployment of school nurses will take as well as the general structure of the provision of all of health services.

CONCLUSION

It is believed that all children in Madison should receive regular healthcare exams as determined by an agreed on periodicity schedule, be immunized at recommended levels, have a primary healthcare home, should not miss school because of an inability to access healthcare, and should have urgent care available to them regardless of setting. It is the hope of the staff that, in the process of determining how to best meet these goals for the children of Madison, other community public and private healthcare providers will join in the efforts to meet these goals. It is hoped the use of technology will be incorporated into this framework also, to ensure that children receive continuity of care.

Nursing care in the Madison Metropolitan School District is surprisingly intense and complex. Expanded healthcare services provided by a differentiated nursing staff can and do make a tremendous difference in students' ability to succeed in school and in growing and developing in all domains (Madison Metropolitan School District, 1994).

References

American Association of Colleges of Nursing. (1991). *Special report on institutional resources and budgets, 1990–1991* (Publication No. 90-91-4). Washington, DC: Author.

American Association of Colleges of Nursing. (1992, January). *The emergence of nursing centers* (issue bulletin). Washington, DC: Author.

Aydelotte, M. E., Barger, S. E., Branstetter, E., Fehring, R. J., Lindgren, K., Lundeen, S., McDaniel, S., & Riesch, S. K. (1987). *The nursing center: Concept and design.* Kansas City, MO: American Nurses' Association.

Barger, S. E., & Bridges, W. C. (1989). Academic nursing centers: An assessment after a decade. In National League for Nursing, *Nursing centers: Meeting the demand for quality health care* (Publication No. 21-2311, pp. 153–167). New York: National League for Nursing.

Barger, S. E., & Bridges, W. C. (1990). An assessment of academic nursing centers. *Nurse Educator, 15*(2), 31–36.

Barger, S. E., Nugent, K. E., & Bridges, W. C. (1993). Schools with nursing centers: A 5-year follow-up study. *Journal of Professional Nursing, 9*(1), 7–13.

Carnegie Council on Adolescent Development. (1989). *Turning points: Preparing American youth for the 21st century.* Waldorf, MD: Author.

Children's Defense Fund. (1994). *The state of America's children: Yearbook 1994.* Washington, DC: Author.

Donaldson, M., Yordy, K., & Vanselow, N. (Eds.). (1994). *Defining primary care: An interim report.* Washington, DC: National Academy Press.

Elsberry, N., & Nelson, F. (1993). How to plan financial support for nursing centers. *Nursing and Health Care, 14*(8), 408–413.

Green, L. W., & Kreuter, M. W. (1991). *Health promotion planning: An educational and environmental approach.* New York: Mayfield Publishing.

Higgs, Z. R. (1988). The academic nurse-managed center movement: A survey report. *Journal of Professional Nursing, 4*(6), 422–429.

Higgs, Z. R. (1989). Models of academic nurse-managed centers. In National League for Nursing, *Nursing centers: Meeting the demand for quality health care* (Publication No. 21-2311, pp. 103–110). New York: National League for Nursing.

Hunter, J. K., Crosby, F. E., Ventura, M. R., & Warkentin, L. (1992). A national survey to identify evaluation criteria for programs of health care for homeless. *Nursing and Health Care, 12*(10), 536–542.

Kaplan, T. (1993, June). Madison's children. *Wisconsin Council on Children and Families, Inc., Madison, WI,* 11.

Madison Metropolitan School District. (1994). *Health services report: 1983–1993.* Madison, WI: Author.

National Commission on the Role of the School and the Community in Improving Adolescent Health. (1990). *Code blue: Uniting for healthier youth.* Alexandria, VA: National Association of State Boards of Education.

National Health/Education Consortium. (1990). *Crossing the boundaries between health and education.* Washington, DC: National Commission to Prevent Infant Mortality.

Richmond City Health Department. (1991, September). *SJR 179: Primary care needs assessment—Final report.* Richmond, VA: Author.

Richmond Community Action Program. (1993). [Richmond Community Action Program Head Start programs]. Unpublished background materials.

Richmond Department of Mental Health, Mental Retardation, and Substance Abuse Services. (1993, March). [Homelessness in Richmond]. Unpublished fact sheet. Richmond, VA: Author.

U.S. Department of Health and Human Services, U.S. Public Health Service (1990). *Healthy people 2000: National health promotion and disease prevention objectives* (DHHS Publication No. PHS 91-50213). Washington, DC: U.S. Government Printing Office.

U.S. Department of Health and Human Services. (1992). *Healthy people 2000.* Boston: Jones and Bartlett.

U.S. Department of Health and Human Services. (1994). *Put prevention into practice.* Washington, DC: U.S. Government Printing Office.

U.S. Preventive Health Services Task Force. (1989). *Guide to clinical preventive services.* Baltimore: Williams & Wilkins.

United Way of Dane County, Madison, Wisconsin. (1993). *Community assessment for health and human services planning in Dane County: 1993.* United Way of Dane County, Madison, WI: Author.

Virginia Coalition for the Homeless. (1993, January). *1992 shelter provider survey.* Richmond, VA: Author.

Virginia Commonwealth University, Medical College of Virginia School of Nursing, Community Nursing Organization. (1993, Spring). [Interviews with homeless service providers, Churches Around Richmond Involved to Assure Shelter, shelter guests, and Downtown Community Ministries lunch program participants]. Unpublished raw data.

Walker, P. H. (1991). The community nursing center. *Rochester Nursing,* 18–19.

Weinreb, L. (1992). Preventive medical care for homeless men and women. In D. Wood (Ed.), *Delivering health care to homeless persons* (pp. 61–75). New York: Springer.

Wood, D. (Ed.). (1992). *Delivering health care to homeless persons.* New York: Springer.

18

Management of High-Risk and Vulnerable Populations

Introduction: Ruth M. Ouimette

The delivery of primary care to vulnerable populations is one of the most important challenges for healthcare providers. The three exemplars in this chapter personify the Institute of Medicine's definition of *primary care* given in Chapter 17 (see p. 255). Many more innovative practice models that serve as exemplars of healthcare delivery could be included in the text. Gerontologic practice initiatives are one such category (Strumpf, 1994). The selected exemplars describe clinical practice roles of advanced practice nurses who are positioned *and* prepared to meet the complex primary care needs of high-risk and vulnerable populations.

Faust provides an exemplary caring approach to understanding and enhancing the advanced practice nurse's ability to care for patients cross-culturally. The interaction between a patient and a provider is more dynamic with an understanding of the individual's migration history. As a result, the provider can offer higher quality care. Faust guides both the new and the experienced clinician on an invaluable journey of discovery about healthcare delivery across cultures. She puts into perspective the importance of understanding non-Western healthcare practices. She also assists the reader to maintain an open mind while working to understand the significance of alternative health beliefs to people from other cultures—beliefs that may differ from the healthcare provider's.

Henderson has been an innovator of advanced practice since the mid-1970s, when she developed a nurse practitioner role designed to provide care to an elderly population. She was able to build relationships between professionals and within a local community to develop what is now a prime example of healthcare for older people: the continuing care retirement community. Henderson's exemplar of advanced nursing practice demonstrates the complexity of her role organizationally and the integrated balance she is able to maintain as she provides individualized care to a large patient population. The care she provides ranges from promoting health and disease prevention to assisting patients and their families to manage complex health problems including completion of life with dignity.

Dick and Burns-Tisdale provide a broader community-based model of advanced nursing practice: home healthcare. Beth Israel Hospital in Boston has long been a pacesetter for mod-

Hickey JV: ADVANCED PRACTICE NURSING: Changing Roles and Clinical Applications © 1996 Lippincott–Raven Publishers

els of care, and this exemplar is no exception. Since 1970, nurse practitioners have been an integral part of providing community-based care to underserved and at-risk populations. According to Dick and Burns-Tisdale, "Nurse practitioners can provide ongoing primary medical aspects of care, serve as case managers, provide linkages to the greater healthcare system, and provide direct hands-on nursing care" (p. 307).

The models and roles described in the exemplars have stood the test of time. After 20 years, they are viable and growing, and are consistent with recommendations for how nursing must approach healthcare to prepare for the 21st century. Each of the exemplars represents what Goeppinger means when, in Chapter 5, she describes the "new" primary care as an opportunity for nursing.

Providing Inclusive Healthcare Across Cultures

Shotsy C. Faust

It is very difficult to know people and I don't think one can ever really know any but one's own countrymen. For men and women are not only themselves; they are also the region in which they were born, the city apartment or farm in which they learnt to walk, the games they played as children, the old wives tales they overheard, the food they ate, the schools they attended, the sports they followed, the poets they read, the god they believed in. It is all these things that have made them what they are, and these are the things that you can't come to know by hearsay, you can only know them if you lived them. (Maugham, 1944)

More than 50 years ago, the English writer Somerset Maugham underscored the difficulty of trying to understand people from different backgrounds and experiences. In clinical practice, nurse practitioners encounter many kinds of patients who present with languages other than English and come from a variety of cultures. When confronted with this diversity, the nurse practitioner might question how to best meet patient needs safely and with sensitivity. This exemplar outlines the following three goals: (1) to examine the process of migration and how it affects clinical care, (2) to explore ways of identifying and incorporating the patient's health belief system into the therapeutic regimen in a culturally sensitive and clinically effective manner, and (3) to evaluate the effect of the bilingual interpreter on the patient–practitioner relationship. Achievement of these goals will enhance the practitioner's ability to care for patients cross-culturally. These goals are presented in the form of the problem-oriented model geared toward the practicing clinician: the SOAP (Subjective, Objective, Assessment, Plan) process.

The traditional Western medical model teaches healthcare practitioners to identify pathophysiologic processes that cause the patient's complaint. Frequently, this disease focus fails to consider the broader context of the patient's health beliefs or practices. When working cross-culturally, it seems simpler to focus on the quantifiable, measurable processes of the body because there are so few guidelines or experiences to assess the context or culture of the patient's complaints. Unfortunately, a focus on the disease itself to the exclusion of its context can lead to frustration for both patient and practitioner. Symptoms and conditions that cannot be explained by our medical tradition and are not readily quantifiable by examination or laboratory testing are easily overlooked or dismissed.

A disease focus also reinforces the view of newcomers as victims, rather than as individuals with strengths and resources as survivors (Meucke, 1992). Most practitioners attempt to understand the cultures of newcomers they see in practice. Practitioners often assume, however, that there is a degree of homogeneity among groups who share the same ethnicity or language. For example, Southeast Asians represent different countries, languages, religions, and cultural identities but are sometimes viewed as being the same. Each patient who comes to a clinic for care brings an individual worldview that is formed by education, class background, urban or rural upbringing, and exposure to Western healthcare (Nydegger, 1983). Newcomers also vary in their motivations to emigrate. Thus, although patients may share language or ethnicity, each patient brings a unique set of beliefs and expectations to the clinical setting.

CLINICAL CARE PLAN: INTEGRATING THE MIGRATION PROCESS INTO CLINICAL CARE

This section addresses the two essential aspects of eliciting the history or subjective information from the patient. Understanding the newcomer's migration status and the psychological stage within the migration process are critical to the provision of appropriate care.

Newcomer's Status

It is useful to understand the difference between *immigrants* and *refugees*. Immigrants and refugees leave their homeland for different reasons and have different experiences of flight and resettlement (Westermeyer, 1990). Immigrants come to a new land seeking opportunity for a better life. They may have the time to plan the emigration; choose the country in which to settle; and bring material goods, resources, and family with them. Although immigration can be overwhelming and stressful, immigrants move toward a perceived goal and future. Conversely, refugees flee persecution or death. Having little or no time to plan for their flight, they often leave everything, including family, behind. They spend considerable time, sometimes years, in a refugee or detainment camp awaiting asylum in a country not always of their choosing. Refugee patients commonly will have been imprisoned or tortured or will have lost other family members to a violent death (DeLay & Faust, 1987). Their focus is to flee from something or someone, rather than to reach for a new goal. Refugee patients, therefore, are at higher risk for physical and emotional crises after arrival than are immigrant patients. It is often at this time that refugee patients first come to the clinic.

At the first visit, the nurse practitioner should ascertain, without exploring details, whether the patient is a refugee or immigrant and how long he or she has resided in the United States. The practitioner's description of the patient as an immigrant versus a refugee should be based on the newcomer's motivation for migration and his or her emotional status, rather than on the patient's political or legal qualifications. Many undocumented newcomers or illegal aliens fear that questions about immigration status could result in deportation or reprisal. Consequently, it is important that the nurse practitioner explain that legal status is not germane to the clinic visit, and will not be reported or documented. Patients should be reassured that information about the circumstances of their immigration is only used to gauge the stress or duress they have experienced.

Migration History

Carlos Sluzki, a physician who has worked extensively with migrant families, developed the Migration History model of migration (Sluzki, 1979, 1992). The Migration History is a helpful tool in the collection of historical information from the patient and is a useful predictor of potential patient distress experienced during each stage in the migration process. Practitioners can also use it as a predictor of physical and emotional distress after the newcomer's arrival.

However, practitioners must evaluate each patient individually. This tool is meant to provide general guidelines for assessing the stresses of migration. Practitioners should not use the Migration History to generalize about all individuals who migrate from one country to another. When applied judiciously, the Migration History can help practitioners understand the individual patient's psychology and craft a care plan that is specific to individual patient needs. Sluzki divided migration into the following five stages; (1) Planning Stage, (2) Act of Migration, (3) Period of Overcompensation, (4) Period of Decompensation, and (5) Resolution Stage or Stage of Intergenerational Support.

The Planning Stage may be a prolonged one for immigrants. During this stage, immigrants make their plans to emigrate to the country of destination. The time between recognition of the need to flee to the act of migration itself often is abbreviated to minutes, hours, or days.

The Act of Migration refers to the duration of transit from the country of origin to the country of destination for immigrants. For refugees, migration is a time of intense stress and uncertainty because their destination is unknown. Refugees may spend from months to years in a refugee or detention camp waiting for permanent placement in a third or permanent country of asylum.

Soon after arrival (the Period of Overcompensation), both refugees and immigrants begin to learn the essentials of daily life in their new country. They focus on obtaining housing, using public transportation, receiving welfare assistance, enrolling children in school, and finding healthcare. Psychologically, newcomers are often relieved at "having arrived," and are hopeful about prospects in the new country. Worries or concerns about past experiences and losses are supplanted by the mastering of tasks necessary for survival in their adopted country. In addition, a newcomer's social services agency or individual sponsor may arrange for a health screening. Nurse practitioners complete typical screening for tuberculosis or hepatitis as well as immunization updates; newcomers often have few health concerns or complaints.

The Period of Decompensation occurs when the newcomers have mastered basic skills, usually 6 months to 1 year after arrival, and the reality of making a life in their new country becomes more apparent. Newcomers typically speak little, if any, English and have few transferable job skills. Housing might be limited to overcrowded rooms in a low-income area. Memories of the homeland, of dead loved ones or loved ones left behind, or of the flight experience itself may surface. Hopelessness and despair frequently ensue. It is often at this point when patients come to a clinic for care. Their complaints are commonly somatic, including headache, weakness, dizziness, fatigue, or exacerbations of preexisting conditions (Westermeyer et al., 1989).

The Stage of Intergenerational Support is related to resolution of migration crises. Families are able to come together to provide strength and support to members, and the process of adjustment or acculturation continues. Practitioners do not often witness the Resolution Stage or Stage of Intergenerational Support because their patients frequently are not in crisis. Patients may reexperience the psychological crises of migration in various stages if other life stresses intensify.

First Clinic Visit

The following discussion addresses how practitioners use the Migration History model during the first three clinic visits. The patient may come to the first clinic visit (Table 18-1)—unless it is a screening visit that was not arranged to address a complaint—because he or she has been experiencing symptoms of crisis, which may present as multiple somatic complaints, vegetative symptoms of depression, or symptoms of posttraumatic stress disorder.

In addition to the symptom-focused medical history, the practitioner elicits information about migration in the reverse order of occurrence, starting with the present living situation only, unless the patient volunteers more. Illustrative questions are, Where are you living? Do you live alone or with family or friends? Do you have any means of income or assistance?

TABLE 18-1 **Format for Three Sample Clinic Visits**

Visit No.	Subjective	Objective	Assessment	Plan
1	Obtain medical history Obtain migration history Apply the explanatory model	Provide a complete or focused exam Look for signs of folk treatment	Perform a differential diagnosis Relabel diagnosis using patient's terminology	Include family in treatment Provide treatment (including symptomatic or over-the-counter) Explain test, lab results Advise on diet Discuss appropriate nontraditional therapies Schedule follow-up visit
2	Follow up complaints Add immediate past of migration history (arrival to USA) Obtain more extensive psychosocial history	Assess blood pressure, pulse, other vital signs Check lab tests results	Hone differential diagnosis Begin to consider psychiatric diagnosis, if appropriate	Adjust medications or treatments; consider other therapies Refer, if needed, to support groups and so forth Schedule follow-up visit
3	Evaluate symptoms Probe migration history/ Premigration flight	Assess vital signs	Continue to assess problems Evaluate healthcare maintenance needs	Adjust medications or treatments Refer, if needed, to specialist (eg, cardiologist) Teach healthcare maintenance Schedule follow-up visit

The patient may view questions about the past or about earlier stages of migration as intrusive and personal because the patient has yet to form a relationship with the practitioner. Furthermore, inquiring about the reasons for fleeing and evaluating torture or abuse may trigger or intensify symptoms.

The patient has come specifically for treatment of particular physical complaints; it is paramount that the practitioner focus on the symptoms at hand because the patient may perceive questions about emotional issues as suggesting mental or emotional disorder. Western culture is unique in its separation of psyche and soma. In other healing traditions, it is uncommon for practitioners to ask probing or psychological questions that seem unrelated to the problem at hand (Westermeyer et al., 1989). Patients and healers in most other cultures do not distinguish so clearly between emotional and physical events, nor do they attribute psychological causes to experience in the Western manner. Patients do not complain of "depression" or "sadness" but rather headache, abdominal pain, or other somatic ailments (Chung & Kagawa-Singer, 1993; DeLay & Faust, 1987). Many cultures equate expression of psychological distress with mental illness or "craziness." A psychiatric diagnosis can reflect and have social consequences not only on that individual but on the family as a group.

Explanatory Model

Western health practitioners often do not understand the value patients place on certain symptoms or treatments; however, patient responses to questions about their health beliefs can be revealing (Patcher, 1994). Practitioners at times may find the patient's description of a symptom (e.g. "hotness in the body") unfamiliar or meaningless. Rather than pursue a fruitless medical evaluation of a misunderstood entity, it is better that they explore the patient's beliefs about the symptom.

Arthur Kleinman, an anthropologist and cross-cultural psychiatrist at Harvard University, developed a series of questions for eliciting the explanatory model that underlies the patient's health beliefs. Practitioners will find it useful to ask these questions (especially 1, 2, and 8) during the first clinic visit when they take the medical history. They should note the patient's phrases or words for describing the symptom (e.g., "hotness") to be used later when the practitioner's health beliefs are joined with the patient's to formulate a shared assessment and plan. It is helpful to use the questions with patients from Western culture as well, because everyone has an explanatory model or system of health beliefs to explain or cope with symptoms. Kleinman's (1978) eight questions are as follows:

1. What do you call your problem? What name does it have?
2. What do you think has caused your problem?
3. Why do you think it started when it did?
4. What does your sickness do to you? How does it work?
5. How severe is it? Will it have a short or long course?
6. What do you fear most about your sickness?
7. What are the chief problems your sickness has caused for you?
8. What kind of treatment do you think you should receive? What are the most important results you hope to receive from the treatment? (p. 256).

Second Clinic Visit

During the second (or follow-up) clinic visit (see Table 18-1), the practitioner reviews the patient's health status, lab test results, and the recommended therapeutic interventions. The practitioner continues the Migration History and explores the act of migration itself. In the case of refugee patients, this may involve discussion of health status or events that occurred in the refugee camp, when symptoms might have emerged for the first time.

Third Clinic Visit

During the third visit (see Table 18-1), the practitioner continues to evaluate the patient's symptoms and assess the efficacy of interventions. It is now appropriate to ask more probing questions about the migration, including the reason for leaving the homeland, the status of family and friends left behind, or specific details of the patient's flight. By now, a trusting relationship has likely been formed, and the patient may feel more comfortable disclosing painful portions of their migration history, such as imprisonment, torture, or other distressing memories. The medical evaluation is well underway, with symptoms evaluated by way of traditional medical, psychological, and cultural approaches.

Physical Exam

The physical exam is an opportunity for hands-on nursing care. Because nonverbal communication is the primary or only mode of communication between the practitioner and patient when they do not speak the same language, the exam allows the nurse to provide touch and reassurance while data gathering. Even in follow-up clinic visits when little new information might be gained from the physical exam, a maneuver that involves touch is helpful. Taking the pulse or blood pressure places the practitioner in direct contact with the patient and reinforces their nonverbal relationship. Otherwise, the pair is forced to rely only on verbal communication, which usually occurs through a third person: the interpreter (Sluzki, 1984).

Folk Treatments

The physical exam also allows the practitioner to examine the patient for the stigmata of folk treatments. In many Southeast Asian cultures, moxibustion, coin rubbing, or cupping are common treatments (Buchwald, Panwala, & Hooton, 1992). Moxibustion involves placing a burning herb stick over or onto an affected area of distress. A small superficial burn typically remains after the treatment, such as two symmetrical burns seen at either side of the umbilicus of young Cambodian children. The patients believe such treatment is useful for diarrhea, but practitioners may mistake the treatment as a sign of child abuse.

In coin rubbing, a coin is rubbed over the back in the linear configuration of the acupuncture meridians. A lubricant, such as tiger balm, facilitates the rubbing and leaves ecchymotic marks across the back. This treatment is common in adults and children, who believe it is useful for upper respiratory complaints. Unfortunately, practitioners unfamiliar with the practice have also mistaken it as evidence of child abuse.

Cupping is a treatment in which a small cup is warmed to create a vacuum and then placed over the area of complaint, usually the forehead, leaving a circular ecchymotic area that lasts for several days. This is a typical treatment for headache; it is not uncommon to see many patients in the waiting room with cupping marks on their foreheads.

Cultures vary in the types of treatments they consider useful. Some patients from Eastern Africa, the Sudan, Ethiopia, or Eritrea use ritual scarification or folk surgery as treatments. Some patients from these cultures believe vertical scars through the eyebrows are a useful treatment for trachoma. Patients consider uvulectomy as a treatment for dehydration. Perhaps the most controversial folk surgery is female circumcision or genital mutilation. Although this tribal custom has been outlawed, it persists, especially in rural areas. Women who have had sexual mutilation surgery may be ashamed and reluctant to be examined for fear of pain during the exam or of the practitioner's judgment. Painful sequelae and complications are associated with this practice, including increased frequency of infection, painful intercourse and childbirth, and decreased sexual sensitivity (El Dareer, 1983; Ntiri, 1993). Other tattoos and scars are visible on patients from many cultures, including our own.

Practitioners should ask patients if marks are for treatment, protection, or beauty. Practitioners must be aware of the marks some treatments leave. Because not all treatments leave marks, practitioners should inquire in a nonjudgmental way about the use of herbs, drugs, or other treatments as part of the assessment. It is important that practitioners present a nonjudgmental attitude about unfamiliar treatments and remember that Western medical treatments may be equally unusual to patients.

Dual Use of Healing Systems

Most patients are dual users of health systems, continuing to consult with folk or traditional healers while seeking help from Westerner practitioners. For example, they may believe Western medicines such as antibiotics are powerful and highly desirable treatments. One way of joining with the patient is to accept and promote the use of harmless traditional healing methods. This acceptance supports and validates the newcomer's health belief system and allows the practitioner to gradually introduce new concepts regarding health promotion, maintenance, or treatment from a Western perspective.

Assessment

At assessment, the practitioner can formulate a differential diagnosis and begin to join the Western paradigm with the patient's health belief system. The nurse practitioner will have completed the history of the patient's illness, using several tools to determine the patient's immigration status and explanatory model or health belief system. The patient will have discussed the complaint and the practitioner will have noted what the patient calls the problem. The completed physical exam will include an assessment for signs of folk treatment. In discussing the assessment with the patient, the practitioner should use both the Western term for the problem along with the patient's terminology; for example, "in this country, what you call "heat in the belly" we call cystitis or urinary tract infection. We believe it is caused by bacteria and is treated in the following manner." Or, "What you call "wind in the back" we call bronchitis or an infection in the lungs." The assessment (and the problem list in the patient's medical record) include the Western diagnostic language along with the patient's terminology for the problem.

Care Plan

For nurse practitioners, the patient care plan includes not only treatment for the patient's problem but also healthcare maintenance, health education, and preventive interventions. When working cross-culturally, the plan is expanded to include interventions that support the patient's health belief system and values. Such support enhances the practitioner–patient relationship and patient compliance and fosters an openness regarding dual healing philosophies. The practitioner should be explicit in discussing each facet of the patient care plan and not assume that the patient or family will understand expectations regarding medications, tests, diet, or consultation with other healthcare providers or folk healers.

Family

It is important to include the family in the care plan whenever possible because diagnoses affect the family as well as the patient. Furthermore, the family is the most important unit of care in most cultures; at times, it is the cohesiveness and integrity of the family unit that gives the patient the hope needed to survive serious illness or depression. The practitioner should ask the patient if particular family members (such as the head of household) need to be present when the practitioner plans to make care recommendations. Including the family according to the patient's beliefs and wishes demonstrates the practitioner's respect for cultural values and enhances the prospects of compliance with the therapeutic regimen or plan.

Medications

Practitioners often incorrectly assume that patients from other cultures have ready access to remedies and over-the-counter medications. Consequently, practitioners may wait until arriving at a firm diagnosis, validated by quantifiable test results, before prescribing a therapeutic regimen. For newcomer patients, simple treatments such as acetaminophen or cough syrup may be unavailable due to the patient's income, inability to read labels written in English, or inability to speak the same language as the store clerk. For these reasons, it is helpful to provide the patient with simple over-the-counter remedies when possible. This demonstrates the practitioner's intention to care for the patient and to give help readily available to others.

Patients who do not speak or read English also have difficulty remembering medication instructions given verbally; practitioners can provide those patients with medication cards (Fig. 18-1). Each medication card has an illustration representing morning, noon, early evening, and night. Medications are affixed to the cards with tape or glue under the appropriate time illustration, and the card is enclosed in a plastic envelope for protection. Patients are encouraged to bring the medication cards to each clinic session for review and revision with their practitioner. Use of medication cards illustrates a concrete way of educating patients how and when to take their medications, even if they cannot read.

Blood Tests and Other Procedures

Blood tests present a particular problem in patient compliance. Because many patients may believe blood embodies the life essence, they are fearful they will become weak from blood loss or that their blood might be used for sinister purposes. It is helpful for the practitioner to

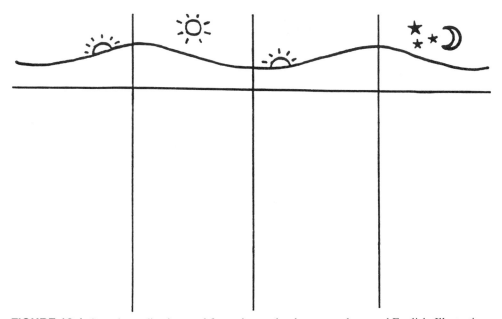

FIGURE 18-1 Sample medication card for patients who do not speak or read English. Illustrations represent morning, noon, early evening, and night. Medications are affixed under the appropriate time illustration.

explain that the body reproduces blood and to give the patient juice or water to help replenish fluids. The practitioner should reassure the patient that only clinic professionals will have access to the blood for testing.

Many highly technical medical tests used in the United States are unavailable in developing countries, so there may not be any equivalent terminology in the patient's language. To allay anxiety, the practitioner should take time to explain why the tests are being ordered and how the procedure will be done. The practitioner should also schedule a follow-up appointment soon after a test or any specialty referral to discuss further information, answer questions, and monitor compliance.

Diet

Diet interventions are common the world over, especially when other treatments are unavailable. Patients will often ask for dietary advice if the practitioner does not offer it. Cultures vary in their beliefs about what constitutes a healthy or therapeutic diet. Hot and cold theories abound, but differ in which foods are assigned "hot" or "cold" status. Rather than memorize specific regimens for each culture, it is helpful for the practitioner to use sound nutrition information available in the United States, noting that some foods may be especially useful for a particular condition in the patient's culture. The practitioner should ask the patient about these foods and accommodate the patient's beliefs when making dietary recommendations that are sensible for the patient.

Folk Healers

Patients may also wish to continue to see folk healers or may choose to augment Western treatment with a religious ceremony or ritual (Shepherd & Faust, 1993). Continued use of folk healers and rituals can be especially helpful when patients suffer from unresolved grief or bereavement for the many losses they have endured (Eisenbruch, 1984). Nurse practitioners encourage patients to participate in their care as much as possible, including using familiar, alternative therapies that are not harmful. The practitioner does not have to endorse an alternative therapy to acknowledge that the patient uses it. During each visit, the practitioner should discuss the patient's response to both the folk and Western treatments.

COMMUNICATION THROUGH INTERPRETERS

Because most practitioners and newcomers do not share a common language, it is necessary to communicate through interpreters. Some clinics and hospitals maintain a staff of trained interpreters, whereas others use volunteer staff or rely on family and friends to provide this service. Medical interpretation, however, is different from word-for-word translation or from having a conversational familiarity with a language. The trained interpreter works not just as a translator of words but also conveys, across cultures, concepts for which there are no words. The interpreter also works as a "culture broker," bringing the patient's beliefs and cultural context to the provider (Faust & Drickey, 1986). Through the interpreter, the nurse practitioner can explore personal and intimate concerns with patients who may be anxious and unfamiliar with English as well as the language and culture of healthcare.

In newcomer families, a school-age child often has the best grasp of English, and the family may proudly suggest the child be the interpreter. Using a child as an interpreter, however, reverses the established parent–child roles and places unnecessary and often inappropriate responsibilities and burdens on the child. For this reason, it is recommended to use a trained interpreter when possible.

Cultural values make it difficult for patients to discuss issues of intimacy in the presence of interpreters, especially if the interpreters are of the opposite gender. To enhance reliability and respect, the best match apparently occurs when the interpreter is of the same gender and is older than the patient. The nurse practitioner should reassure the patient during the first visit that the clinical encounters involving an interpreter are confidential, especially when the interpreter may also be a member of the patient's community.

It is often helpful for the practitioner to review the case with the interpreter before beginning the clinical encounter. They can exchange information about the patient's history and the goal of the visit. With pertinent information, the interpreter will be able to guide the visit, and a useful practitioner–interpreter alliance can be enhanced. It is helpful for the practitioner to face the patient and interpreter together. The practitioner will then be able to maintain eye contact and establish important nonverbal communication with the patient while checking easily with the interpreter. The practitioner can also ask the interpreter for a cultural explanation of the patient's beliefs or practices. For instance, it is common for an interpreter and patient to engage in lengthy conversations in which the provider cannot participate. If requested, the interpreter will explain to the practitioner the cultural context of the discussion that may have concerned a test or treatment unfamiliar to the patient or a healing practice commonly practiced by the patient's culture.

 ## CASE VIGNETTES

The following clinical vignettes use the methods of cross-cultural care discussed in this exemplar. The Western medical tradition is not discussed in depth because it is assumed that the nurse practitioner reader has considerable experience with this tradition.

Vignette I

A 48-year-old Russian woman, K, came to the clinic with a complaint of chest pain. A thorough history was taken to assess for a cardiac etiology of her pain. After listening to the patient's explanation of the symptom, it became apparent that the complaint was not cardiac in nature but rather "heartbreak" over the losses she experienced as a result of migration. The aching pain over the heart began soon after arrival in the United States and now persists for hours or days. The pain did not radiate, and there was no diaphoresis, nausea, palpitation, or dizziness. She described the pain as being worse at night when she "thinks too much" and cannot sleep. She had been taking medicine for "nerves" from Russia, and valerian herbal tea to calm herself. She came to the United States as a refugee fleeing persecution for her Christian beliefs, but wondered if this was the right thing to do. Life seemed so hard in this country. She was here with her husband and eight children, living on welfare and residing in public housing. Her husband had worked as a miner in Russia and she used to operate a machine in a Kiev factory. Neither spoke English. She requested medicine for her heart from the practitioner and perhaps a referral to a "heart specialist."

Her physical exam revealed borderline hypertension and obesity but otherwise was within normal limits. The assessment helped to shape the care plan as well as validated the patient's perception of her complaint. The nurse practitioner's diagnosis included borderline hypertension, obesity and rule/out ischemic heart disease. In addition, the problem list included "heartbreak" and anxiety due to stresses of acculturation. The nurse practitioner ordered appropriate lab tests, an electrocardiogram, and a exercise tolerance test. Furthermore, the practitioner discussed nutrition information and recommended a 24-hour diet recall or diary. Knowing that valerian tea is a harmless and common treatment for "heart pain" and nervousness, the nurse practitioner encouraged the patient to continue its use because it gave some relief. The practitioner referred the patient to a social worker for vocational assessment and help locating an entry-level English class for her and her husband. Her follow-up appointment was set for 2 weeks later.

Vignette 2

A 62-year-old Vietnamese man, V, came to the clinic with a complaint of generalized weakness and fatigue for the past year. A refugee who had resided in the United States for a little more than 1 year, V had been an army officer imprisoned for 10 years in a "reeducation camp" in Vietnam before his arrival. He lost most of his family in the war, but was here with his son and grandchildren, who were able to escape several years earlier. He believed that his weakness was due to a problem with his brain and worried about "cancer."

He requested medicine to cure his problem, because acupuncture treatments had given him no relief. He denied neurologic symptoms but, with further probing, complained of poor appetite, insomnia, nightmares, and intrusive thoughts about past events in prison. During times of intensified symptoms, he had palpitations, sweated profusely, and felt severe panic. Due to these episodes, he felt weak, fatigued, and never seemed rested.

V's physical exam revealed a thin older male who appeared worried and fatigued. His neurologic exam was completely normal and he showed no signs of an endocrine disorder. Aside from being slightly underweight, his physical exam was otherwise within normal limits. Tests were ordered to rule out anemia and endocrine conditions. Benadryl and herbal tea were prescribed for sleep. He was advised to eliminate caffeinated beverages from his diet. A follow-up appointment was set for 2 weeks.

During the third visit, V became tearful while recounting the history of his incarceration in the Vietnamese prison. He had considered taking his own life, but felt he must remain strong for his grandchildren. At the time of the third visit, he had no active plan or means to commit suicide. V's symptoms were consistent with a diagnosis of posttraumatic stress disorder (Hinton; Kroll, Habenicht, Mackenzie, et al., 1989). Because psychiatric terminology such as *depression* might be difficult for the patient to accept or comprehend, the practitioner discussed the "weakness" that the patient felt in terms of the suffering and worry he had endured, in addition to malnutrition. "Pain in the life can lead to pain in the body" was a phrase the practitioner found useful when discussing the patient's symptoms.

The assessment and problem list encompassed Western terminology—posttraumatic stress disorder—and also the patient's perception of the problem—"weakness and fatigue." Symptomatic therapies were recommended at the third visit. The nurse also offered a contract and plan to minimize the risk of suicide. At future visits, the practitioner will discuss other interventions such as antidepressants or support group participation. In addition, the practitioner might advise the patient to see a counselor or psychiatrist, if available, if the patient agrees.

SUMMARY

This exemplar discussed an approach to cross-cultural patient care based on the patient's explanatory model and the Migration History model. By understanding patterns in the patient's migration history and immigration status, the practitioner can become aware of psychological stressors that affect the patient's health. Eliciting the patient's explanatory model of illness and examining for evidence of folk treatment enhance awareness of the patient's worldview and assist with supporting the relationship between the nurse practitioner and patient. Treatment options are expanded to include interventions from the patient's culture as well as Western medicine.

Perhaps the most important aspect of this approach is the acknowledgment of the patient as the cultural expert and as the practitioner's ally. It is critical to remember that, behind each political event, wave of migration, or cultural worldview resides an individual who has come for care. Patterns of culture and migration vary with each person, although some generalizations can be made about groups. Mindfulness of and respect for the individual as well as the cultural group of which he or she is a member can only deepen the nurse practitioner's understanding and practice. The following prose poem illustrates the ability to look to the person for the biography of migration—for the true story.

Tools of the Trade
I turn my back as he unbuttons his shirt, the fifth article taken off (first a heavy coat brought from the old country, under that a new one—light flimsy—given at the point of entry, then a discarded suit jacket, a cardigan, now the flannel shirt).

His fingers, no longer supple, labor down the buttons. Sent to cobalt mines, he worked the Ukraine thirty years, hands curved around a pick and hammer. He tells this to the interpreter who in turn tells me. Something is lost. I imagine caves full of dark blue stone, blue glass that shatters with every hammer brought down.

They all come in with stories: Zina with her tired bones, Nadezda with her cough. Exposed to cobalt, to the regime, he places his body before me, offers it up. Given everything: how did this man survive? With the tools of my trade, a faith in the tangible, I search for clues (a strong constitution? a vigorous heart?), hold the stethoscope in my hands to warm it, to give his body one less shock.

When I turn and lift the gown—hospital regulation, small blue stars against thin white cloth, a picture of the heavens—I find his body covered with faint blue lines, as if the gown were never raised. Looking closer, angels kneel on either side of his chest, face each other, hands clasped over the heart. As he breathes the wings on their backs expand, flutter.

He tells the interpreter the angels were tattooed on long ago to protect him from Stalin. His life has been lifted on their wings. What lesser mystery could have guaranteed his passage to this exam room, my care, the soft rubber hammer at his knees?

(Mirosevich, 1994)

Note: References are cited at end of chapter.

B

Elder Care: One Geriatric Nurse Practitioner's Experience in a Continuing Care Retirement Community

Martha L. Henderson

SETTING, POPULATION, AND CONCEPT OF CARE

In the mid 1970s, a continuing care retirement community in the Piedmont region of North Carolina was being conceived of by a small group of elderly people who had retired to a university town. They wanted to establish a private, nonprofit community that offered comprehensive services, including lifetime healthcare. They also wanted an atmosphere of active and independent elderly people, who were involved in the surrounding town. Many residents were attracted to the concept of maintaining an active life in a community setting that would minimize their day-to-day responsibilities, such as groundskeeping, enable them to have privacy by living in a garden apartment if they wished, and guarantee health services, thus ensuring they would not become "a burden" on others for care in their later years. The planners and eventual residents perceived themselves as having the best of all worlds. Eventually, the retirement community comprised approximately 320 residents who lived independently and 60 individuals who resided in the inpatient facility—the Health Care Center. The population was largely white, middle class, and educated. Approximately half the residents were from regions beyond the local community.

The continuing care retirement community where I practiced provided multilevel healthcare throughout the resident's lifespan. Outpatient care, with both preventive and disease management, was available through the clinic to all new residents and residents who continued to reside in their own apartments. *Sheltered care,* a domiciliary level of care, was available to 30 residents who needed short-term or long-term minimal supervision of health and personal care. *Skilled nursing care* was provided to 30 residents who needed the care and supervision of registered nurses. Residents could stay in the Health Care Center for 60 days without having to give up their apartment and move permanently into the inpatient facility. (Exceptions to this policy were made on an individual basis.)

Acute hospital care for residents was delivered at one of the three regional medical centers. Attending physicians were the attending staff of the hospital, with input from the resident's local primary physician, as available. Care in the continuing care retirement community was coordinated by the geriatric nurse practitioner (GNP), with the goal of returning the resident to the healthcare center for convalescence as soon as medically reasonable. Eventually, services were expanded to included home healthcare—a valuable addition.

OVERVIEW OF HEALTH PROGRAM

The concept of healthcare envisioned by the founding board and guided by a retired visionary physician who chaired the healthcare committee of the board was that of admitting active, elderly residents in good health, who may have stable chronic illnesses, and who were functionally independent. In addition, they envisioned providing comprehensive health services that would enable residents to maintain their health and independence as long as possible. The visionary physician had experience as a medical director of a private, nonprofit retirement community and he also researched what would be the best provider model for this setting. His recommendation to the board was that a GNP would be the best director and full-time primary provider for the healthcare program. His reasons were that the GNP would be knowledgeable about elderly people and specifically educated to provide on-site the majority of primary care needed by this population. The GNP would be comprehensive in focus: he or she would be able to respond to psychosocial needs, would emphasize disease prevention, offer health education, and diagnose and treat acute and stable chronic illnesses. Ongoing physician backup, consultation, and referral services would be provided by local internists and family practice physicians.

Geriatric Nurse Practitioner's Initial Involvement

I heard about the continuing care retirement community when I was on the faculty of a GNP program. The visionary physician on the board of directors had brought a proposed floor plan of the clinic and inpatient facility to the school of nursing for nursing input. A room in the clinic had been labeled "GNP" and the physician explained his commitment to the GNP as the proper role model in this setting and the plan to hire a GNP. I was impressed not only by his apparent understanding of the GNP role and the benefits of using a GNP in those settings, but also by his search for input from the professional group who would primarily be working in the healthcare facilities. A colleague and I, who were earning our master of science in nursing degrees in gerontologic nursing at a nearby university, interviewed for director of health services and assistant director of health services; the assistant director would essentially be the director of nursing for the Health Care Center.

After 1 year of negotiating the terms of the contract, both my colleague and I were hired as director of nursing and director of health services, respectively. I had substantive input in salary negotiations, including benefits and time off for conferences, development of job descriptions, and establishment of the care philosophy. The above responsibilities, including defining the relationship to the medical director and local physicians and obtaining legal practice authority, were all time-consuming tasks that took nearly 1 year to complete.

Geriatric Nurse Practitioner as Administrator

I was initially hired as the director of health services and GNP to enable me to have administrative as well as clinical authority over the health program. I was responsible to the executive director. For the first year, I was the primary administrator of the health program with input from the board, primarily from the founding physician, and some input from the executive director of the retirement community. My specific administrative functions included defining what health services would be offered and developing appropriate policies and procedures. One particular GNP colleague, a consultant in a similar position and setting, was very helpful.

Administrative work was shared with the assistant director of health services, that is, the director of nursing of the Health Care Center. We identified and articulated a care philosophy and developed a new program administratively, which included deciding on and ordering equipment ranging from beds and clinic furniture to medicine carts and medical records. We also defined specific services. The director of nursing and I not only collaborated on nursing policies and procedures for the Health Care Center, but also jointly hired almost all inpatient staff.

The residents' association started early in the life of the community. There was an active health committee of the residents' association that consisted of noted and experienced healthcare professionals, such as a former chief nurse of the U.S. Public Health Service and a former professor of public health education. The committee worked closely with me and provided invaluable advice and support during the start-up phase and in subsequent years. Of course, this group primarily represented residents' views and concerns and was motivated to maintain high standards of care. At times, group members' expectations seemed unrealistically high; for example, they expected staff to respond to call lights instantly, but healthy debate informed all involved.

The financial aspects of the program presented a special challenge for a person educated to be a clinician. Setting up systems of payment for services rendered, whether hospital or physician charges, was difficult because the facility did not have an "expert" in the area of Medicare billing and payment. The bookkeeper and I worked closely together and set up a workable system; I monitored the system closely to see what services were reimbursable, at what rate, at what pace, and so forth.

After approximately 1 year of functioning in the dual administrative and clinical leadership role, I asked to create and assume responsibility for the role of director of clinical services. The reasons were primarily threefold: program and administrative direction had been set, residents were requesting that I spend more time with them clinically, and I felt that the operation deserved an administrator properly prepared in healthcare administration to care for all the details of the day-to-day operation. The administration of clinic services continued to be my responsibility as well as the administration of a home health program that was later added to complement health services (see the section Clinical Services and the GNP's Role).

With the relinquishment of the original administrative authority came some, but not a major, loss of input into administrative decisions. The new healthcare administrator represented health services at the weekly department heads' meeting, so there was less connection with the overall organization and implications for the healthcare program. The healthcare administrator also assumed the role of formally meeting with the residents' health committee, so resident input with the GNP was informal. The retainment of an administrative title—Director of Clinical Services—did ensure that direction for clinical services and decisions affecting clinical care originated with me or had major input from me.

Clinical Services and the Geriatric Nurse Practitioner's Role

My primary clinical role was to provide primary care services on a daily basis to residents in the clinic and in the Health Care Center (see Table 18-2). A service that was highly valued and not always available from community physicians was prompt attention for acutely ill residents; thus, this service had priority. Every morning, there were a couple of slots in the clinic schedule for urgent problems. The other professional staff, including a clinic nurse and, later, a home health nurse, triaged urgent problems and referred to me those needing my level of expertise. I would see residents in the clinic or would visit them in their homes if they felt too ill to come to the clinic. My time at the clinic consisted primarily of interviewing, examining, diagnosing, and managing acute and chronic illnesses. In the state in which I practice, "medical management" is defined as making a medical diagnosis and providing treatment, including prescribing medications. All nurse practitioners have a prescribing number, issued by the state board of pharmacy, and use a book of protocols written by physicians on the nurse practitioner program faculty in the early days of the program to guide prescribing practices (Hoole, Pickard, Ouimette, Lohr, & Greenberg, 1995).

For clinical problems that were beyond the practitioner's expertise, state law required that a physician always be available for phone consultation. If the patient needed to be seen by a physician, clinic staff made transportation arrangements, for example, the patient was transported by car to the physician's office or, rarely, the physician came to the retirement commu-

TABLE 18-2 Schedule of Typical GNP Activities

To Do	Appointments		Notes
1. Review initial health assessment form	9:00 10:00 10:15	Rounds in NH Clinic report New applicant eval	Eval. Mr. R's home situation before D/C
2. Meet with clinic staff about handling walk-ins and emergency procedures	11:00 11:30 12:00	Mr. J. (Memory loss) Mrs. P (Bronchitis f/u) Mrs. T's son (ETOH concern)	Re-eval. dementia screen protocol Call re AA transportation
3. Call pharmacy to set up formulary com. mtg.	12:30	Lunch with dermatologist (Desires clinic here)	
4. Prepare proposal for home care for health care committee	1:30 2:30 3:30	Level of Care mtg. Mr. N's initial home visit Mrs. B (CHF)	Level of Care needs new structure-draft
5. Read chaplain proposal	4:00 4:30 4:45 5:00	Mrs. S. (change una boot) HH nurse report review lab reports finish clinic notes NH rounds	Teach LPN to do una boots

Source: Clinical Practice of Martha L. Henderson.

nity, depending on the urgency of the problem and the physician's schedule. When it was obvious that a resident needed to go to the emergency room, staff called an ambulance, administering appropriate care in the clinic or Health Care Center in the meantime.

Although I felt that there was a need for another GNP for the 60 residents in the Health Care Center (at certain times there was another GNP), there were years during my 10-year tenure that I was the only GNP in the retirement community. During these times, I would check with the charge nurses in the Health Care Center to see if there were any urgent problems with their patients. If so, I would take care of them, whenever convenient, depending on the urgency of the problem. Usually, I responded to acute problems in the Health Care Center early in the morning, late in the afternoon, or when there was a lull in the clinic. I held interdisciplinary care planning and regular rounds routinely. At one time, when the patient care load was unusually heavy, I negotiated to work longer hours to provide care for outpatients and inpatients. By showing the costs that the GNP would save by providing the services instead of paying physicians to provide this care, I negotiated a higher salary until another GNP was hired. These savings could be demonstrated despite the lack of Medicare reimbursement for GNP services. This federal financial discrimination against a competent provider was challenged periodically, but without success.

Although treatment of acute and chronic illnesses was the primary focus of the GNP's service, there were many services that I provided in the clinic that would not fall under a narrow definition of treatment of disease. I offered healthcare and preventive services in the clinic that were broadly defined and seemed to be appreciated by the residents. These included supervision of a weekly routine foot care clinic, listening to accounts of problems with adult children or other psychosocial concerns, supervising allergy shots and immunizations, and referring stressed residents to physical therapy for a massage. In addition, the clinic was perceived as a supportive environment, in which the clinic staff realized they were a friendly "halfway house" for early dementia patients. The article "A GNP in a Retirement Community" (Henderson, 1984) provides more details of the clinical aspects of the role.

I was also involved in providing terminal care to residents. Most important, as soon as was possible and appropriate, I discussed with residents their wishes regarding medical treatment should their prognosis become poor. Many residents had advance directives that directly influenced the treatment they received, including whether they were sent to the hospital. Comfort was always a primary goal of care, whether or not residents wanted aggressive medical treatment. As part of my doctoral research, I interviewed 60 residents, who already had living wills, about their specific wishes regarding end-of-life treatment and care. I found that facilitating the residents' sense of control over the process of dying was significantly related to a decrease in death anxiety (Henderson, 1990).

Geriatric Nurse Practitioner as Case Manager

I functioned as a case manager for all residents at the retirement community. I was the primary professional caregiver who offered multiple services to residents with a variety of needs. These services were given in a comprehensive, coordinated, continuous health program.

The GNP role of comprehensive care provider began with the resident's application process. Originally, the admission process required that the resident undergo a physical exam and that his or her previous physician complete a form within 60 days before entry. Although the form instructed physicians to provide diagnoses and list medications as well as give certification that the patient was functionally independent, it became apparent that, at times, the retirement community staff did not get an adequate picture of a resident. The application process was changed to require that the director of clinical services interview each applicant so he or she could obtain additional data, if necessary.

As a comprehensive care provider, I helped residents obtain whatever health services they needed, whether preventive, acute care, or psychosocial, or help dealing with a family member. There was a definite sense that the retirement community, with the resident, was responsible for providing services to maximize residents' lives until they died. Ultimately, this meant helping residents define what kind of care they wanted at the end of life and trying to provide this care.

Coordination of care primarily involved keeping all caregivers informed about the patient. For example, I may have updated a medicine sheet and noticed a drug incompatibility, sent a progress note to be read and signed by the back-up physician, and ensured that the discharge summary and orders were sent back from the hospital with a patient.

Continuity of care was ensured by reassessing the patient when care needs changed, no matter what the setting. Based on experience, a policy was developed that all residents returning to the community after a hospitalization would spend at least one night in the Health Care Center to ensure they were stable and that all discharge plans were complete and coordinated. (Exceptions to this requirement were individualized.) Patients could be admitted to the Health Care Center from their apartment by me whenever I thought such a move was appropriate, whether to monitor a patient with a head injury after a fall or to support a frail resident through an acute illness. When a patient was discharged from the Health Care Center, the home health nurse was notified and made a home visit to the patient the next day.

Home Health Services

Theoretically, residents would receive outpatient services in the clinic as long as they could. When they were no longer able to be "independent," they were supposed to move into the Health Care Center. As I interviewed patients in the early years about their wishes for health services, most expressed a desire to have services in the home as long as possible. I explored both being certified as a home health agency and contracting with the local private home health agency. The greatest problem with both of these approaches was that many of the services needed were for personal care, not professional services, on an ongoing basis. This meant that many of these services would not be reimbursable by third-party payers. Another advantage of providing the services on-site was that more comprehensive, coordinated, and continuous services could be given by personnel who knew the residents and could document on the resident's health record.

Eventually, an exceptionally bright and experienced licensed practical nurse was hired to provide in-home assessments and care under my supervision. She also provided coordination of care by privately hired aides. The retirement community provided, on a limited basis, home health services to residents as part of their basic service package. However, if residents needed daily visits, for example, for ongoing wound care or to monitor frail residents with acute illnesses, the residents were expected to come into the Health Care Center. Home health was an important and appreciated addition to the health service package.

Acceptance of the Geriatric Nurse Practitioner Role

The most important aspect of acceptance of the GNP role was the initial recommendation by the visionary physician on the board to hire this new provider based on research and a good understanding of the role conceptually. It was helpful to have administrative authority incorporated into the new position to set the direction for the healthcare program.

Most of the residents at the retirement community were educated, demanding of the "best" in healthcare services, and accustomed to using specialists, based on their own judgment, whether or not they needed them medically. I decided my informal public relations campaign would be based on early welcoming and assessment of the residents' health status, information about the nurse practitioner role, a contract with residents about their goals and approach to health needs, and a commitment to meet their health needs by the on-site staff, or others, in a timely manner. My partnership with the residents' doctors to meet the residents' needs competently and in a holistic and caring manner was the norm, which was explicitly stated. I helped residents unfamiliar with the community choose a physician, based on their healthcare problems and other preferences. Residents were amazingly open to and accepting of a new type or provider: the GNP. That I was the only primary provider available, on-site, added to my popularity. The residents expressed appreciation about the time made available to be heard by a provider who responded to any problems.

For the physicians, acceptance of the GNP provider role initially was slow. Because I was part of the staff in the new retirement community in which physicians wanted to acquire new patients, the physicians were open to being educated about the new provider. I met with all involved physicians individually in their offices to explain the GNP role, show them the book of guidelines for practice including medicines the GNP could prescribe, and obtain their participation in the state approval process. The mechanism established for reviewing and co-signing progress notes, including orders, was to send them by courier daily for physician signatures. Although the physicians were polite and agreed to comply with regulations and the collaboration, there was lack of knowledge and expected reticence in supporting the role wholeheartedly. I consulted with the physicians frequently by phone in the early days to keep them informed about "their" patients and to facilitate a relationship based on knowledge of each others' competencies and preferences. Over time, mutual respect grew and, finally, the physicians deferred routinely to my judgment. They knew that a consultation or referral was important and needed their attention promptly. The physicians were glad to have a provider they trusted to see their patients on-site in the Health Care Center and to save them a visit for routine or minor problems or consult with them on more serious ones.

The number of individual primary care services provided by the patient's physician and by me varied greatly. I provided primary care for most residents. Some healthy residents saw their physician once a year for a checkup. I would see these residents for a more functionally oriented assessment midyear. For other residents with chronic illnesses, I provided ongoing management, consulting with the physicians as needed.

SUMMARY

The evolution of the GNP at a continuing care retirement community started on sound footing and won the credibility of residents, administration, and physicians over time. The services of a holistic provider with clinical competence who was available and caring proved to be valuable and valued. The persistent lack of Medicare reimbursement for outpatient services was the only serious constraint in the GNP's otherwise successful role. The retirement community seems to be an ideal site for the continued development of this role.

 ## CASE VIGNETTE

J came in for an interview to enter the retirement community just 2 months after his wife died. J and his wife had planned to come together. After reviewing the medical data sent by J's physician and satisfying myself that the applicant was capable of independent living, I spent time listening to J reminisce and grieve over his wife's recent death. I ascertained that J's wife had been involved in helping J manage his medications and treatment for chronic obstructive pulmonary disease and congestive heart failure and that her missing role in his care created a real void. I explained my role as a GNP and told J that the clinic was there to help him, in any way possible, from day one, and that he should come, meet the staff, and get checked in the first week of his arrival.

The first week of J's arrival, I was notified and arranged a home visit to his apartment to welcome him, assess his home situation, begin his orientation to health services, and continue his database collection. After this visit, I suggested that J come to the clinic, meet the clinic staff, and complete his database with vital signs, weight, any necessary lab work, and so forth. Because he was from out of town, I helped him select a physician who would provide backup for me. An appointment was set up for J to meet his new physician. As early as this first visit, J said he had a living will and would not want life support if he became terminally ill. I noted the advance directive and wondered if it were part of his grief reaction to his wife's death. I encouraged J to discuss this issue with his physician as well. I told J about another resident who had just lost his wife and who was a naturally supportive individual. I made sure J knew how to take all of his medications. Another visit was scheduled for 2 weeks to see how J was settling in.

J did well; he was welcomed by the hospitality group on his hall and spent time with his local daughter's family. After he had been at the retirement community just 6 months, J developed a purulent cough, fever, and increased shortness of breath. He came to the clinic. Based on the history-taking and an exam that revealed dullness and rales at the left base, I suspected pneumonia. Because of J's chronic obstructive pulmonary disease and congestive heart failure, the primary physician I consulted agreed to send J to the emergency room for further evaluation and probable admission. J reminded me that he had a living will and he would not want to go on a respirator if he got worse. I clarified that sometimes a person with chronic obstructive pulmonary disease and an acute infection may need temporary support from a respirator. The patient was adamant about not wanting mechanical ventilation and said his family was aware of his wishes. When I called the emergency room to give admitting information, I passed along information about the advance directive and included a copy with transfer papers. I helped J call his daughter to inform her of the transfer to the hospital, but we realized his family had left town for a week. J was quite anxious but felt better once the oxygen was started in the clinic. The daybed in the transcriptionist's room in the clinic served as an observation area until the rescue squad came.

On the way home, I stopped by the hospital to confirm that J did have pneumonia and that he had been admitted. During that visit, J said he hated being in the hospital and wanted to get back to the Health Care Center as soon as possible. I reassured him and told him I would call his physician in the morning. I also made sure he knew that the retirement community had a skilled nursing facility that could administer oral antibiotics, pulmonary toilet, and supervision, whenever J was stable enough to come back. In just 3 days, J was back in the Health Care Center, and in 3 more days, he was ready to return to his apartment under the supervision of the home health nurse and me. He continued to do well and recovered to his baseline.

After 3 months, J came in to see me complaining of forgetfulness and weight loss. After doing a thorough history and physical and screen for dementia, including a neurologic exam, a Folstein mini-mental test, and appropriate lab work, I felt J had pseudodementia because of depression stemming from grief over his wife's death and relocation to a new community away from old friends. I discussed this tentative diagnosis with the patient and back-up physician and started an antidepressant. I did supportive counseling with the resident and recommended he join a new widower's support group started by the social worker from the Health Care Center. The depression slowly improved as well as the memory.

Gradually over the next 2 years, however, the cognitive problems worsened. During this time, J would stop in to the clinic to share a story about his grandson, to get directions to the dining room, or to get clarification on his medications. He said he just felt more secure knowing the clinic staff were there. As his cognition declined, he resisted the idea of coming into the Health Care Center to live in sheltered care. He wanted to stay in his apartment and felt a move was premature. I called a family conference with J and his daughter, the social worker, and home health nurse. It was negotiated that every morning, a privately hired aide would come in to be sure J got his bath and breakfast and morning medications. He would get an alarm wristwatch to prompt him to take his medications the rest of the day. The home health nurse would monitor his medicine box, which she would prepare weekly. The dining room host would ensure that J came to supper each night, unless J or his daughter notified the host that J would be out with his family. I would see J every month in the clinic and on an as needed basis per patient or other provider request. Everyone agreed to this plan and a 2-month trial period. At the end of that period, the plan was working and J was happy and fairly independent in his apartment. Whenever the aide had concerns, she would consult with the home health nurse or me. The daughter accepted the inherent risk in this situation so that her father would be happy.

This plan lasted 3 more years. Another flare-up of chronic obstructive pulmonary disease necessitated a Health Care Center stay. When J tried to go home, his confusion had increased and he was unable to recover the tenuous independence he had managed for several years. J and I had a poignant conversation in which I stated the unsafe nature of the present situation and promised returned independence if it became possible. I managed to persuade J to come back to the Health Care Center. In concert with the interdisciplinary team, I came up with a new care plan for J that included going to the main dining room each night with a friend and going out with his aide every morning for a walk. I visited this resident on a regular basis to reassure him of his importance and support his feelings as he dealt with a world of fewer options and more structure and safety. J eventually had a small improvement in function: he could bathe independently and attend a gardening group. J's daughter was pleased with his care and continued to meet with me periodically for support and information.

After 3 more years of cognitive and physical decline in the Health Care Center, including recurrent trouble with swallowing and aspiration pneumonia, J's family decided, with my support, not to send him back to the hospital. His confusion had worsened in that setting and he seemed unhappy. J and his family had decided some time ago that he did not want a feeding tube. When his bout of pneumonia came, oral antibiotics did not reverse the process, and dehydration became problematic, J gradually drifted into a coma. The family gathered with the minister, me, and the two aides most involved in his care as the minister gave a blessing. The blessing affirmed the life of a gentle man who was ready to leave this world. It affirmed an environment that could support him and also let him go.

Note: References are cited at end of chapter.

C

Beth Israel Home Care:
A Model for Practice

Karen L. Dick ▪ *Susan Burns-Tisdale*

The delivery of home health services is changing in response to changes in the larger health-care system. Services historically viewed as hospital based are now routinely provided in the patient's home. Almost every treatment modality that can be made portable is a possible home care service (Council on Scientific Affairs, 1990). These modalities include caring for the ventilator-dependent patient, administering intravenous therapies, monitoring the patient with a high-risk pregnancy, and a variety of other care services. The expertise and equipment required to treat and sustain patients have been successfully applied in the home, where patients, families and diverse healthcare professionals work together in a less formal, structured environment (Mehlman & Younger, 1991). Care at home spans the continuum from prevention to rehabilitation to long-term maintenance. The most prevalent type of home health service is care of the older adult with a disabling chronic illness or illnesses.

Older people have long been the focus of home healthcare. The Medicare Home Health Benefit, introduced during the Johnson administration in 1965, ensured access for older adults to home health services. The intent of the benefit was to cover patients' short-term needs, generally following a hospitalization. There are a few exceptions in which limited longer term needs are addressed. Patients must be homebound and under a physician's care to qualify for services under this benefit. Other recipients of home health services include younger, homebound patients with disabling illnesses. These may include patients with illness related to the human immunodeficiency virus (HIV), cancer, or multiple sclerosis. Patients requiring short-term intervention, following surgery or other invasive procedures, also require home health services. Most home health programs care for sick children and postpartum mothers and their infants.

In the late 1980s, most insurance plans began to offer home care as part of their healthcare benefits package, thus increasing access for a wider population. There has been a proliferation of both private and nonprofit agencies that offer an array of specialized services and programs and compete for patients with complex medical and nursing needs. The growth of managed care systems may limit the number of home care services that patients may receive for a specific episode of illness. Managed care companies often hire internal case managers who, based on their review of the patient's medical record, dictate the type and frequency of home care services offered. These companies also subcontract with specific home care companies to deliver home services, often at the most competitive price. Many patients may be at risk of compromised care when assessment and care delivery focus on specific reimbursable services rather than on the establishment of a holistic care plan (Benson & McDevitt, 1994).

Expenditures have risen significantly in recent years. The home health benefit is often viewed as an area in need of reform. Home health providers have argued that expenditures have risen only modestly compared with Medicare-financed hospital and physician expenditures during the same period. Clearly the demand for home care services will continue to increase due to prospective and capitated payment systems, early discharge from acute care, and the continued use of advanced technologies at home. Simultaneously, home care programs are dealing with the realities of decreasing access as a result of managed care, Medicare-capitated senior plans, and the possibility of a prospective payment system for Medicare patients who are not in a capitated system.

Nurses have had a long history of providing care in the home. The basic assumptions underlying community health nursing practice, as described in the 1970s, still hold great relevance in the practice of home care nursing in the 1990s. The emphasis on the environmental, social, and personal health factors influencing health status, as well as the care of the individual who is experiencing disease or disability, characterizes this practice. Nurses are most often the formal case managers for patients receiving home health services. The nurse completes an assessment, develops a care plan, monitors the patient's care needs, and adjusts the plan accordingly. He or she must give time and attention to supporting and teaching the patient and others about how to care for the patient and effectively deal with issues related to patient care. The burden of care falls on the patient and family. Nurses and other health providers need to pay close attention to patient and family's ability to manage the many overwhelming components of care. The professional nurse best coordinates this type of family-centered care, with interdependent relationships among the patient, family, and environment.

BETH ISRAEL HOME CARE: A DESCRIPTION OF SERVICES

Beth Israel Home Care Department has been providing care for patients at home since 1954. In the late 1970s, nurse practitioners were integrated into the department with a physician practice called the Urban Medical Group. This independent, nonprofit group practice of primary care physicians and midlevel providers had been providing individualized care to chronically ill, elderly, homebound patients and nursing home residents in urban Boston. Their care was characterized by the elements of personalization and continuity. The group was committed to working with other providers, including nurse practitioners, to meet the complex needs of vulnerable populations (Master et al., 1980).

Nurse practitioners brought to the homes of generally frail, sick elders services that had previously required a trip to an ambulatory center. This arrangement was particularly important for this group of patients who had great difficulty leaving home and therefore had limited access to care. Although the program has grown in recent years to encompass a more diverse patient population, most of the patients continue to be older than age 75 years and have several chronic illnesses. This patient population continues to require ongoing monitoring and evaluation of the interplay of acute and chronic disease, social factors, function, and safety. The nurse practitioner model based on the Beth Israel Professional Practice Model of Primary Nursing seems to provide for care delivery that best meets the needs of this vulnerable population. Nurse practitioners can provide ongoing primary medical aspects of care, serve as case managers, provide linkages to the greater healthcare system, and provide direct hands-on nursing care (Burns-Tisdale & Goff, 1989). This care delivery model is in keeping with the need for the development of alternative programs and approaches to meet the needs of the underserved and at-risk populations. Nurse practitioners have provided this type of primary care service for many years and have skill in triaging, coordinating, and managing healthy and unhealthy populations in primary care settings. This care equals and sometimes exceeds that of physicians in the same setting (Office of Technology Assessment, 1986).

It is clear to us that the need for the advanced practice nurse in the home setting will continue to grow to meet the needs of increasingly complex and challenging patient care situations, particularly without a consistent physician presence. We continue to expect to see the demand for primary care for homebound elders with multiple chronic illnesses increase over the next several years. The HIV patient population also presents care providers with many challenges for meeting patient needs for skilled monitoring of medical conditions, the integration of technology for specific therapies, caring and restorative interventions, and end-of-life support. It is the advanced practice nurse who has the well-developed collaboration and communication skills necessary to ensure the delivery of safe, quality care to both these populations.

Beth Israel Home Care is a certified home health agency that provides the customary skilled nursing and home health aide visits, physical, occupational, and speech therapies, social services, and physician visits. Although most nursing staff are nurse practitioners, baccalaureate-prepared nurses also provide care and work collaboratively with the nurse practitioners. The major differentiation between the two nursing roles is that nurse practitioners provide primary care. Primary nursing serves as the practice model for care delivery, with each nurse accountable for the coordination and provision of care to his or her primary patients. Both the clinical nurses and nurse practitioners serve as both primary and associate nurses for patients in the practice. The nurses, physicians, therapists, social worker, students, and other providers meet weekly at a team meeting to discuss problematic patient situations, explore alternative interventions, and pursue joint problem solving. Clearly there is a high degree of trust and shared values in the group as the team comes together to plan for patient care. All agree that promotion of function, safety, and quality of life is the principle that underlies and guides care decisions.

A hospital-wide on-line electronic mail system, cellular telephone, and the use of fax technology have greatly eased the communication between Beth Israel Home Care staff and physicians and other providers. The staff also has access to on-line patient information that includes information regarding past hospitalizations, medication histories, discharge summaries, and functional health pattern assessments. This type of information sharing in a centralized database supports patient care continuity.

Most of the referrals come from the inpatient setting, with patients who are referred for posthospital services following the exacerbation and treatment of acute medical or surgical problems. Beth Israel Home Care also receives referrals from physicians, community agencies, and other providers. Our program has a reputation for providing a high level of coordinated care, focusing on promoting and maintaining patients' comfort, dignity, and function. Department staff care for many terminally ill patients who choose to die at home. They often require nontraditional, innovative caring practices that are integrated and provided by both clinical nurses and nurse practitioners. We have seen a need to respond quickly to the earlier hospital discharge of patients who may require a higher level with intervention. This includes the availability of more nursing visits, specific technologies such as intravenous therapy, complex medication regimes, and the need for intensive patient and family education that was not completed during the acute-care stay.

Because we are hospital based, nursing staff can visit patients before discharge to help ease the transition to home, particularly when there are specific therapies, equipment, or wound care protocols to follow. Often just meeting with the home care provider while the patient is hospitalized serves to ease patients' fears and anxieties about their impending discharge. Home Care staff also consult with various program-based, advanced practice nurses who may have been involved with patients in the inpatient setting and who work with the department in planning for discharge. For example, the rehabilitation nurse specialist has been helpful in planning care for patients with significant wound problems. There is a spirit of partnership as we share knowledge and resources to optimize patient care. We have also had situations in which we have had these inpatient resources accompany us on home visits for help in problem identification and care planning for specific patient problems.

The home care department also works collaboratively with the nurse practitioners in the hospital-based ambulatory practice. We often receive referrals from them for patients who become terminally ill or homebound or who need additional supportive home services. We may share patients with them, or entirely assume the care. Again, colleagueship is fostered and promoted through our professional practice model, as is the recognition of the scope of responsibility and expertise of each practice.

 ## CASE VIGNETTES

We are often asked to delineate how care provided by nurse practitioners differs from that provided by clinical nurses. There is much interest in the cost, efficiency, reimbursement mechanisms, and feasibility of this model, particularly in today's climate that emphasizes controlling spiraling healthcare costs. Although we have no definitive data, we strongly believe that our patients have fewer hospitalizations and emergency room visits and that patients are hospitalized with lower acuity rates compared with patients managed by other community nursing providers. We further believe that nurse practitioners are effective in sorting out patients' physical, emotional, and social needs and are skilled in assessing the multiple complicated illnesses and the interaction among individual patient, illnesses, and therapies (Burns-Tisdale & Goff, 1989). Patients and families rate their satisfaction high as measured by our unit-based survey programs; physician satisfaction also is high, as suggested by the increasing number of physician referrals. Although we will need to continue to defend our practice model from a fiscal perspective, care examples from our practice give us a rich illustration of the kind of care that nurse practitioners provide. The following is one example of a critical incident as told by a Home Care nurse practitioner.

Vignette 1

I admitted W, a 45-year-old woman who was HIV-positive to Home Care in late fall 1993. It was another busy Thursday, and I did not get to her third floor loft apartment until late afternoon. She had returned home the previous afternoon after a 1-week Beth Israel Hospital stay for evaluation of fatigue and severe jaundice. The diagnosis of viral hepatitis C was compounded by another dismal diagnosis—immunoblastic lymphoma—confirmed by a bone marrow biopsy. Diagnosed with HIV in 1987, it had become clear during this recent admission that her prognosis was very poor.

W had been placed on high doses of prednisone (100 mg every day) the day before her hospital discharge to address the lymphoma and was not a candidate for chemotherapy. When I climbed the stairs to her apartment, I found W with a friend. Her friend had arrived only a couple of hours earlier to welcome her home. W had been alone all night and morning and was not verbally communicative beyond an occasional "no." She mostly shook her head and sighed deeply. Her mouth and lips were extremely dry. I suggested her friend make some soup, but W seemed not to know how or what to do with a spoon or a glass of water. She had been discharged home with approximately four medications, but indicated that she was very confused about how to take them. They were all scheduled to be taken every day. I made her a new medication chart, but she still did not understand. Was this delirium or dementia related to acquired immunodeficiency syndrome? I did not know at first.

W's referral made no indication of mental status changes. The pink intake sheet from Home Care noted that her insurance had approved her for skilled nursing visits only once a week. Her very quiet friend was not much help either beyond stating that W "didn't seem herself." I called the floor at Beth Israel Hospital where she had been discharged. The primary nurse had left for the day, and no one who knew W was on the floor. I called her physician who was unavailable by page. I spoke with the nurse case manager at the community health care center where W received her care; she said if I had to send W back to the emergency unit I could, but she knew that W did not want to go back to the hospital. And, no, her behavior was not baseline per my description. Finally some information! My assessment was a steroid-induced psychosis. Unfortunately, I did not have any idea of the patient's real baseline.

I was somewhat incredulous that W had been discharged less than 24 hours earlier and no one had seen this mental status change. I had never before been the first clinician on the scene to make the assessment of a new psychosis. I knew that W could not be left alone. I also quickly assessed that her friend was overwhelmed and could not manage the situation. I knew I wanted to avoid W's landing in the emergency unit within 24 hours of discharge, if possible. W's friend had left the apartment within 30 minutes of my arrival. I was awaiting the supposed visit of W's sister, H, late in the afternoon. Fortunately, at 5:30 P.M., H, a nurse, did arrive and agree to spend the night. H was clearly torn between her role as a nurse versus a sister who was seeing her sibling slip away. I spent the next 30 minutes talking with H about who her sister was while she cried and hugged W. I gently broached the role of nurse with H, trying to focus her and outline a care plan, with a primary emphasis on safety issues. I felt that H was up to the task, despite her ambivalence, fear, and sadness. I asked H not to administer any more prednisone until I spoke with the physician the next day, presumably to start a taper; that was what happened. H was adamant that she would "pinch hit" during this crisis, but she had no intention of becoming the primary caretaker. She had to leave the following day. I had a crash course in case management issues with W's managed care plan. I worked hard to negotiate for 8 hours of home health aide time and skilled nursing visits every day. I instituted this plan on W's second full day at home, and within 1 week, her delusions cleared, mental status returned to baseline, and I finally got to know my patient.

My initial feeling when I walked out of her loft after that second visit was that I had been lucky. On further reflection, I realize I had taken a lot of clinical information, cross referenced with a geriatric knowledge base of dementia versus delirium, and used my ability to work with families to pull together a plan that gave the patient her best shot at remaining home. Months after our initial meeting, W would often laugh about how crazy she had been those first days at home. She had vivid recollections of her delusions. In an effort to acknowledge it had been a shared experience, I told her I was a little scared not having sent her back to the hospital. She responded by telling me it was neither fear nor bravery, that I was a professional who knew what I was doing. "Ah, fooled again," I told her, but I knew I had been paid a wonderful compliment.

This case is an illustration of the various functions that nurse practitioners practicing in the home are called on to carry out. In this case, the nurse used an advanced knowledge base to assess a medical condition, communicate with other providers, negotiate with third-party payers for increased services, and formulate a workable plan with a family member. She also provided emotional support and prevented a readmission to the acute-care setting. This case illustrates the role of the nurse practitioner as an autonomous provider who successfully intervened for a vulnerable patient.

Vignette 2

This second vignette describes a case of a woman who, without a Home Care nurse practitioner, would have lacked care. A had a lifelong history of avoiding healthcare, especially physicians. She also had a long and active problem with alcoholism. Ten years before her home care admission, A's daughter found her unconscious at home. She was admitted to the hospital, diagnosed with a left cerebrovascular accident that had occurred in the setting of an acute anemia caused by gastrointestinal (GI) bleeding due to portal hypertension. She was treated and discharged, but never returned for follow-up. Ten years of continued drinking followed. A began to have severe foot pain from gout and to self-medicate with aspirin. She also developed a large venous ulcer on her chronically edematous legs. Her daughter felt frantic and did not know where to turn for help because her agoraphobic mother refused to go out and see a doctor. At this point, her daughter approached me as I was visiting other patients in an elderly housing building. I agreed to meet the daughter at her mother's apartment, with the goal of providing care.

On the appointed day, I arrived and was greeted by a frightened, elderly woman with severe ascites and mobility limitations who was shouting in an abusive manner that she would never, under any circumstances, come to the hospital. Using many different therapeutic approaches, I finally persuaded A to allow care. It would be a long process to convince her to accept a physician, and ultimately she saw the physician only twice over a 2-year period marked by significant medical instability. Initially, I persuaded her to allow venipuncture, which revealed a severe anemia and a probable active GI bleed that needed to be assessed and treated in the hospital. She refused. I worked long and hard with her to encourage her to stop drinking and taking aspirin. I consulted with her physician and began treatment with a H$_2$-

blocker and iron for the GI bleed and diuretics for the edema from the cirrhosis. I made daily visits to treat the venous ulcer.

Providing personal care required much therapeutic negotiation and limit setting, because A was choosing self-neglect out of her fear. I consulted the Home Care social worker, who provided invaluable assistance and support with this difficult situation. Home health aides and the physical therapist provided maximal support as well. Ultimately, after another acute period of deterioration with a rebleed treated and managed at home, an unstable fluid status managed at home, and marked immobility supported by appropriate provider interventions, A reached a level of optimum health and function for her. She had 2 good years before I found that she had a nonhealing mouth lesion that eventually was diagnosed as malignant. At this point, she was finally ready to see a physician and accept hospitalization. But treatment options for her malignancy were limited, and she died peacefully on intravenous morphine in a coma induced by liver failure.

This case is an example of a patient whose only access to healthcare occurred through her contact and relationship with her Home Care nurse practitioner. A is another example of the complex medically ill patient who can be managed primarily by a nurse practitioner with appropriate consultation from a supportive physician. The nurse practitioner working in the home care setting has an autonomous practice and must be confident in managing the full scope of responsibility for patient care. It is the nurse who initiates discussion to implement or change a treatment plan and directs the physician. If the nurse's assessment suggests a need for multidisciplinary interventions, the nurse consults the physician for a concurrence of orders. It is a nurse-driven system in which the nurse functions as manager, advocate, caregiver, decision maker, and facilitator. The nurse practitioner must enjoy a high degree of independence, be comfortable with independent decision making and actions, supervise other caregivers in the home, interact and plan with other professional providers, and keep current with regulatory and fiscal constraints that influence patient care.

Vignette 3

This case example describes collaboration between a clinical nurse and nurse practitioner when the clinical nurse sought help with a problematic patient situation. This case was referred to me by a clinical nurse. She was having difficulty managing the patient, the patient's two daughters, and private help hired to assist with care at home. The patient had been a wealthy, prominent woman. When I met her, she was extremely agitated and demented, and most probably terminally ill with a recurrent bowel cancer. On assessment, it was clear that I could provide little care to the patient without establishing a trusting relationship with the daughters. I spent as much time as the daughters wanted on the phone, responding promptly to their frequent phone calls and numerous questions. One daughter could describe the mother's life before illness, her abuse of drugs and alcohol, her frivolous relationships with men outside her marriage, and her behavior that was not only a disappointment at times but also a source of embarrassment to this daughter. The daughter wanted her mother to look and act respectably in whatever time she had left. As it was, the patient had developed a total body rash with no clear diagnosis after many referrals. She had open sores from the constant, frantic scratching and rubbing. Using physician consultation, we first tried antihistamines and anxiolytics, but the patient became too sedated and continued to scratch. After weighing all the risk and benefits involved, I suggested to the primary physician a course of steroids. Before initiating the plan, I discussed it extensively with the identified daughter.

The results were remarkable. The patient now takes a very low dose and the daughters are pleased that they can visit with their mother with some semblance of a social interaction. The phone calls are infrequent and the visit frequency for nursing has changed to once a month instead of twice a week. The success of this consultation is demonstrated in several ways. The patient is clearly comfortable and her problem is under control. The daughters feel that their concerns were taken seriously and they understand that their concerns are our concerns; their goals our goals. Of interest is that the daughter thought that I would become the primary nurse. With assistance, she has become comfortable with the present arrangement, knowing that I am a consultant and that the original nurse continues to be her mother's primary nurse. This example shows the importance of the nurse practitioner consultant role in helping to determine a plan that brought comfort to the patient, family, and primary nurse.

THE FUTURE

When we think about the future of the nurse practitioner model in home care, it may become feasible to consider two alternative approaches. One is a care team model, including a nurse practitioner, a clinical nurse, and a physician. When the nurse practitioner is the primary nurse, the clinical nurse will be the associate nurse; and when the clinical nurse is the primary nurse, the nurse practitioner will be the associate. Our sense is that this model will provide patients the best of what we have to offer in knowledge and skills. In addition, this model will ease coordination of complex patient care and intradisciplinary and interdisciplinary collaboration. Case Vignette 3 reveals a primary nurse–nurse practitioner partnership that resulted in a positive patient outcome.

In another type of program, nurse practitioners can be paired with primary care physicians together in teams and collectively decide how to best follow a caseload of homebound patients. Unlike the nurse practitioners in the Beth Israel Home Care program, these nurse practitioners do not provide all the required nursing care. The practitioner may complete the assessment, develop the care plan, and then refer the patient to a local visiting nurse association for skilled nursing. The visiting nurse associations have a contractual agreement to the hospital-based program. The nurse practitioner may then work closely with the visiting nurse association and depend on them to notify him or her of changes in the patient's condition (Mitiguy, 1994). This model has the advantages of accessing expert consultation and supervision at the individual case level, ensuring a mechanism for early referral of patient problems, and potentially decreasing the incidence of serious complications and hospital readmissions by this linkage to an advanced practice nurse (Soehren & Schumann, 1994).

We believe that the nurse practitioner is the provider who can best meet the needs for comprehensive, skilled, dignified, cost-effective patient care for vulnerable individuals and populations. The practitioner not only provides early detection and treatment of disease, health promotion, and casefinding, but also provides for safe, optimized function, and even a comfortable death in compromised, frail, chronically ill individuals.

Our future task will be to support our claims with outcome-based research that can demonstrate specific indicators. We are currently working with a graduate nursing program to develop partnerships between clinicians interested in research and students who are required to complete a research project. In addition, Beth Israel Hospital is developing care models that more closely link care delivered with critical paths and, it is hoped, the resulting outcomes.

References

Benson, E., & McDevitt, J. (1994). When third party payment determines service: The elderly at risk. *Holistic Nursing Practice, 8*(2), 28–35.

Buchwald, D., Panwala, S., & Hooton, T. M. (1992). Use of traditional health practices by Southeast Asian refugees in a primary care clinic. *Western Journal of Medicine, 156*(5), 507–511.

Burns-Tisdale, S., & Goff, W. (1989). The geriatric nurse practitioner in home care. *Nursing Clinics of North America, 24*(3), 809–817.

Chung, R. C., & Kagawa-Singer, M. (1993). Predictors of psychological distress among Southeast Asian refugees. *Social Science and Medicine, 36*(5), 631–639.

Council on Scientific Affairs. (1990). Home care in the 1990's. *JAMA, 263*(9), 1241–1244.

DeLay, P., & Faust, S. (1987). Depression in Southeast Asian Refugees. *American Family Physician, 36*(4), 179–184.

Eisenbruch, M. (1984). Cross cultural aspects of bereavement: II. Ethnic and cultural variations in the development of bereavement practices. *Culture, Medicine and Psychiatry, 8*(4), 315–347.

El Dareer, A. (1983). Complications of female circumcision in the Sudan. *Tropical Doctor, 13,* 41–45.

Faust, S., & Drickey, R. (1986). Working with interpreters. *Journal of Family Practice, 22*(2), 131, 134–138.

Henderson, M. (1984). A GNP in a retirement community. *Geriatric Nursing, 5*(2), 109–112.

Henderson, M. (1990). Beyond the living will. *Gerontologist, 30*(4), 480–485.

Hinton, W. L., Chen, Y. C., Du, N., Tran, C. G., Lu, F. G., Miranda, J., & Faust, S. (1993). DSM-III-R disorders in

Vietnamese refugees: Prevalence and correlates. *Journal of Nervous and Mental Disease, 181*(2), 113–122.

Hoole, A., Pickard, G., Ouimette, R., Lohr, J., & Greenberg, R. (1995). *Patient care guidelines for nurse practitioners* (4th ed.). Philadelphia: J.B. Lippincott.

Kleinman, A., Eisenberg, L., & Good, B. (1978). Culture, illness, and care: Clinical lessons from cross-cultural research. *Annals of Internal Medicine, 88*(2), 251–258.

Kroll, J., Habenicht, M., Mackenzie, T., et al. (1989). Depression and post-traumatic stress disorder in Southeast Asian refugees. *American Journal of Psychiatry, 146*(12), 1592–1597.

Master, R., Feltin, M., Jainchill, J., Mark, R., Kavesh, W., Rabkin, M., Turner, B., Bachrach, S., & Lennox, S. (1980). A continuum of care for the inner city: Assessment of its benefits for Boston's elderly and high risk populations. *New England Journal of Medicine, 302*(26), 1434–1440.

Maugham, W. S. (1944). *The razor's edge* (Introduction). New York: Farrar, Straus & Giroux.

Mehlman, M., & Younger, S. (Eds.). (1991). *Delivering high technology health care.* New York: Springer.

Meucke, M. (1992). New paradigms for refugee health problems. *Social Science and Medicine, 35*(4), 515–523.

Mirosevich, T. (1994). Tools of the trade. *Seattle Review, 17*(1), 44.

Mitiguy, J. (1994). Caring for the elderly at home. *Boston Nurse, 2*(9), 1–6.

Ntiri, D. W. (1993). Circumcision and health among rural women of Somalia as a part of a family life survey. *Health Care for Women International, 14,* 215–226.

Nydegger, C. (1983). Multiple causality: Consequences for practice. *Western Journal of Medicine, 138*(3), 430–436.

Office of Technology Assessment, U.S. Congress. (1986). *Nurse practitioner, physician assistants and certified nurse midwives: A policy analysis.* Washington, DC: U.S. Government Printing Office.

Patcher, L. (1994). Folk illness beliefs and behaviors and their implications for health care delivery. *JAMA, 271*(9), 690–694.

Shepherd, J., & Faust, S. (1993). Refugee health care and the problem of suffering. *Bioethics Forum, 9*(2), 3–7.

Sluzki, C. (1979). Migration and family conflict. *Family Process, 18*(4), 379–390.

Sluzki, C. (1984). The patient provider translator triad: A note for providers. *Family Systems Medicine, 2*(4), 397–400.

Sluzki, C. (1992). Disruption and reconstruction of networks following migration/relocation. *Family Systems Medicine, 10*(4), 359–363.

Soehren, P. M., & Schumann, L. L. (1994). Enhanced role opportunities available to the CNS/nurse practitioner. *Clinical Nurse Specialist, 8*(3), 123–127.

Strumpf, N. E. (1994). Innovative gerontological practices as models for health care delivery. *Nursing and Health Care, 15*(10), 522–527.

Westermeyer, J., Bouafuely, M., Neider, J., & Calleis, A. (1989). Somatization among refugees: An epidemiologic study. *Psychosomatics, 30*(1), 34–43.

Westermeyer, J. (1990). Motivations for uprooting and migration. In W. H. Holtzmann & T. H. Bornemann (Eds.), *Mental health of immigrants and refugees* (pp. 78–89). Austin, TX: Hogg Foundation for Mental Health.

19

Managing Acute and Chronic Illness Across Settings

Introduction: Joanne V. Hickey

When we are ill, we seek help from the healthcare system in accordance with our particular circumstances. The circumstances may include our location (e.g., rural), our job circumstances (e.g., military service), the particular nature of our illness (e.g., terminal illness), or the episodic nature of the acute stages of our illness (e.g., as with diabetes). These and other similar circumstances often circumscribe the setting in which our care will be provided.

In this chapter, several authors discuss examples of practice settings that reflect this reality and in which advanced practice nurses (APNs) function successfully to provide quality care designed specifically for the particular circumstances of the patients attracted to that setting. Access to care as well as quality of care is influenced by the circumstances of the settings in which patients find themselves. For example, populations such as those living in rural areas or those in federal employment have limited access to healthcare because of where they reside or work. Hanson and Murphy describe the diverse populations and variety of health problems for which care is provided in the rural system and federal systems, respectively. Access to care may also be compromised by barriers that appear during transitions in illness as patients recover, deteriorate, or prepare to die from a terminal illness. Richmond and Keane, who discuss acute-care nurse practitioners, and Koesters, who discusses hospice care, address transitions in care across physical boundaries such as hospital to home and across transitions in illness from recovery to peaceful death. The common, uniting theme in Exemplars A through D is the APN's ability to provide access to healthcare, improve access to care that is sensitive to the needs and wishes of patients and their families, and provide for transitions in care as the course of an illness changes.

In Exemplar A, Richmond and Keane comment on the fluidity of boundaries in and among healthcare providers that contributes to the new and rapidly evolving role of the acute-care nurse practitioner. Paradigm shifts and new models of collaborative practice provide opportunities for acute-care nurse practitioners that transcend institutional barriers and cross

Hickey JV: ADVANCED PRACTICE NURSING: Changing Roles
and Clinical Applications © 1996 Lippincott–Raven Publishers

healthcare delivery boundaries for transitional care. Transformation in healthcare is providing new opportunities, resulting partly from the anticipated decrease in hospital residents and partly from the redesign of healthcare providers' roles to include knowledge and skills for furnishing cost-effective and quality care.

In Exemplar B, Koesters discusses the home as the primary site for hospice care, where APNs are an integral part of the coordination and administration of care. The goals of hospice care are to support a high quality of life—as defined by the patient—that neither hastens nor postpones death, but reaffirms life; to relieve suffering; and to allow for a peaceful death. Using an interdisciplinary team approach, the patient and family are assisted in making decisions and supported through the multiple losses along the journey to the expected death.

In Exemplar C, Hanson points out that the rural nurse practitioner must understand the culture as well as the healthcare needs of the people in the area in which he or she is practicing. The needs of patients and the severity of their acute and chronic illnesses are exacerbated by poverty, limited regional resources, and lack of basic preventive care. Because patients range from infants to elderly people, the rural nurse practitioner is challenged to understand the developmental and special needs of each age group. In addition, the practitioner must manage a wide range of health problems, which requires that he or she have broad knowledge and skills.

In Exemplar D, Murphy reminds us that the military healthcare system is the largest single healthcare organization in the world, providing care during peacetime and wartime. It services military, embassy, and other federal employees, their dependents, and retirees in many national and international settings. Service includes all age groups from infants to elderly people, and spans the continuum of care from disease prevention and health promotion to acute and chronic illness management. This is the ultimate in comprehensive care. In addition, the military APN may become involved in humanitarian missions in foreign and hostile environments. The challenging role of the military APN means providing care anywhere in the world.

The authors of the exemplars in this chapter share substantive vignettes depicting the exciting and innovative practice and holistic care models. These practice models are meeting the needs of multiple and diverse populations in a diverse range of settings and circumstances.

Acute-Care Nurse Practitioners

Therese S. Richmond ■ *Anne Keane*

Acute-care nurse practitioners (ACNPs) are nurses prepared at the graduate level who are expanding their scope of practice to incorporate both the caring paradigm of nursing and parts of the therapeutic paradigm of medicine. To this end, ACNPs draw on the strengths of the primary care nurse practitioner, but focus specialized knowledge and skill on the management of select patient groups who often have acute and specialized healthcare needs. Although the title *acute-care nurse practitioner* implies that individuals in this role practice exclusively within the walls of acute-care hospitals, their actual practice may extend beyond hospital walls. Exemplar A focuses on the evolution and implementation of ACNP roles. Exemplars derived from interviews with currently practicing ACNPs highlight important themes and issues that should be considered as the ACNP role continues to evolve.

THE CHALLENGE

As a result of changes in society and current and anticipated changes in healthcare, boundaries within and among healthcare providers are increasingly fluid, and roles are evolving rapidly (Keane, Richmond, & Kaiser, 1994). As we move into a system that is responding to pressures to lower the high cost of care and grappling with the feasibility of delivering acute care with fewer physicians, the opportunities for advanced practice nurses (APNs) are numerous. As the system transforms, the way of doing business and the delivery of healthcare will have to change as well.

Society, legislators, and members of the healthcare team agree that the healthcare system, as currently designed, does not adequately meet the needs of millions of Americans. The system must change to meet the primary and preventive care needs of all Americans. The challenge is to meet these needs without compromising the strengths of the current system and the continuing acute-care needs of the population.

With the predicted downsizing of medical residency programs, the reallocation of more residency slots to primary care settings, and the current difficulty in filling existing acute-care residency slots, the management of patients in acute-care hospitals (especially teaching hospitals) will have to change drastically (Richmond & Keane, 1992). In the face of diminishing lengths of stay and changing patterns of medical education, nurses must offer efficient and complex nursing services to provide a system of seamless services. The need for seamless services is further driven by the economic reality that results in the rapid transit of acutely ill patients through the various phases of care. For years, we have realized that business must be done differently, when the period of convalescence no longer occurs within the hospital setting. Patients are discharged while still in the acute phase of illness. The ability to coordinate multiple services such as nursing, medical, home health, social services, and various other therapies is a critical skill for any individual who is primarily responsible for the management of the acutely ill patient. These skills have always been the strength of nurses. Diminishing lengths of hospital stay drive the system to identify healthcare providers who can simultaneously manage the patient's medical problems and manage the human responses to the illness or injury at a personal, family, and community level (Keane & Richmond, 1993). The ACNP is a healthcare provider who is uniquely qualified to meet these needs.

CURRENT STATUS

Nurse practitioner (NP) forms of practice have evolved and have been integrated into the acute-care setting for years. This happened in two ways: primary care NPs moved into the acute-care setting and clinical nurse specialists responded to the changing demands of specialized populations. Although primary care NPs are not educated to manage acutely ill patients with specialized needs, they often acquire knowledge and skills required for this management under the mentoring of physicians in specialized practice. Similarly, clinical nurse specialists are prepared to manage patients with specialized needs, but they are not prepared to assume NP roles nor are they recognized as NPs within the healthcare system. However, many clinical nurse specialists' practices have changed in response to the needs of patients and systems, and they have assumed many practitioner functions under the tutelage of specialized physicians or NPs.

Nurse practitioner practices in the acute-care setting vary considerably. Unit-based neonatal NPs have been practicing for many years and demonstrate a successful model for the APN who focuses on highly specialized populations needing intensive technological support. Another practice model includes NPs who are population based (e.g., cardiopulmonary service) and who focus on groups of patients with specialized needs throughout the continuum of care. Currently, the population-based model focuses on inpatient management, but these practices are now beginning to extend beyond the traditional walls of hospital settings. Other APNs use a problem-based approach to care delivery; these APNS include practitioners who provide specialized wound care, manage urinary incontinence, manage acute and chronic pain, and provide nutritional support. Their responsibilities are not necessarily limited to acute-care settings, because these complex problems require the provision of care to patients outside the hospital. The problems of patients with complex nonhealing wounds, urinary incontinence, or chronic pain are rarely completely resolved within the confines of a single hospitalization.

To date, little consideration has been given to determine where these ACNPs fit within the existing organizational system. Typically, they have been placed in existing organizational niches within clinical ladder systems, within the management component of the nursing system in an effort to reflect their extended range of responsibilities, or, alternatively they work in an existing physician practice plan. These may be convenient solutions within the current organizational structures, but they also create challenges and potential barriers to the full scope of advanced nursing practice.

EXEMPLARS AND THEMES

Exemplars describing the range of role responsibilities, challenges, satisfactions, and serendipitous opportunities were gleaned from interviews with seven ACNPs currently in practice in acute care hospital settings. The narratives helped us identify recurrent themes, validate perceptions, and understand the modifications of the role required in different settings, organizations, or by the varying demands of specific patient populations. At the time the ACNPs were interviewed, they were practicing in adult and pediatric tertiary care hospitals in three major Middle-Atlantic metropolitan areas—Washington, D. C., Delaware, and Pennsylvania/New Jersey. These practitioners identified major themes that exemplify the evolving role, challenges and opportunities related to ongoing practice, and system and personal barriers that must be addressed.

Expansion of the Advanced Practice Nurse Role

The scope of the APN role is recognized by all of the healthcare providers but some components are recognized more than others. All ACNPs interviewed stated that their role had greatly expanded and that this expansion was driven by patient needs and the type of practice. Increased responsibility for practice, decision making, and outcomes accompanied role expansion. Outcomes were predominately patient driven and only secondarily system driven. This variety of roles was reflected in the interviews.

> I do a lot as a clinician . . . with both inpatients or outpatients. [I do] histories and physical assessment in terms of the patient's general condition, the diagnosis (whether it is medical or adaptation to the problem). I do consultations. I admit patients; I can admit directly from the clinic to the hospital setting. It can be set up as outpatient ahead of time. I can work through the emergency department after a decision has been made whether the patient needs to be admitted. [The decision is made] in collaboration with the MD.

There were common threads throughout the interviews. All of the ACNPs reported responsibilities for H&Ps [histories and physicals] including an assessment of the health status; everyone reported making clinical decisions and prescribing studies, treatments, and medications.

> I went over and did the cardiac consult—wrote it on the chart, wrote my recommendations, ordered an echocardiogram. The MD in our practice went by when the patient was getting the echocardiogram, read the report, made suggestions, called me and suggested a VQ [ventilation/perfusion] scan to rule out a pulmonary embolism. I then called the referring MD and suggested the VQ scan.

The majority of the ACNPs talked about managing the psychological needs of patient and family, including teaching needs.

> I spent time with them and their care and concerns. We get a lot of patients far from home, families can't always come. I . . . deal with their anxiety. . . . [My patient] was upset. I went back later and . . . asked him about his family and if I could talk to them later (usually I leave my card, since the families aren't there when I make my rounds). I found that his wife was housebound. He didn't want to bother his children. I encouraged him to tell the children. I called his wife to let her know what was happening. I called her after the surgery. I think I was able to bring her there even though she couldn't come. I think he did better because of it. I feel that I make a difference.

Most ACNPs talked about admission and discharge responsibilities. Almost all of the ACNPs interviewed talked about responsibility for consultation and collaboration. The need to practice within the interdisciplinary healthcare team was a common role component. Another emerging role responsibility was the need for advocacy for third-party payers.

> I negotiate with the insurance carriers. I have to justify the reason for the stay. Through watching the physician, I learned certain cue words that you need to get the patient through the system.

Ongoing management of chronic, unresolved problems may be a key component even in delivery of care to acutely ill patients. Other ACNP roles not identified by the ACNPs interviewed include serving as a first assistant in the operating room (Gates, 1993).

Importance of the Nurse Practitioner in the Provision of Continuity of Care

Continuity of care is increasingly difficult to assure in today's healthcare environment. The ACNP whose practice spans inpatient and outpatient settings can deal with the multiple transitions in care (Richmond & Keane, 1992). Many of the ACNPs interviewed described the importance of providing stable, continuing care for their patients as they moved through different settings or were seen by different team members.

> The continuity with the cerebral palsy kids—we know them as outpatients—we know their background, when they get into trouble and the kinds of situations that get them into trouble. I provide continuity. At the CP [cerebral palsy] team meeting, the orthopods [orthopedic physicians] say who is coming in next week. If we have the information ahead of time, we can go to the staff and say who is coming in—set them up. It is a full circle.

From a different perspective, continuity within the inpatient setting is an important aspect of the NP role.

> I am responsible for patients from the minute they walk into the door until discharge. . . . We have 10 physicians in the practice [and two NPs]. We [the NPs] are the continuity—if it's Tuesday, it must be Dr. X. Physicians come in for 1 or 2 days. The patients often only remember us, since they see many different doctors during the week of hospitalization.

Acute-care nurse practitioners expressed firm beliefs in the value to their patients of their continuing presence.

> The care is better with NPs because of the continuity. It is often a revolving door because of organ rejection. I think that the continuity is important. It is appreciated by patients—to see a familiar face, to know that they don't have to wait for the attending [MD], to know that the NP will be there—to know . . . and trust [him or her]. With the residents, they come and go. There are different ones all the time. When you affiliate yourself with a hospital—you see the same attending and same NP. . . . It's going to be better for patients and the hospital.

Many of the ACNPs were able to identify situations in which their practice made a difference to patient care outcomes.

> I had a man who had been in and out of the hospital waiting for a heart transplant. He came in on a dobutamine drip waiting for a transplant. We had developed a special relationship; I had followed him from his very first hospitalization, and I was able to see the daily changes. He took a turn for the worse and ended up in the CCU [coronary care unit] very near death. They kept discussing the LVAD [left ventricular assist device], . . . but at this institution, they had used it before and both patients died. I kept hearing it and hearing it and no one was willing to make a decision. Finally, I sought out the transplant coordinator . . . and said, . . . "What are we waiting for? This physician is saying one thing, this one is saying another. In the meantime, we are forgetting the patient: he is dying." She looked at me and said, "You are right, we are getting clouded." Within 2 hours, he was on the schedule and within 4 hours, he was on the LVAD. . . . He had a rocky course, but now he comes back [for follow-up] 3 years later. Because I was in an unusual role, I could cross over boundaries and I could see what was happening and that we were forgetting. . . . The surgeons were too concerned about their mortalities, the CCU [coronary care unit] staff didn't know him that well—he was one more transplant. But I knew him and I was there.

The following exemplar extends this idea:

Where there were difficult family situations that needed organizing and coordinating interdisciplinary meetings, I was able to identify that we were not all on the same wavelength. I was able to bring some of the different services together and make sure that we could get these patients discharged a lot sooner than we might have. I make a difference where there are complex patients.

Collaboration as an Essential Component for Role Success

Acute-care nurse practitioners clearly understand the value of collaboration with other team members. Although ACNPs are expected to collaborate with residents and attending physicians, they can enhance the involvement of the staff nurse in the daily management and decision making concerning patients (Gates, 1993).

I work very strongly with the MD—joint decisions for the plan of care. Once the patients are in house, I round on them on a daily basis, get a feel for what happened overnight, how the plan is progressing. And then I work as an intermediary between the MD and resident and MD and nurses in making sure the plan is working.

Limitations in Independent Practice as Barriers

In addition to identifying strong satisfaction with their practice, the ACNPs repeatedly identified frustrating limits or barriers.

My frustrations are time issues. We have several general surgeons but only one is here per day. When you need something you need it now, but you can't always get it. Do I stay down in the clinic and watch the sick kid, get the IV [intravenous drip] started or do I have the staff monitor the blood pressure? . . . Do I admit him without an attending [physician]? I can. If I'm wrong, it would be okay . . . the surgeons would rather be safe than sorry. I don't like to admit without an attending seeing the kid. I think it is an insecurity for me. What if I'm wrong? They could be home. It's expensive.

Another example of lack of independence—not seen as a barrier, but rather an example of the closeness that develops in the collaborative relationship—follows.

Everything (H&P, et cetera), has to be co-signed by the attending . . . . The closeness . . . of the surgeons who work with you, their supervision, not only for me, but of the residents, is important. In this department, you have an attending who sits down with you and talks about the patient and does "hands on" rounds. This occurs every day in a collaborative fashion.

Contrasted with the limits of enforced dependence are the gains and concerns related to increased autonomy.

I think this is a great role—you can be involved with many different aspects of the patient's care. You get to work with lots of different departments. There is a lot of autonomy, more than any other previous nursing role.

Yet, sometimes the autonomy hurts:

Sometimes they rely on me too much . . . for convenience rather than confidence. I'm still nervous dealing with sick patients, being the ultimate decision maker.

These comments suggest the need for a phased period of levels of supervision as suggested by Snyder and colleagues (1994). The ACNP postgraduate apprenticeship should progress through phases of direct, proximate, general supervision, and independent function as the ACNP progresses and matures in role capabilities and decision making.

I ordered all the tests, invasive or not, in my previous practice. With this practice, I would order echocardiograms and one of the [medical] partners got down on me the first couple of months. One of the partners said, "Why did you do this? Did you call anyone?" It was establishing my rationale and credibility. Now they have no problem.

Substitutive Nature of the Nurse Practitioner Practice

The ACNPs describe many of their activities as substitutive of physicians' work.

Rather than hire another fellow, they hired an NP [me] who could fill the fellow's role. . . . I manage people daily, assess them, write H&P, write their orders, and basically follow them from admission to discharge. I work in collaboration with the attending , but I do everything unless I have a question.

Is the substitutive role just the physician extender—a miniresident—or advanced nursing practice? Some described their role as purely substitutive, whereas others understood how their background and preparation permitted them to contribute much more broadly to patient care demands. The difference may rest in organizational structure, in personal factors, or in philosophical perspectives.

The differences between the resident and I are none—except experience. I equate myself with a first- and second-year resident. The fourth-year residents can educate me, but I can educate them as well.

But they are different. Acute-care nurse practitioners must have clinical expertise in both nursing and medical management of the patient. However, it is clear that they must have a strong nursing identity. As Gates (1993) stated, they "must know who they are and not be trapped as 'physician extenders' in the medical model" (p. 51). One ACNP's comments reflect Gate's insight:

I know their history as far as nausea and vomiting. I know what works. I know these patients and families over the long haul. And the residents don't. They are here for 1 to 2 months. My database for that patient is much broader. There have been situations, more with chemotherapy, when a kid has a side effect, that I know the kid had before and I know he needs this, instead of trying another treatment. I've developed patient profiles and said to the staff, they need them, they need to know nuances. My hope is that the residents will use this information.

Lack of Mentors

The practitioners were asked to identify those who served as professional mentors for them. Invariably, they identified the attending physician as their mentor:

The attending is the only person who serves as a mentor.

Although many of the ACNPs interviewed could not identify a mentor, some talked about role models:

No provision [for a mentor] is available to me. The practice doesn't do anything, because my role in the practice is new. They and I are still learning. I went to an established NP for the CT surgeons. . . . I sought out the CNS [clinical nurse specialist] for her educational focus.

I have to say I don't [have a role model] and I miss not having one. I don't have a mentor at this time.

The need for continuing education to keep up with the demands of the ACNP role was clearly identified. Some ACNPs, however, indicated that continuing education programs in nursing did not fully meet the needs of their expanded practice. One of the challenges of being on the cutting edge role in the transformation of the work force is that there are limited educational programs available to them and no established mentors.

> My professional development is self-motivated. I rarely go to nursing conferences. I find I don't learn what I need. I take advantage of grand rounds, weekly echocardiogram conferences. I go to one or two continuing education programs a year, usually in cardiology but sometimes something else in adult health.

Increasing Physician Acceptance of Acute-Care Nurse Practitioners

The importance of establishing collegial relationships with medical colleagues was a common theme in all NP interviews. One advantage of this role is that ACNPs not only achieve immense personal and professional satisfaction but earn true respect and collegiality from medical colleagues who come to rely on them (Edmunds & Ruth, 1991).

> If a physician comes on board—let's say there is a new specialist and they see all their colleagues have an NP/CNS—they want their own advanced practice nurse. We are established. We have been able to prove our worth. Many times I will call the outside referring physician to discuss the case. I have never had the doctor say, "I want to talk to the doctor." I give them the information, I send the dictations. Most say great, wonderful, thanks for calling me. That's another thing we do—maintain the communication. They love it. They know if we weren't there, no one would call them.

Barriers

The lack of admission and discharge privileges was repeatedly identified as a frustrating problem. None of the NPs interviewed had formal admission and discharge privileges. Few NPs have admitting privileges to hospitals (Iazzetti, 1992).

> I wouldn't be the one to initiate the admission or discharge. If I had someone who needed to be admitted, I would consult with the attending . . . . I write the discharge order, but it's in the name of the physician. But it is definitely a team plan.

While a common problem, all of the ACNPs had devised methods to circumvent this barrier.

> It's all informal. I admit patients under Dr. X. I just happen to pick whatever physician happens to be in the hospital that day. I discharge the patient and write it as a verbal order of Dr. X.. Usually it's a joint decision, but it could be my independent decision. Oftentimes, it is so routine. All charting in this hospital has to be written as a verbal order. It causes a lot of extra charting. They [the orders] never get signed in 24 hours. I go down to medical records with a signature stamp and stamp them all.

Lack of independence in writing orders was also identified as a barrier to practice. Few hospitals have developed systems that permit ACNPs to write direct orders. Many have developed a shadow system of verbal orders and include the use of protocols to guide the ACNP and others in the range of orders appropriate for specific situations.

> I'm involved in computerizing chemotherapy order sets and developing order sets. The residents don't write chemo orders. We have no fellows. I write the chemo orders and

the attending has to cosign. I establish the protocols in collaboration with the attending, but I can't order them.

The barrier of limitations of writing orders is driven in some ways by state practice acts. Although prescription privileges are nonexistent in some states, in other states, these barriers are falling.

I write verbal orders from the physician. They have to co-sign them before the chart can be closed for good. Until I get my certification, they have to. Once I get my certification number, they have to cosign [only] the first orders on the chart that I have written under my name and numbers.

Because many patients are referred from other geographical areas to the hospitals in which the ACNPs work, the issue of writing discharge prescriptions is complex. Some patients are discharged to jurisdictions in which the ACNPs' prescriptions will be honored. Others are discharged to settings in which the prescriptions are deemed invalid.

I write my own prescriptions under my own name. They are filled in Maryland, the District of Columbia, and Virginia, but not Pennsylvania and Florida. National Blue Cross/Blue Shield mail orders will not fill them.

Another barrier identified related to the difficulties posed by the lack of recognition among insurance companies of ACNP status as reimbursable providers. As Edmunds and Ruth (1991) stated, NPs are considered "shadow providers" when functioning within a hospital, because they cannot generate revenue or direct contributions to healthcare apart from physicians and the institutions. However, many ACNPs frequently perform CPT [current procedural terminology]-coded services for which physicians or the group practice are reimbursed (Griffith & Robinson, 1991). One ACNP's comments reflected a sensitivity to these issues:

Because of length of stay issues and reimbursement issues, insurance carriers say that if the patient is sick enough to need a hospital bed at $350 a day, they are sick enough to see a physician.

It is unclear how reimbursement schemes will play themselves out over the coming decade. However, we are moving into an era of capitated payment for patient groups, and one might argue that even direct reimbursement of physicians for care provided in hospital settings will be a thing of the past.

Lack of Technological Aspects of the Role

The technological components of the role are still early in their development. Many ACNPs identified a lack of interest in involvement in this part of the role. Most had not been prepared for high-technology tasks in their educational program and hesitated to incorporate this component of the role.

Passing A-lines [insertion of arterial lines]. That's a technical thing. Anyone could do that.

I don't do biopsies. But if I wanted to, I could learn. Same thing with central lines. The only thing we had in school was learning to suture. I prefer not to put in central lines because it is just a technique. It is the same thing over and over again. It would be so easy to get rid of our technicians, and the residents need the experience.

Are these attitudes couched in the past? Do ACNPs have to be house residents? Is the antipathy toward involvement with technology an attitudinal barrier? Edmunds and Ruth (1991) have expressed reservation about the development of positions in which APNs, especially those in acute-care settings, would focus on technical procedures. They proposed that a nursing background is not needed in such roles. We concur that focusing on technical procedures alone is not an effective way to use the ACNP's knowledge and skills. However, as the boundaries of practice continue to evolve and change, nurses must be open to acquiring technical skills that have been the purview of physicians. Historically, nurses have successfully incorporated tasks exclusively associated with physicians, such as taking blood pressure measurements, monitoring electrocardiograms and treating dysrhythmias, and monitoring cardiovascular variables. We caution that an attitudinal barrier against the technological components of the role is short sighted and may be a major barrier to ongoing expansion of the ACNP role.

> I didn't learn central venous access in my program. I wasn't able to build the experience into my fieldwork. The one thing I wanted to learn was lumbar punctures and bone marrows. I still don't do it. The oncologists don't think I need it. But I will need it with outpatients. Had I learned lumbar punctures and bone marrow aspirates, they would probably have let me do it.

Reeducation and Socialization of Physicians

Acute-care nurse practitioners commented on their developing relationships with physicians and physicians' need to respect and trust them.

> MDs need to become more comfortable with allowing APNs to do what they can do and not redoing what they do. They have to understand we have the knowledge and ability to take care of these patients and they have to trust us and not feel they have to go back in and do what we did. I think with healthcare reform they are going to have to start to let go, whether they want to or not.

We are moving in that direction. In their discussion of the use of ACNPs in critical care, Snyder and colleagues (1994) state, "We believe that when ACNPs can function safely without direct and immediate supervision, as determined by their knowledge, skill, patient need, and severity of illness, these professionals are likely to increase the efficiency of critical care physicians in patient care management" (p. 303).

Importance of Support and Reporting for Role Functioning

The importance of physician support and respect was clearly identified by the ACNPs. Approximately half ($n = 3$) of the ACNPs interviewed reported directly to a physician with no organizational linkages to nursing. In general, the ACNPs identified the importance of physician support as critical to the effective implementation of their role, even more so than support from nursing administration. This finding differs from those of a recent study of 288 master's-prepared clinical nurse specialists, in which McFadden and Miller (1994) found that the majority ($n = 53.2\%$) of respondents indicated the need for nursing administrative support, whereas fewer (11.7%) identified physician support and acceptance as important.

Some ACNPs saw the value of reporting to nursing administration with organizational matrixes to physicians.

> The physicians don't have total control over us. If they do, we would be closer to a physician's assistant role. I think they would push it to the limit. Especially those who need you out there seeing patients, [doing] H&Ps, and writing orders. The department of nursing has said there are more things nurses can offer than just being a physician extender. When I first came here, I was upset I didn't report to the physicians; I thought they would protect me. I now realize it's better to be in nursing. You get a bigger picture. . . . It affects how we are viewed here.

The ACNPs who held joint reporting mechanisms were clear on their reporting responsibilities to physicians, but less clear on the content of their reports to nursing.

> I report to the associate director of nursing; my position is paid by their budget. I have an allegiance to the physician division head of the gastroenterology department, although he doesn't pay my salary. I look to his direction in terms of my activities and performance.

In general, the ACNPs who reported directly to nursing reported primarily on system-related issues rather than their daily role responsibilities.

FUTURE CONSIDERATIONS

As nursing grapples with the transformation of the workforce, it is apparent that we and other professions must be willing to shake up the old models of care and create new paradigms. This will not be easy. Care systems are changing daily, and no period of stability appears to be in the foreseeable future. Although primary care and prevention are critically important, people will continue to have acute and chronic health problems that require a full array of services in all phases of care. We believe the evolution of the ACNP is an appropriate and timely response to the changing needs of healthcare in the United States.

When any one player within the system changes, other players and the system itself must change as well. It is time that we reconceptualize the system as a whole to more effectively meet the needs of patients and their families. How might this occur? As Naylor and colleagues (1994) have pointed out, we need a different model of care than we have now if we are to respond effectively to these changes. The ACNP must be able to focus on the entire spectrum of the illness or injury and not be bound by the artificial boundaries of the current systems. Rather than limiting practice to the acute-care system or within the community, the ACNP must be able to transcend institutional and other boundaries to provide care for patients across systems of care.

Naylor and colleagues (1994) have been able to demonstrate that the use of APNs who followed elderly patients across systems of care (i.e., acute, rehabilitative, and home maintenance) served to improve patient outcomes, reduce costs, and decrease the number of readmissions. The APNs in their study were part of a research team and received their salaries through a research grant.

How might ACNPs create a position that permits and indeed facilitates the care of acutely and chronically ill patients throughout the entire spectrum of their illness? To whom would ACNPs report and from whom would they obtain a salary? Most of the ACNPs we interviewed were salaried by the acute-care hospital, and their practices either were limited to the inpatient setting or extended only to the outpatient clinics of the hospital. Even those ACNPs who were salaried through a physician practice plan had practices focusing exclusively on patients within the acute-care setting, with no responsibilities once the patient was discharged.

As ACNPs cross care delivery boundaries, an organizational paradigm shift will be necessary. Nurse executives, physicians, and administrators with whom the ACNPs work must be visionary and assist in influencing the system as it undergoes dramatic changes. Acute-care nurse practitioners and their patients may be best served by reporting to nursing administration with a matrixed line to physicians, as was the case with some of the ACNPs we interviewed. As Gates (1993) has argued, a reporting model to nursing administration with reporting matrixes to physicians allows for the development of strong alliances with collaborating physicians and staff nurses alike. If this is the path chosen, it is important for nurse executives to recognize the value of cultivating a practice pattern that extends beyond the hospital walls if ACNPs are to manage patient care throughout the entire spectrum of the illness, be it in the hospital or the home.

Acute-care nurse practitioners will require additional knowledge about how to effectively navigate these systems—specifically knowledge about insurance carriers, community-based support, and the artificial boundaries that directly influence patient outcomes. Are there other models of reporting in which this can be accomplished? Acute-care nurse practitioners hired within physician practice plans may experience fewer constraints when it comes to system boundaries such as in-hospital versus out-of-hospital care. However, based on our interviews, this is not necessarily the case. Perhaps ACNPs will be salaried through insurance companies that will assume increasing responsibilities for patient management throughout the spectrum of the illness. Whatever the reporting mechanism and from wherever the salary is obtained, we believe the critical issue is that ACNPs need to break out of the current mold and work toward creating new paradigms of care.

Once the extension of care boundaries into the community has been endorsed, ACNPs must determine the scope of care to be provided to patients. The ability to work collaboratively with other care providers in both the acute-care and non–acute-care settings must be cultivated. Acute-care nurse practitioners will need to examine their unique role within this changing system of care. How ACNPs play out their roles will be determined by their own unique background, interests, knowledge, and skills. It will be important for ACNPs to examine how their roles support the goals of new paradigms of care and enhance continuity across the entire spectrum of illness.

Acknowledgment: The authors of this exemplar would like to acknowledge the participation of the following APNs in the interviews on which the exemplar was based: Janeen Constantine, RN, MS, PNP, ANP-C, Certified Adult Nurse Practitioner, Cardiology Associates, P.C., Washington, D.C.; Linda DeNavas, NP, Nurse Practitioner, Transplant Unit, Transplantation Services, Washington Hospital Center, Washington, D.C.; and Betty Hart RN, MSN, CRNP, Cardiac Nurse Practitioner, Heart Institute of Southern New Jersey, Camden, NJ. Also, the following APNs from the Alfred I. Du Pont Institute of the Nemours Foundation in Wilmington, DE: Alexis Perri, MSN, RN, Gastroenterology Advanced Practice Nurse–Nurse Practitioner, Gastroenterology and Nutrition Services; Jennifer Sullivan, RN, MSN, Surgical Advanced Practice Nurse–Nurse Specialist; Cathy Trzcenski, RN, MSN, Pediatric Advanced Practice Nurse–Nurse Practitioner, Cerebral Palsy Program; and Jean Wadman, MSN, RN, Oncology Advanced Practice Nurse–Nurse Practitioner, Oncology Service.

Note: References are cited at end of chapter.

Hospice Care

Susan Koesters

The transition from life can be every bit as profound, intimate and precious as the miracle of birth. (Bylock, 1994)

ROOTS OF HOSPICE CARE

The term *hospice* comes from the Latin word *hospes,* meaning both "guest" and "host." In medieval times, *hospice* was used to describe a place of shelter and rest for weary and sick travelers or pilgrims on long journeys. Mostly run by religious orders, hospices were often way stations on the way to the Holy Land. In the late 1800s, the Irish Sisters of Charity opened a hospice in Dublin; they later opened one in London as a home for the dying, that is, for those in the last stages of life's journey. Today, *hospice* refers to a coordinated program of compassionate care for people with terminal illnesses and their families provided by a team of professional care providers and volunteers.

Hospice, the modern movement in caring for the dying, had its beginnings in England under the leadership of Dame Cecily Saunders, a nurse, social worker, and physician. In the late 1940s, she sat at the bedside of a dying man as he related to her how and where he would like to die. Her vision of a special home for the dying began to develop. From 1958 to 1965, Saunders worked at St. Joseph's Hospice in London, where she learned how management of distressing physical symptoms, counseling, and spiritual care could ease the suffering of the dying and their families. She began St. Christopher's Hospice as an inpatient care program and initiated programs to teach nurses, physicians, social workers, chaplains, and volunteers how to work together to improve the dying person's quality of life. The first hospice in the United States was established in Connecticut in 1974; programs then spread throughout the country. Hospices are now located around the world.

Patients served in early U.S. hospice programs had a diagnosis of terminal cancer, whereas patients now served in most hospices include those with any incurable condition with a life expectancy measured in months, not years, if the disease runs its expected course. Hospice care recipients today may have endstage cardiovascular disease, kidney failure, neuromuscular disorders, chronic obstructive pulmonary disease, acquired immunodeficiency syndrome (AIDS), or genetic conditions incompatible with life. Care recipients range in age from newborn to very elderly. Some hospice programs in metropolitan areas specialize in the care of people with cancer or of children or adults with AIDS. Most smaller communities, however, have programs that are not restricted by diagnoses. Mountain Area Hospice in North Carolina, for example, provides care to people in all age groups with a diagnosis of a terminal illness and a life expectancy of fewer than 12 months.

The primary setting for hospice care in the United States has shifted from inpatient care to home care. The goal is to enable terminally ill people to live out their remaining days in comfort and die at home with family present. Home may be the traditional house or apartment for most people, but home also includes assisted living and skilled nursing facilities. Short-term inpatient care is also provided in the hospital or hospice unit. For example, Mountain Area Hospice has a 12-bed, freestanding inpatient unit called Solace. Patients may be admitted for short-term management of symptoms such as pain or nausea unmanageable in the home, with the goal of returning home when the symptoms are controlled. Several days of respite care are also available to enable caregivers to have a rest from the demands of 24-hour care. Some beds are also available for residential care when there is no available or able caregiver.

THE CONCEPT OF PALLIATIVE CARE

Underlying all aspects of the hospice concept is a philosophy of care that neither hastens nor postpones death but affirms life. Dying is regarded as a normal process. Care is directed toward promoting a high quality of life, the relief of suffering, and a peaceful death. Hospice care is also described as palliative or "the active total care of people whose disease is not responsive to curative treatment" (World Health Organization, 1990, p. 3). Diagnostic procedures and treatments such as chemotherapy, radiation, and surgery may have a place in palliative care if the benefits in providing relief of symptoms outweigh the disadvantages. The goal of any intervention is to improve the quality of life for the person, not to control or cure disease.

Not all care for the dying is hospice care. Hospice care takes a particular holistic approach to the entire family, not just the person with the terminal illness, is the focus of care. *Family* is defined broadly as the support system—those the patient identifies as significant, not necessarily the traditional family. One or more people are designated as primary caregivers. They may live with the patient and provide care or be responsible for arranging care. Spouses, children, and significant others may provide care.

As mentioned earlier, the focus of hospice care is on maintaining quality of life and promoting a peaceful death. Physical, psychosocial, and spiritual needs of patient and families are addressed. Hospice programs use an interdisciplinary approach to providing care including the physician, nurse, social worker, chaplain, therapist, counselors, volunteers, patient, and family. Hospice care also continues after death, with bereavement follow-up by counselors trained to assist with the grieving process and to recognize and coordinate treatment for people with abnormal grief responses. Continuity of care is promoted; services continue with changes in the care setting, whether it be home, hospital, extended-care facility, or hospice inpatient unit.

Because people with endstage illnesses and their families have special needs, a new field of palliative medicine is evolving. It is now recognized as a specialty in the United Kingdom; perhaps American medical education will follow suit. Hospice care is now a nursing specialty with certification available through the Hospice Nurses' Association.

Palliative care focuses on the relief of suffering when the underlying disease cannot be cured. In his article "The Nature of Suffering and the Goals of Medicine," Eric Cassel (1982) defined *suffering* as "a state of severe distress associated with events that threaten the intactness of the person"(p. 640). Suffering is broader than physical pain; it involves the whole person—body, mind, and spirit. Hospice care seeks to palliate or relieve the sources of physical, psychosocial, and spiritual distress. A local oncologist (Michael Messino, MD, personal communication, July 1995) concerned about the label "routine terminal care" applied to patients in the hospital has pointed out that there is nothing "routine" about terminal care. It involves active listening, careful assessment, skilled intervention, and constant reevaluation.

SYMPTOM MANAGEMENT

Physical symptoms vary with the kind of endstage disease affecting the patient. An estimated 75% of people with cancer experience pain at some time during their illness (U. S. Department of Health and Human Services, 1995). Other endstage conditions associated with pain include heart disease, AIDS, decubitus ulcers, and neuropathies. Besides pain, other physical symptoms may include the following:

neurological: seizures, paralysis, or changes in mental status such as lethargy, confusion, agitation, or hallucinations; sensory and perceptual changes may also occur

cardiovascular: edema, syncope, hemorrhage, or angina

respiratory: dyspnea, cough, or congestion

gastrointestinal: nausea, vomiting, anorexia and cachexia, constipation, diarrhea, or hiccup

genitourinary: incontinence, retention or dysuria

musculoskeletal: weakness and fatigue and pathologic fractures

skin and mucous membranes: pressure ulcers, ulcerative lesions, dry mouth, oral lesions and infections, or pruritus.

The hospice movement has made a major contribution in the area of pain relief. A holistic view of pain and its management includes attention to physical, emotional, social, and spiritual needs. Adequate availability and doses of analgesics, including narcotics, around-the-clock scheduling, and the use of co-analgesics and other nondrug interventions have made the control of pain an attainable goal.

Depression, anxiety, and sleep disorders may also be present and may reflect physical or emotional etiologies. Furthermore, unique psychosocial issues accompany terminal illness. Emotional responses such as denial, anger, sadness, acceptance, and hope may vary from day to day and may differ in the patient and family members.

PERSONAL, CULTURAL, AND LEGAL ISSUES FACED BY HOSPICE CARE PATIENTS AND FAMILIES

Hospice patients and their families face many issues. They experience and try to cope with multiple losses along the journey to the expected death. As their disease progresses, patients' lost time from work becomes permanent disability, perhaps resulting in little or no income. Consequently, chronic illness stresses family finances. Even if insurance is available, most insurance policies do not cover 100% of costs, and there may have been years of bills for medicines, physician services, surgery, diagnostic procedures, hospitalizations, and chemotherapy or radiation.

Losses may also include loss of support systems or the ability to carry out roles and outside activities. Actual and anticipated losses all result in a grieving process for the ill person and for the family. Isolation and loneliness can occur. People with AIDS may be estranged from family; also, a supportive family for the person with AIDS may be isolated from their support systems because of the stigma attached to the disease.

Coping skills may be limited in some patient/family systems and strained at some time or another during a terminal illness. Sexual and intimacy issues often are not addressed. For example, a 32-year-old married woman with terminal cervical cancer who was receiving fluids as well as pain medication intravenously and who had a gastric tube for abdominal decompression expressed her distress because her husband no longer would hold her. He was able to provide her complicated medical care but had difficulty talking with her about her dying and meeting her need to be touched and feel loved.

Finding meaning and purpose in the midst of suffering and loss are spiritual issues dying patients and their families face. Cultural issues are also important. Culture defines roles, expectations, behaviors, and attitudes toward illness and death. A sick or dying person's culture influences whether he or she will be comforted or isolated, accepted or rejected.

Patients in hospice care and their families must also confront and resolve legal issues early. Once in hospice care, they are encouraged to resolve power of attorney, wills, advanced directives, guardianship for dependents, and other related issues.

HOSPICE CARE: THE PROCESS

The needs of terminally ill people and their families require a holistic, integrated approach to care. The hospice care process begins with a referral, usually from the primary care physician. Initial contact may also be made by other healthcare professionals, patients themselves, family members, or clergy; the patient then obtains a physician referral before care is initiated.

A specially trained admissions nurse and social worker may make an initial visit to the hospital before discharge, if requested by the patient, but, in most circumstances, they visit the patient's residence. They explain the hospice program to the patient and family. If the patient elects to receive services, he or she signs consent forms and an initial assessment is conducted. To develop a care plan with a patient and family, it is important to have the patient and family tell the story of the illness and describe significant events in their life history. The nurse and social worker can then identify and begin to address physical, psychosocial, and spiritual needs.

Hospice services are available around the clock, 7 days a week. The specific services are decided on with the patient, family, primary care physician, and the interdisciplinary hospice team, which includes the nurse, medical director, social worker, and chaplain. Services that must be available are defined by licensure and and Medicare certification guidelines.

Intermittent nursing care is given by or under the supervision of a registered nurse. The nurse manages and supervises the care plan. During home visits, the nurse provides direct physical care, monitors the disease process, and assesses symptoms such as pain and dyspnea and the patient's response to medications and other nursing and medical interventions. The nurse provides instruction and emotional support, supervises the nursing assistant care, acts as liaison with the physician and other care providers, and communicates with other hospice team members. Physician services by the primary care physician or medical director include office visits, home visits, inpatient care, phone consultation, and participation in the interdisciplinary team process.

The social worker provides social services to the patient and family. He or she assists the patient and family to deal with issues of loss, current and future role changes, communication problems, financial needs, isolation, and legal and care-giving concerns. The social worker also provides assistance in coordinating resources and making referrals to other community agencies.

Chaplain services are provided as requested by patient or family. The chaplain is available to address spiritual concerns and act as a liaison with community clergy.

Other interdisciplinary team members offer services as well. Certified nursing assistants provide personal care. They assist with activities of daily living and help maintain a safe environment. They may also relieve the caregivers in some housekeeping tasks such as meal preparation, cleaning, and laundry. Volunteer services are provided as part of the care plan. Volunteers may run errands, provide transportation for an outing for the patient or a family member, and make visits to provide emotional support.

In addition, physical, occupational, and speech therapy services are provided to assist in maintaining mobility and performing activities of daily living for as long as possible. Medical supplies and durable medical equipment such as hospital beds, oxygen, and wheelchairs are also provided.

Nutritional counseling is an integral part of care. As most endstage diseases progress, patients experience expected anorexia and weight loss. Food is closely associated with love and caring, and family and social activities; food is about feelings, not just feedings. The quality of food eaten is often used by caregivers as a barometer of the patient's well being. Family members often voice concerns that the patient is starving while patients often report that they eat because they feel pressured by family. Teaching and emotional support are equally important as goals change from trying to maintain adequate nutritional intake to food and fluids for comfort.

Nutritional counseling is also an integral part of care. Initial counseling is designed to determine the patient's basic daily nutritional needs, adapt dietary intake to meet any limitations imposed by illness, incorporate the patient's personal food preferences, and assist the caregiver in preparing and serving the diet to meet the nutritional goals set for the patient. Recommendations may also include the best route for nutritional intake based on special patient circumstances. For example, a gastrostomy tube may be appropriate for a patient with esophageal cancer. Over the course of the illness, there will most likely be a need to modify consistency and amount and also to manipulate time intervals of dietary intake. Not only will the caregiver need to make these decisions with input from the interdisciplinary team, but he or she will need support and education about these changes.

During periods of crisis, a registered nurse, licensed practical nurse, or certified nursing assistant provides continuous home care. Appropriate laboratory and diagnostic services are given as ordered by the physician and needed to manage the patient's symptoms.

Short-term inpatient care is provided for symptom control, respite care, or terminal care (when death is imminent). Bereavement care includes supportive, educational, and counseling services for up to 24 months following the patient's death. Support groups are available for both children and adults as are telephone contacts, personal visits, individual counseling, and educational materials.

Although each discipline providing care has its area of expertise, assessment and interventions overlap. For example, team members from physician to volunteer carry out the interventions to control the various causes of pain. The chaplain is not the sole guardian of spiritual life. The certified nursing assistant may spend the most time in the home, perform the most personal care, and be privileged with special insight into the patient's physical, emotional, and spiritual concerns.

Throughout the care process, the patient is central in making decisions about his or her pain management. Judicious use of prescriptive and nonprescriptive drugs can greatly enhance the quality of life by providing relief from pain and other symptoms such as nausea, vomiting, and diarrhea. Analgesia includes not only drug therapy, but also nonpharmacologic strategies such as imagery, massage, therapeutic touch, music therapy, and meditation. The goal of therapy is to keep the patient comfortable, as defined by the patient, without overly clouding mental and cognitive function that would interfere with participation in life activities. Needless fears of addiction are frequently a concern to patients and families. Thus, teaching and facilitating expression of feelings about the use of medications are critical interventions if medications are to be used effectively.

ROLE OF THE ADVANCED PRACTICE FAMILY NURSE PRACTITIONER

The role of the advanced practice family NP in hospice care has been evolving over the past few years. Responsibilities include direct patient care, clinical consultation and collaborative care, and education. The hospice medical director or hospice physician supervises the NP's medical acts. For other responsibilities, the NP reports to the executive director.

Direct Patient Care

The NP completes histories and physicals and provides follow-up care for patients followed by the hospice medical director, usually the family physician in private practice. Hospice patients may reside in their home, an extended care facility, or a hospice inpatient facility. Both medical and nursing care are provided, with particular attention paid to symptom management and physical care. Counseling and instruction are also provided. Following consultation with the primary care or supervising physician, referrals are made if specialists are needed to assist in managing symptoms. On admission to the hospice program, many patients are seen by specialists, especially medical and radiation oncologists, gastroenterologists, and pulmonary physicians. Contact with consulting physicians and other healthcare providers is made to coordinate care following the interdisciplinary plan.

Clinical Consultation

The NP may evaluate those people who have been referred to the hospice program in any care setting to determine their appropriateness for hospice care. The practitioner may consult the medical director if there are concerns about the diagnosis, prognosis, or palliative care plans. The NP also makes visits, sometimes with other team members, to assist patients in managing symptoms and to ensure that all reasonable, necessary care is provided. The NP also provides hospice staff and primary physicians with current information on palliative care; assists in developing and evaluating policies and procedures, care plans, and care standards; and consults with nurses, physicians, social workers, chaplain, therapists, and certified nursing assistants regarding particular patient problems.

Collaborative Care

Working with other members of the hospice team, community physicians, their associated NPs and physician assistants, and other healthcare providers is an integral role of the hospice NP. Responsibilities include participating in weekly interdisciplinary team conferences during which new patients are presented and patient care plans are developed and reviewed, attending hospital patient care conferences as needed when hospice patients are admitted to the hospital, and communicating with the nurse managers for home care and with the inpatient unit regarding clinical care. Other responsibilities involve participating in the utilization review process with the medical director and other disciplines for patients in the hospice inpatient facility and serving on committees within the hospice organization as assigned by the executive director.

Education

The NP helps educate staff, community physicians, and other healthcare providers regarding quality palliative care. The practitioner reviews current literature and resources on palliative care, makes information available, and assists in the development of educational programs. The NP acts as a preceptor to medical students and family practice residents during site visits to the hospice inpatient facility or home services. Instruction is provided at team training and in-service programs on palliative care issues and for other hospice program staff and healthcare providers. The NP also identifies available resources for patient and family education. As a member of the hospice organization education committee, the nurse helps plan educational opportunities for all hospice disciplines, from physicians and nurses to volunteers.

Nurse practitioners working with hospice are responsible for using appropriate research findings to improve medical and nursing care for hospice patients and their families. In the future, there undoubtedly will be opportunities to participate in research studies on specific palliative care issues such as pain management.

CONCLUSION

Like most healthcare agencies, hospice programs are currently developing models to provide a mechanism for continuous quality improvement. Quality assurance programs have been inadequate to accurately determine care outcomes. They have traditionally involved chart audits to determine, for example, if all patients had an initial and ongoing pain assessment. However, the care outcome—pain relief—was not necessarily measured.

Studies have shown reimbursement for hospice, which emphasizes home care, to be a cost-effective alternative to costly, end-of-life hospital care (Mitchell, Hunter, Blackhurst, Strand, & Lee, 1994). Hospice care is covered under Medicare and under Medicaid in some states. In addition, hospice care is covered by an increasing number of private insurance companies. Military personnel and their dependents may be covered by the Civilian Health and Medical Program of the Uniformed Services or the Department of Veterans' Affairs. In some hospice programs, when skilled services are provided and no health insurance is available, a sliding scale fee is used to reflect the circumstances of each individual family. To the maximum extent possible, hospice will provide services based on need rather than ability to pay. Services may be reimbursed on a cost-per-visit or by a per-diem rate. With a per-diem rate, the program manages all aspects of the patient's care with a designated fee per day. The author's hospice is a nonprofit agency that receives additional funding from the United Way and from donations. Mechanisms are being pursued to reach underserved populations in the area through the development of a minority task force.

The advanced practice nurse in hospice has a unique role as part of the team providing care. Each day brings different responsibilities. Visits are made to patients in the hospital and inpatient unit to provide ongoing assessment and management of the care plan. Patients are seen at their residence (i.e., home or extended care facility) for follow-up or consultation about specific problems, either symptom management or caregiver and support system concerns. Patient/family conferences are also held. Time is spent attending weekly interdisciplinary team conferences and various committee meetings and providing consultation to other hospice team members: nurses, social workers, chaplain, and volunteers. Hospice care offers the opportunity and special privilege to be a midwife to dying people, to participate in the transition at the end of life's journey, and to help provide a safe passage. It is not all sadness and suffering; it can also be a place of joy and peace.

You matter because you are you.

You matter to the last moment of your life and we will do all we can not only to help you die peacefully, but to live until you die.

(Saunders, 1994)

Note: References are cited at end of chapter.

C

Rural Nurse Practitioner

Charlene M. Hanson

RURAL COMMUNITY

Since the 1960s, nurse practitioners (NPs) have been seen as viable primary care providers who could enhance access and quality of care to people living in isolated or underserved rural areas. There are many barriers to quality healthcare in rural settings that intensify the need for NP care. Nearly one in four rural citizens lives in poverty; lack of transportation to health services is a major factor for poor and elderly people; high-risk special populations are often aggregated in rural areas; and there is a severe lack of healthcare providers in rural communities. For many of these reasons, providing healthcare in the rural community offers the rural NP unique opportunities to care for clients within a broad practice environment with high potential for autonomy and job satisfaction. Although rural NP practice is demanding, it also allows for flexibility and innovation and gives the NP an excellent opportunity to care for a caseload of families and individuals as the primary provider of healthcare.

The focus on national healthcare reform has enhanced the role of advanced practice nurses (APNs) overall. As NPs enter their 30th year as primary care providers, the role has become more stable and recognized by the professional and lay public. The 1990s have been watershed years for both education and practice of all types of APNs in a myriad of settings. The use of NPs in rural communities has been of long duration. The trend toward community-based primary healthcare and away from hospital-based care has further identified the rural community as a major setting for NP practice.

The essence of rural health nursing, in general, is that rural nurses, and most specifically NPs, are generalists and need expert skills in physical assessment, clinical decision making, and in work with community resources. All levels of rural-based nurses need to have a well-grounded community and public health orientation. Nurse practitioners must be, first and foremost, excellent community health nurses who have added the additional skills necessary to provide primary care diagnosis and treatment, as well as sound preventive care to their repertoire. Preventing illness presents a particular challenge to the rural NP because health promotion programs are severely lacking in many rural areas. This is due in large part to the lack of funding in the current American healthcare system (Anderson & Youhos, 1993).

The ideal team of providers practicing in a variety of rural and frontier settings is the interdisciplinary primary care team comprising the physician, NP, midwife, social worker, and mental health provider; others may be added as necessary. Communities vary in the type of healthcare providers they can attract. For example, each community is unique with regard to lifestyle, spousal employment opportunities, schools, and churches. The rural community offers a unique blend of community leaders from various disciplines, resources, and population groups who set the tone for healthcare in that community. A physician in a particular county often serves as a referral physician for outreach teams working in adjoining rural counties. These factors lead to a positive component of rural healthcare practice that is evident in the close camaraderie between healthcare providers. Isolation and lack of support systems may bring health providers closer together, regardless of hierarchy and turf. The NP is often the mainstay of the healthcare team in outreach settings because of the broad generalist and community-based model within which nurses are educated. This background allows the NP to bridge gaps in care offered by other disciplines. Distance and transportation are the most crucial factors for receiving healthcare. For example, the availability of a rural hospital and or nursing home within the community typically is important to the elder population, the distance to obstetric and neonatal services is a concern of families planning to have children, the accessibility of adult day care or respite care may be important to families caring for members with chronic illnesses, and the distance to the local pharmacy cannot be discounted.

Rural healthcare is difficult to define because of the unique characteristics of individual rural communities. For example, the population mix, culture, and healthcare needs are vastly different in Mississippi than in the remote Rocky Mountains of Montana and Wyoming. It is critical that NPs planning to undertake a rural practice consider the importance of understanding the sociocultural factors that will lead to success or failure within the rural community. For example, in the rural Southwest, which has a large population of Hispanic people, bilingual NPs who can communicate well with the Hispanic population are helpful in facilitating the acceptance of NPs and the care they provide. In addition, NPs caring for Native Americans need a careful awareness of various tribal customs to build trust and appropriate communication. Nurse practitioners who are practicing in predominantly southern African-American communities need to understand and accept that population's healthcare beliefs and practices, especially among the elderly members of those communities.

Nurse practitioners need to fully immerse themselves into the culture of the rural setting in which they will be practicing to be able to understand health beliefs and values that differ from their own. Insight into the southern African-American healthcare belief system is a must in the rural South, just as the awareness of Native American customs is crucial for NPs who staff the clinics supported by the Indian Health Service. Nurse practitioners planning a career with a unique high-risk rural population find that knowledge and understanding of diverse cultures is one of the most useful attributes that they bring to their practice (Bigbee, 1993). Rural practice requires a willingness to live within the culture and mores of the community to gain the trust and confidence of the people who make their homes in the particular setting. It takes time for people in other cultures to accept care from someone who is different from them, but once this trust is established, it allows for an excellent level of healthcare delivery.

NEEDS ASSESSMENT

A community-based assessment that lays out the broad healthcare strengths and weaknesses of the community is invaluable. It is important to understand fully who makes decisions within the community. To whom does the community look for direction and guidance? How will you gain the trust of the population? What are the demographics of the area? For example, the predominant age group of the community greatly affects the mix of services needed. What is the percentage of elderly people in the community compared with that of adolescents? What are the special needs of the subgroups in the particular community? What is the literacy rate? Are their special diseases endemic to the region, such as the "stroke belt" of the rural Southeast where large numbers of rural elders suffer from coronary artery disease and hypertension? Is there a high rate of teenage pregnancy? Acquired immunodeficiency syndrome (AIDS)? Substance abuse? Mental illness? (Hanson, 1992.) Often, these community characteristics have been collected and analyzed; they typically are available at the rural court house or health department. Information about the rural setting is an important precursor to choosing a rural community for practice.

FOCUS OF CARE

The focus of care offered by an NP in a rural setting is most often primary care that is community based and generalist in nature. Family nurse practitioners (FNPs) are the most sought after nurse providers in rural settings because they are able to see families and individuals across the life span and interface with other provider team members to supply broad-based comprehensive healthcare. FNPs frequently care for high-risk populations who live and work in rural communities. They may care for mobile migrant farm workers who move with the seasons across the United States. The migrant care model varies from state to state so that the NP may be providing migrant care within the health department, in a rural community health clinic, or a mobile van that goes into the migrant camp to meet the workers.

Nurse practitioners may work in federally funded rural health clinics where they provide primary care to, for example, pregnant teenagers or to young adults who have contracted sexually transmitted diseases or AIDS. Rural AIDS patients are the fastest growing cohort of AIDS patients in the United States (Carwein et al, 1993). Rural NPs may practice in private practice settings, either as a satellite outreach clinic or as a member of a solo physician practice team. Table 19-1 is a partial listing of common practice settings in which NPs provide care.

In many states, NPs who work in county health departments are the mainstay of primary care delivery in rural communities. These nurses provide a continuity of preventive and primary cares services in addition to assisting families who need referrals to healthcare specialty services and support services.

COST/REIMBURSEMENT MECHANISMS

Healthcare providers who practice in rural and underserved areas often receive financial incentives for their rural practice. The federal government defines *rural* according to population density, geographic barriers, and access to healthcare providers.

At present, Medicare and Medicaid reimburses rural NPs more broadly than NPs who work in nonrural settings. Nurse practitioners working in clinics classified as rural are allowed by law to bill directly for their services. Legislation currently before Congress would remove the preferential "rural only" language; however, currently, rural APNs are able to bill more easily for their services. State merit system plans reimburse NPs who work within the state-driven public health system in some states. The numbers of other private insurers who reimburse NPs for rural practice vary from state to state and from plan to plan. Furthermore, spe-

---

TABLE 19-1   **Common Settings for Practice**

Migrant clinics	Rural health clinics
Nursing homes	Private practice
Ambulatory care centers	Community health clinics
Public health departments	Health maintenance organizations
School based clinics	Hospitals
Prisons	Wellness centers
Indian Health Service clinics	Home health clinics
Occupational health clinics	Mobile van clinics

cial initiatives that address the needs of rural high-risk populations fund salaries for NPs working with migrant farm workers, Indian Health Service projects, and for those NPs who care for rural teenagers who are pregnant or abusing alcohol or drugs. School-based and after-school clinics in rural communities staffed by NPs offer a variety of educational, diagnosis and management, and counseling services to high school students. The number of federally and privately funded healthcare projects that target high-risk populations is considerable.

The education of rural NPs is also the target of many state and federal funding initiatives. Data clearly show that healthcare workers who are recruited from their rural hometown are more likely to return and stay there to work (Fowkes, Gamel, Wilson, & Garcia, 1994; Hanson, 1991; Keller, Hosokawa, Bruce, Huntington, & Lassiter, 1985). These students are culturally "comfortable" returning to the rural setting. Schools of nursing may receive trainee-ship funds for rural-based students as well as money to develop or expand programs that are targeted to rural and underserved populations. These programs offer specialized curricula and study programs that offer a strong foundation in rural families and communities, cultural diversity, and generalist primary care concepts.

The National Health Service Core offers both a loan payback and scholarship program for APNs (i.e., NPs and nurse midwives) who agree to practice in an underserved area for at least 2 years of service. Many educational funding sources require payback to the community in terms of rural placement based on the dollars borrowed. In addition, an excellent resource for educational loans or scholarships is the rural community itself. Rural communities are well aware that supporting a local "landlocked" individual—someone who has ties to the community through family commitments—to return to school offers the best chance of recruitment and retention over time.

PRIMARY CARE

Rural NPs serve as generalist providers of primary care and interface closely with the subspecialist physicians to provide comprehensive care to individuals and families. The rural community is an optimal setting for NPs who want to provide basic healthcare, across a continuum of time, based on a firm foundation of prevention and wellness. The autonomy that is afforded by the isolation of rural practice makes it possible for rural NPs to implement holistic nursing and medical care regimes (Bigbee, 1993). Routine episodic care and chronic ambulatory care compose the largest portion of the NP's time in a rural practice. That a NP lives in a rural community increases the likelihood that the patient will return for follow-up care. Compliance is often contingent on the ability of the patient and the caregiver to interact outside of the clinic setting. Rural NPs have reported that interactions and chance meetings that occur in the grocery store or on the street give them a great deal of satisfaction and that this is an important dynamic for them to remain in their job. Within rural cultures, it takes time to build this type of trust in a relationship; unless the NP is a local, homegrown product, he or she will have to earn the "insider" status (Bigbee, 1993).

Public health clinics are often the mainstay of the rural community. The state government employs NPs to do the greater part of the healthcare for childbearing women and children in rural and underserved areas. High-risk teenage pregnancy and high infant mortality rates continue to plague the rural South, and certified nurse-midwives serve to care for these populations both in public and private rural settings. Together, with NPs, they offer the family planning, pregnancy, postpartum, and newborn care for rural poor and underserved women and their families.

The mental health clinical nurse specialist is sorely needed as a consultant to rural primary care providers. There is a dearth of mental health services in rural and frontier communities, even though the incidence of home violence and substance abuse is high. Currently, the generalist nature of rural NP care and the severe lack of mental health personnel in the small rural community place the burden of caring for the "walking wounded" patients who suffer from a wide range of mental and emotional health problems within the NP's domain. However, reimbursement mechanisms to fund mental health clinical nurse specialist care continues to be of paramount importance.

Rural NPs are often asked to follow stable, chronic patients of all types who need frequent monitoring of their treatment regimen. One example is that of cancer patients who are undergoing chemotherapy or radiation. These patients need daily support between visits to the oncologist. Nurse practitioners are also key members of teams who are caring for home-based hospice patients. Because of their keen abilities in coordinating care and services, they are able to interface extremely well with volunteer teams and family groups who are working through serious health problems. Assisting AIDS patients and their families in rural areas is increasingly becoming more difficult, and the rural NP is often the primary provider of counseling and monitoring services for patients with AIDS or AIDS-related complex.

ACUTE-CARE NURSE PRACTITIONERS AND OTHER ADVANCED PRACTICE NURSES IN RURAL SETTINGS

With the advent of healthcare reform and as one of the outcomes of diagnosis-related groups, rural hospitals are changing the way in which they offer services. There is a need to improve communication between the hospital and community. In addition, funding for resident physician house staff often does not extend to the rural hospital. Rural hospitals are finding it both cost-effective and quality-effective to use NPs in the role of house staff and to staff the emergency room. This role, if offered within a nursing model, allows nurses to direct both the hospital and discharge planning to include nursing problems and a comprehensive care plan for patient and family. Educational programs to prepare acute-care NPs are springing up around the country at a rapid rate.

Many rural hospital emergency departments are changing their focus away from sole emergency care to ambulatory care clinics with a wellness component to better meet the community's needs. Small emergency departments have transitioned into rural health clinics that offer a wide range of primary care and health maintenance services to the local community. Often support groups for abuse, mental health, or cardiac rehabilitation are a part of the hospital-based primary care clinic. In this type of rural practice setting, nurse practitioners need good skills in triage and the judgment to know when to care for the patient and when to provide emergency transportation to the closest larger hospital or trauma center. Some NPs are hired by the hospital to provide discharge planning and to collaborate with home health nurses and families.

Other APNs are often providing care within the rural setting and serve as colleagues and an excellent support system for the rural-based NP. For example, the certified registered nurse anesthetist is the backbone of surgery in the rural hospital. Overall, small rural hospitals would be unable to conduct surgery without the rural nurse anesthetist because few anesthesiologists practice in small rural hospitals. Rural nurse anesthetists contract their services to rural hospitals under the direction of the attending surgeon. Certified nurse-midwives are serving in birthing centers and teaming up with rural-based obstetricians to provide maternity care. The payment mechanisms for both rural certified registered nurse anesthetists and certified nurse-midwives can be either direct payment for services rendered or salary through the hospital or clinic in which they are employed.

TELECOMMUNICATIONS AND DISTANCE LEARNING

One of the most exciting expansions of telecommunications in rural healthcare is the ability of the isolated rural community to interact with members of the nearest university. With the advent of personal computers, modems, and interactive television, it is possible to provide excellent two-way communication between rural-based NPs and precepting physicians, university-based researchers, and academicians. It is now possible for health researchers to form teams with other researchers in isolated areas to carry out projects without face-to-face interaction.

It is also possible to include rural nurses in distant continuing education offerings by up-links to urban programs. Cohorts of students who live in small rural towns can access direct classroom experiences by interactive television. The system allows students to see the teacher and distant classmates and to dialogue with them during class. Visuals are transmitted by television screen and written materials are sent by fax. Students in the field who are carrying out distant preceptorships can interact with faculty through personal computers fitted with modems on the Internet. It is possible for students to transmit clinical logs and assignments and for faculty to respond within a designated time frame. These communications tools allow students to access clinical training in rural sites distant from the university.

NURSE PRACTITIONER AS COMMUNITY LEADER

One of the most positive aspects of practicing in a rural community is the respect that the NP receives from other professionals, community leaders, and patients. Small communities allow for an unusual continuity of care that occurs both professionally and informally, for example, in the church or in the park. Social interaction with long-term patients and their families offers another dimension to the healthcare offered. Continuity of care is facilitated and long-term relationships allow for exceptionally high-quality primary care. Nurse practitioners are perceived as knowledgeable teachers and counselors as well as rural community leaders. In addition, they are sought for directing educational experiences centered around health and wellness and primary prevention for serious illness.

 ### CASE VIGNETTES

Vignette 1: Family Nurse Practitioner Who Cares for a Rural Grandmother

I have lived in rural Mississippi all of my life. I was born and grew up in the town in which I now practice as an FNP. After working at the local public health department as a community health nurse for 5 years, I returned to school to earn a master's degree in nursing and to become nationally certified as an FNP. I currently am employed in the district healthcare system and "ride the circuit" from county to county to conduct hypertension and diabetes clinics in the six county health departments in my health district. I work in collaboration with local physicians and care for poor and elderly people who have poor access to healthcare for their chronic illnesses.

One of my patients is O, a 68-year-old African-American grandmother with poorly controlled hypertension and non–insulin-dependent diabetes (type II diabetes mellitus), which is now controlled by insulin. O also has trouble with her "arthritis" and doesn't see "as well as she used to." She keeps her appointments at the health department twice a month where she is followed by me, her FNP healthcare provider.

On O's initial visit to the NP-run clinic, and once annually thereafter, I perform a complete physical examination including pelvic examination and pap smear, breast examination with return demonstration for teaching, stool for occult blood screen, and a hypertensive blood panel including blood sugars and urine creatinine. I also check to ensure that O is up to date with her immunizations and offer her influenza and pneumococcal vaccine during the winter months.

On a biweekly basis, I do a modified physical examination in which I check blood pressure, blood glucose, peripheral pulses, and liver, auscultate heart and lung sounds, and perform an ophthalmoscopic examination. O has had one episode of congestive heart failure for which she needed hospitalization, so I carefully evaluate her for subtle cardiovascular changes, such as tachycardia, that might be clues to impending cardiac decompensation. I also monitor O's blood and urine sugars and counsel her about her diet, trying to adapt the 1600-calorie American Dietetic Association diet (Rakel, 1994) to the foods that O has access to in town. O does not drive and relies on her daughter to shop for her in the rural community.

O is scheduled for biweekly visits to give her the support she needs to monitor her chronic illnesses. She knows that she could replace insulin injections with oral hypoglycemic agents if she could maintain her weight within normal limits. She needs encouragement in terms of dietary choices, getting enough exercise, and taking her medications faithfully.

I help O to make an appointment with an ophthalmologist who offers care to indigent patients and tell her about the Lions Club program that will help her to obtain new eyeglasses. I also make plans for O to see the visiting podiatrist to have the calluses on her feet treated and to have him work with her about trimming her toenails. I help O fill out the paperwork so that she can get the refund for elderly customers on her heat and electric bills; we also complete the forms that will allow her to get county food supplements of cheese and rice and milk products. O and I discuss the need for her to join a group of older women who meet before church services two nights a week to walk in the local park for exercise and meet for social support. I work out arrangements for O to get a ride to the clinic with two other patients who live near her on the same rural road.

At each visit, I review the medications that O has been instructed to bring with her. Then, I refill them from the prepackaged state system supply that the pharmacist has left for these patients. I have ordered these prescriptions through a collaborative system that has been worked out with local physicians, using medications that are within the state formulary.

Usually, O brings two "grands" (i.e., grandchildren) for whom she cares when she comes to clinic. She tells me that she gets plenty of exercise chasing after them most days. I also review health department records on the two preschoolers and monitor their well-child exams and check to see that they receive their immunizations on time. Last week, the younger child had an otitis media infection that I treated. I am seeing the child with the grandmother in follow-up today and will send home instructions for O's daughter to follow to prevent another ear infection.

Over the years, my relationship with O has been fostered by the warmth of living within the small rural community, close to my patients. I have developed a trusting relationship with O that has grown over the several years we have worked and lived close together. I have helped to keep O's health in stable condition and have enabled O to live at home in her later years.

Vignette 2: The Nurse Practitioner Who Provides Care in a Rural After-School Clinic

Another NP who lives and works in the same rural community is employed by the county board of education to conduct weekly after-school health clinics for teenagers who are using contraception and for pregnant teenagers. The school system has rented two rooms in the senior citizens building, which is down the street from the high school, to hold the clinic. The waiting room has an abundance of literature and videotapes that help the students to better understand their sexuality and associated concerns about pregnancy, contraception, and sexually transmitted diseases. Clinic hours are scheduled for the students' convenience, and students are encouraged to bring their friends to the clinic for support.

Adolescent girls receive a full physical examination with pap smear, breast exam, and screening blood work on admission to the clinic. This assessment includes time for teaching self–breast exam and for clients to ask questions and learn about their changing bodies. Screening for sexually transmitted diseases and AIDS is offered on a routine basis, as necessary. Pregnant teenagers are jointly followed by the NP and the visiting obstetrician, who attends clinic once a month to assist with complex problems. The physician preceptor reviews the NP's records, and both the physician preceptor and NP make plans with clients for delivery in the hospital. Prenatal classes are held weekly during the evening and offer a further opportunity for interaction with significant others and labor coaches. Counseling is available with or without an appointment. Students are encouraged to include their parents in their care, and special parent–daughter support groups have been a popular component of the clinic. The NP finds this rural clinic a rewarding place to work and has developed excellent rapport with both students and teachers in this setting.

Note: References are cited at end of chapter.

D

Federal Healthcare Nurse Practitioner

Patricia C. Murphy

I felt as if I was signing my life away. I signed papers stating that I assumed responsibility for a helmet, flak jacket, sleeping bag, metal pan, eating utensils, first aid kit, canteen, air crew chemical warfare bag, and gas mask. My destination was classified but the bottle of sunscreen gave it away. The last item was a .38 revolver. Reality hit hard. (Glendon, 1993)

This Air Force nurse practitioner (NP) survived 26 SCUD missile attacks in Operation Desert Storm in 1991. She is one of thousands of NPs in federal service.

Federal NPs include those commissioned in the Army, Navy, and Air Force. As commissioned officers in the U.S. Public Health Service (PHS), NPs may be assigned to the Indian Health Service, U.S. Coast Guard, Immigration and Naturalization Service, National Oceanic and Atmospheric Administration, Federal Bureau of Prisons, National Health Service Corps, and other government agencies. Furthermore, they may be employed by the Department of Veterans' Affairs and the State Department.

The origins of federal nursing can be traced to the Revolutionary War. In the past 200 years, from the Revolutionary War to Operation Desert Storm, more than 2 million women have served in the Armed Forces; until recently, most of these trailblazers were nurses (Vaught, 1994). This wartime history of federal nurses is recounted in striking detail by Vaught. More than 1500 nurses served in the Spanish-American War and their presence led to the formation of the Army Nurse Corps in 1901 and the Navy Nurse Corps in 1908. During World War I, 23,000 Army and Navy nurses "served in field, mobile, evacuation, base, and convalescent hospitals, as well as on troop trains and transport ships" (Vaught, 1994, p. 89). Military nurses in World War II, joined by other military women, made up a volunteer force of more 400,000.

Military nurses were never spared the dangers of wartime. When the Japanese invaded the Philippines, 77 nurses became prisoners of war. Days after the Korean conflict began in 1950, nurses were on duty close to the war zone and at significant risk for injury and death. In 1969, while evacuating Vietnamese orphans from Saigon, Air Force nurse Captain Mary Klinker was killed when her C-5A Galaxy strategic transport aircraft crashed during takeoff (Holm, 1982). Likewise, in Vietnam, Navy nurses were in the path of enemy fire and became the first women recipients of the Purple Heart when they were injured by a by a Vietcong terrorist bombing. Army nurse, First Lieutenant Sharon A. Lane, was killed in 1969 by a rocket attack on her hospital in Chu Lai and is among eight women whose names are inscribed on the Vietnam veterans' memorial in Washington, DC (Vaught, 1994).

The role and presence of military NPs must be understood in the context of the military healthcare system, which is the largest, single healthcare organization in the world. Annually, the U.S. military cares for more than 10 million people with a budget of more than $15 billion. Each year, in more than 500 hospitals and 900 ambulatory care facilities (Lanier, 1993), 1 million patients are admitted and 50 million receive outpatient services (Legters & Llewellyn, 1992). The "mission" of military medicine in peacetime is to ensure the optimal health and medical readiness of the active duty population. Providing medical care for military families as well as for retirees and their families is of secondary importance. During wartime, the medical focus moves to the immediate care of injured and ill military personnel and their rapid return to duty, if feasible. The prevention of injury and disease is a daily goal.

Active duty personnel make up 30% of those eligible for healthcare in the military system; the remaining 70% of beneficiaries are families of active duty, retirees, and their families. Military healthcare resources (the number and type of medical personnel, facilities, and training programs) are based on the number of active duty military—only 30% of the population served. In 1992, there were 170,000 active duty medical staff, including doctors, nurses, NPs, physician's assistants, technicians, and other healthcare professionals (Legters & Llewellyn, 1992). For healthcare providers, this chronic shortage of personnel and resources contributes to ongoing frustration and pressure to "do more with less."

In the event of war, it is projected that active duty medical forces would need to be augmented as much as 60% by military reserve members (Legters & Llewellyn, 1992). The more than 200,000 civilian professionals in the medical reserve arm of the military train regularly for their contingency roles in wartime.

UNIFORMED NURSE PRACTITIONERS

The history and development of NPs in the uniformed services parallels that of the civilian world. The physician shortage in the military resulting from the end of the draft and poor recruitment in concert with an increasingly skilled, independent nurse corps established both the need and the role for NPs.

In the early 1970s, the military began its own training programs for NPs, sometimes in conjunction with civilian academic programs. These 6-month long programs provided a certificate to practice as an NP. As master's preparation became increasingly vital for professional practice, the certificate programs were eliminated and replaced with graduate education at civilian universities. In 1993, the Uniformed Services University of Health Sciences in Bethesda, MD, began its own master's program for family NPs. This graduate program is available to nurses in the Army, Navy, Air Force, and PHS.

Like other healthcare systems, the military recognizes that NPs provide competent, compassionate, cost-effective, accessible medical care, with high levels of patient satisfaction as well (Brodie, Bancroft, Rowell, & Wolf, 1982; Goldberg, Jolly, Hosek, & Chu, 1981; Nice & Hamilton, 1990; Selby & Gonzales, 1978). From their inception, uniformed NPs have functioned with autonomy, including prescriptive authority, and respect. Unlike other healthcare systems, there is no basis for conflict between physicians and NPs in the military for economic reasons. Physicians have generally welcomed, although sometimes merely adjusted to, their NP colleagues.

Uniformed NPs, like their civilian peers, see a multitude of patients of all ages and maladies. They, too, manage heavy caseloads, working through lunch and staying late to complete charts. They are required to be nationally certified and credentialed and may work in hospitals or ambulatory care settings. They teach patients, staff, NP students, and residents. They are members of state and national nursing organizations and conduct research as well as publish. They are parents and community volunteers. Like their civilian counterparts, military NPs are entrepreneurs who establish wellness clinics and health promotion programs (Schafer et al., 1990). They develop novel approaches to healthcare aboard Navy ships with mixed-gender crews. They carve out creative roles within a regimented military environment.

Unlike their civilian counterparts, military NPs accept orders to remote duty stations, foreign countries, ships, humanitarian missions, and war. Moves are frequent—as often as every year. Assignments may be in the United States or overseas, in Cuba or Korea, in Sasebo or Sardinia, in Alaska or Iceland, and on land or at sea. Nurse practitioners may be separated from their family members during deployments. Children and spouses are uprooted unexpectedly. The personal and financial stresses are evident. Their sacrifices are relatively unknown and unspoken.

Uniformed NPs are often called on to participate in humanitarian medical missions. In 1975, after the fall of South Vietnam, NPs worked in refugee camps in Guam and California, caring for populations of up to 30,000 Vietnamese . In 1987, two Navy and one Air Force NP deployed on the *Mercy*, the Navy's newest 1000-bed hospital ship, spent 6 months in the Philippines and South Pacific island nations providing medical and surgical care to the poorest of the poor populations. Nurse practitioners were assigned to Guantánamo Bay, Cuba, in 1991 to care for the influx of Haitian refugees, with 12,500 people encamped at one time (Lukasik, 1993). Although rarely publicized, military medical professionals often aid medically indigent people or disaster victims throughout the world. From their beginnings, military NPs have been part of these humanitarian ventures.

For military nurses, wartime duties take precedence over all. The U.S. military NPs in Southwest Asia were the first NPs to serve in wartime. Many ashore recall being blasted from sleep several times nightly by sirens heralding impending missile attacks, donning head-to-toe protection from nuclear, chemical, and biologic weapons, and then seeking shelter in bunkers. A more recent example is that of a Navy NP, who, having received orders to Fleet Hospital 5 in Jubail during the Gulf War, left her 6-month-old daughter in the care of her active duty husband. She boarded a military transport plane and celebrated her birthday by learning how to don a gas mask on the flight to Saudi Arabia.

It is true that many NPs labor under difficult conditions. Few, however, find themselves working in temperatures of more than 120°F, filling sandbags to deflect incoming projectiles, sharing a tent with 13 women with only 12 inches between cots, and anticipating missile attacks and an onslaught of wounded and dead people (Glendon, 1993). Army, Navy, and Air Force active duty and reserve nurses and practitioners ashore and at sea shared similar trials during the Gulf War.

> BOOM! BOOM! BOOM! The noise was incredibly loud and I thought I was going to die. I said a prayer and thought—this is it. Out of the corner of my eyes I could see flashing lights. I couldn't believe the SCUDs were landing as close as they were. ALARM BLACK. This meant contamination was expected from nuclear, biologic, or chemical agent. (Glendon, 1993, p. 247)

Even the NP's predecessor in military nursing, Florence Nightingale, who took care of Crimean War casualties did not face quite the same terrors.

Army, Navy, and Air Force NPs are the vanguard of military nursing. Juggling their roles as military officers as well as NPs is an incredible challenge accepted by those who choose this profession. As of 1994, more than 550 active duty Army, Navy, and Air Force NPs were in specialties such as family practice, adult health, pediatrics, obstetrics/gynecology, psychiatry, and community health.

U.S. Public Health Service

In 1798, when the Marine Hospital Services cared for merchant mariners, the Public Health Service was born. A commissioned corps was established in 1889; in 1912, it was named the U.S. Public Health Service (PHS). Among the numerous officers in the PHS, "perhaps one of the most important—and least heralded—of these are the primary care professionals" (U.S. Department of Health and Human Services, 1988, p. 1).

The goal of the PHS, the major health agency of the U.S. government, is "to improve the health of our Nation's people" (U.S. Department of Health and Human Services, 1988, p. 1). The PHS is part of the U.S. Department of Health and Human Services and is under the authority of the assistant secretary of health. The Agency for Health Care Policy and Research, Agency for Toxic Substances and Disease Registry, Centers for Disease Control, Food and Drug Administration, Indian Health Service, Health Resources and Services Administration, and National Institutes of Health, and Substance Abuse and Mental Health Services Administration are all part of the PHS. The PHS employs a sizable number of NPs in a variety of its organizations.

Indian Health Service

Since the late 1700s, the U.S. government has participated in the care of Native Americans and Alaska Natives. The Indian Health Service became the newest agency of the U.S. Department of Health and Human Services in 1988. The goal of the Indian Health Service is to "ensure the equity, availability, and accessibility of a comprehensive, high-quality health care system for American Indians and Alaskan Natives" (Indian Health Service, 1993, p. 1). Working alongside tribal communities, the Indian Health Service attempts to assist with the identified needs and priorities in community healthcare.

Nurse practitioners work for the Indian Health Service as commissioned PHS officers as well as federal employees. In more than 50 hospitals, 139 health centers, and 305 clinics managed by the Indian Health Service and tribal groups, more than 1 million Alaska Natives and Native Americans receive comprehensive medical services (Indian Health Service, 1993).

Issues of particular medical concern for these peoples include unsafe water supplies and sanitation, inadequate nutrition, poor dental health, alcoholism, diabetes, accidents, and family violence. As increased medical care has become available in these communities, the infant mortality rate and infectious disease prevalence have clearly been reduced (Indian Health Service, 1993).

U.S. Coast Guard

Nurse practitioners from the PHS contribute to the healthcare of more than 150,000 active duty and retired U.S. Coast Guard personnel and their families as well as the patients they rescue. Healthcare occurs in 31 shore medical facilities located on the East, West, and Gulf coasts as well as Alaska, Hawaii, and Puerto Rico (PHS, 1994).

Immigration and Naturalization Service

The Immigration and Naturalization Service, an agency of the U.S. Department of Justice, "enforces the law regulating the admission of foreign-born persons to the United States" (PHS, 1994, p. 32). Each year, this enforcement involves temporarily confining more than 200,000 people who often require medical services. Nurse practitioners from the PHS provide ambulatory care, medical screening, acute care, health education, and referral services to detainees when necessary. Additional duties for NPs and nurses may include evaluating patients before flights as well as managing inflight medical concerns when people are returned to their countries of origin (PHS, 1994).

National Oceanic and Atmospheric Administration

The largest agency in the U.S. Department of Commerce, the National Oceanic and Atmospheric Association, was established in 1970. The responsibilities of this agency are myriad. They include forecasting the weather and climate, compiling nautical and aeronautical charts, surveying coastlines and adjacent waters, observing and documenting the effects of marine pollution, and protecting certain endangered marine species (U.S. Department of Commerce, 1992).

Again, the PHS assigns medical personnel, including NPs, to take care of the more than 400 scientists and their families as well as other seagoing personnel. Nurse practitioners serve on research vessels, with a physician available only by radio contact. National Oceanic and Atmospheric Administration ships and crews may deploy for as long as 7 months in vessels as large as 300 feet with crews of 100. Shipboard assignments may be temporary or permanent, ranging from weeks to 2 years; NP assignments are generally 2 years. Officers may spend 180 days to 250 days a year at sea (U.S. Department of Commerce, 1992) and research deployments may take crews from Seattle to Honolulu, Tahiti, Chile, and Antarctica.

Federal Bureau of Prisons

Nurse practitioners in the PHS may work in the Federal Bureau of Prisons health service. Although the Federal Bureau of Prisons is part of the U.S. Department of Justice, the PHS assigns medical support personnel to some prison facilities. Nurse practitioners may be employed in infirmaries as well as hospitals from coast to coast in both rural and urban settings. One example of a prison medical center is a medical and psychiatric referral center for approximately 1800 female inmates in Lexington, KY. In addition to the usual medical services, that center also offers obstetric and gynecologic care (U.S. Department of Justice, 1994).

Health concerns of particular significance for federal prison populations and their healthcare providers include acquired immunodeficiency syndrome, substance abuse, infectious disease, wellness, and geriatric care. Although, at first glance, employment in prison healthcare may seem dangerous, it is likely that these facilities are "safer than many city hospitals" (U.S. Department of Justice, 1994).

National Health Service Corps

The National Health Service Corps was established in 1970 with the passage of the Emergency Health Personnel Act. The Corps places healthcare providers in areas where there are critical shortages of medical resources "for those whose access to primary care has been limited by socioeconomic, geographic, language, and cultural factors" (Trible, 1993, p. 264). As of 1993, at least 38 million people resided in more than 2200 sites designated primary care shortage areas. More than 16,500 healthcare providers, including NPs, have worked in shortage areas since 1973. In 1990, the National Health Service Corps Revitalization Amendment was passed, allowing for continued federal financial support until the year 2000 (Trible, 1993).

An NP in the National Health Service Corps may work in Appalachia caring for women who otherwise would have to travel more than 100 miles for prenatal care. Migrant or seasonal farm workers and their families may receive care from a Corps NP. An inner-city clinic frequented by an elderly, poor population may have an NP on staff (Trible, 1993). The PHS clearly uses NPs in exceedingly creative, independent, and varied roles.

The National Health Service Corps has various enticements to service. Scholarship and stipends are available for nurse practitioners in exchange for a minimum of 2 years of work after graduation. Federal and state loans are reduced while working for the Corps. Community scholarship programs are available to those people who wish to return to their underserved communities of origin. Since the early 1970s, scholarship programs have trained more than 10,800 healthcare providers, including nurse practitioners. The Corps plans to hire more than 4400 primary care providers by the turn of the century (Trible, 1993).

Veterans' Administration

The Department of Veterans' Affairs (DVA) medical system is responsible for the healthcare of men and women who have been in the Armed Services and who have sustained a service-connected injury or illness, as well as veterans who are medically indigent (i.e., have an income of less than $19,000 per year). Nurse practitioners are part of this "largest centrally managed health care delivery system" (Cramer, 1994, p. 6). More than 170 medical centers, 300 clinics, and 130 nursing home units managed by the DVA employ 35,000 nurses. Among those nurses, 760 are nurse practitioners.

In addition to taking care of veterans, the DVA medical facilities and staff provide primary medical backup to the Department of Defense during wartime or national emergency (Cramer, 1994). Of recent interest is the rapid increase in women veterans. The DVA is expanding services to these women; services now include cervical and breast cancer screening, contraceptive counseling, education, and evaluation of gynecologic concerns ("Women's Health, Other Benefits Subject of Vets Bills," 1993).

The mission of the DVA is formidable. One can imagine that the DVA, as "any chronically under-funded system serving a disproportionately impoverished, elderly, and ailing population, will have its flaws" (Cramer, 1994, p. 6). The diversity of inpatient and ambulatory care roles makes the DVA an attractive place of employment for nurse practitioners.

State Department/Foreign Service

"Getting ill in a primitive place is a frightening and potentially dangerous experience" (Noyer, 1989, p. 12). The approximately 45 nurse practitioners working in the Foreign Service for the State Department know this well. For example, one nurse practitioner in Khartoum, Sudan, was the sole caretaker for 350 American Embassy personnel and their families. The "100 degree plus temperatures, . . . contaminated water, and disease carrying insects can have catastrophic effects on health. . . . Diarrhea may be dysentery and febrile seizures may signal malaria" (Noyer, 1989, p. 11).

The evening of her first day of work in Khartoum, the nurse practitioner found herself paged back to the embassy for an emergency. She recounted the emergency as follows:

> Terrorists bombed a hotel frequented by British nationals . . . seven people had been killed in the explosion with 15 wounded . . . casualties were brought to our health unit that was turned into a mini-emergency room as local doctors and 2 British nurses assisted in bandaging the wounded, administering antibiotics and assessing the extent of injuries. (Noyer, 1989, p. 10)

Since 1978, Foreign Service nurse practitioners have worked for the State Department in one of 256 posts throughout the world "providing primary medical care, evaluating the local health care facilities, advising management of significant health problems in the area, establishing and conducting preventive health classes, recommending and effecting medical evacuation of seriously injured or ill patients" (U.S. State Department, 1993, p. i). Embassy posts are located in Europe, Africa, North and South America, Asia, and the Near and Far East in such cities as Paris; Tokyo; Abidjan (Ivory Coast); Yaoundé (Cameroon); Managua (Nicaragua); Quito (Ecuador); Kuwait City; and Ankara (Turkey).

Only a quarter of the nurse practitioners work with a Foreign Service medical officer. The majority have assignments independent of physicians, and all are on duty 24 hours a day. Foreign Service nurse practitioners spend almost 60% of their careers abroad and the remainder of their time in the Washington, DC, area. Initial tours are for 2 years, with reassignment to new posts every 2 years to 4 years (U.S. State Department, 1993). Nurse practitioners looking for independence and excitement will certainly find it in the Foreign Service.

NURSE PRACTITIONERS IN CIVIL SERVICE/OTHER GOVERNMENT SERVICE

A multitude of federal nurse practitioners work in agencies other than the uniformed services, DVA, or Foreign Service. The greatest number of nurse practitioners working for the U.S. Department of Health and Human Services as well as the Army, Navy, Air Force, and National Health Service Corps are civilians in government service. Hired by the federal government, these nurse practitioners may work in military treatment facilities, Indian Health Service sites, National Health Service Corps underserved areas, federal prisons, or other government agencies. Civil service nurse practitioners even work in some overseas positions.

One family nurse practitioner in civil service who worked at Portsmouth Naval Hospital in Virginia, for example, took care of patients in the endocrine clinic. She was also the diabetic educator for the hospital and clinic. Although she has worked in the civil service system for 14 years, she also has worked as a nurse practitioner in other military clinics in the Tidewater area of Virginia. Autonomy, prescriptive authority, job security, salary, and retirement benefits may attract nurse practitioners to civil service employment.

The federal nurse practitioner community is rich with uniformed and nonuniformed colleagues. Truly, the lives of nurses and nurse practitioners who serve and have served in the Army, Navy, and Air Force are "stories of courage, dedication, sacrifice, and valor that are part of the fabric of the nation's history" (Vaught, 1994, p. 87). Similarly, nurse practitioners in civil service in the PHS, DVA, Foreign Service, and other government agencies have careers of remarkable challenge, complexity, and service that "involve uncommon commitments and occasional hardships, as well as unique rewards and opportunities" (U.S. State Department, 1993, p. 30).

References

Anderson, J., & Youhos, R. (1993). Health promotion in rural settings: A nursing challenge. *Nursing Clinics of North America, 28*(1), 145–153.

Bigbee, J. L. (1993). The uniqueness of rural nursing. *Nursing Clinics of North America, 28*(1), 131–143.

Brodie, B., Bancroft, B., Rowell, P., & Wolf, W. (1982). A comparison of nurse practitioner and physician costs in a military out-patient facility. *Military Medicine, 147,* 1051–1053.

Buttery, C. M. (1992). Provision of public health services. In J. M. Last & R. B. Wallace (Eds.), *Maxcy-Rosenau-Last public health and preventive medicine* (pp. 1113–1128). Norwalk, CT: Appleton & Lange.

Bylock, I. R. (1994, January 17). Kevorkian: Right problem, wrong solution. *Washington Post*, p. A23.

Carwein, V. L., Sabo, C. E., & Berry, D. E. (1993). HIV infection in traditional rural communities. *Nursing Clinics of North America, 28*(1), 231–238.

Cassel, E. J. (1982). The nature of suffering and the goals of medicine. *New England Journal of Medicine, 306,* 639–701.

Cramer, G. R. (1994). How secure is VA health care? *VFW Magazine, 81*(5), 6.

Doyle, D., Hanks, G., & MacDonald, N. (Eds.). (1993). *Oxford textbook of palliative medicine.* NY: Oxford University Press.

Edmunds, M. W., & Ruth, M. V. (1991). NPs who replace physicians: Role expansion or exploitation? *Nurse Practitioner, 16*(9), 46–49.

Fowkes, V. K., Gamel, N. N., Wilson, S. R., & Garcia, R. D. (1994). *Effectiveness of educational strategies preparing physician assistants, nurse practitioners, and certified nurse-midwives for underserved areas.* (Vol. 109, No. 5), 673–682.

Gates, S. J. (1993). Continuity of care: The orthopaedic nurse practitioner in tertiary care. *Orthopaedic Nursing, 12*(5), 48–51.

Glendon, M. T. (1993). Point of view. Saudi, SCUDS, and survival. *Journal of the American Academy of Nurse Practitioners, 5*(6), 245–248.

Goldberg, G. A., Jolly, D. M., Hosek, S., & Chu, D. S. (1981). Physician's extenders' performance in Air Force clinics. *Medical Care, 19*(9), 951–965.

Griffith, H. M., & Robinson, K. R. (1991). Survey of the degree to which critical care nurses are performing current procedural terminology-coded services. *American Journal of Critical Care, 1,* 91–98.

Hanson, C. M. (1991). The 1990's and beyond: Determining the need for community health and primary care nurses for rural populations. *Journal of Rural Health, 7*(Suppl. no. 1), 413–426.

Hanson, C. M. (1992). Care of clients in the rural setting. In M. J. Clark (Ed.), *Nursing in the community* (2nd ed., pp. 676–696). Norwalk, CT: Appleton & Lange.

Holm, J. (1982). *Women in the military.* Novato, CA: Presidio Press.

Iazzetti, L. (1992). Extended role allows growth, creativity for NPs [Letter to the editor]. *Clinical Nurse Specialist, 17*(3), 15.

Indian Health Service. (1993). *Professional opportunities for nurses in the Indian Health Service.* (Available from Indian Health Service, Nursing 6A-44, Rockville, MD 20857)

Keane, A., & Richmond, T. S. (1993). Tertiary nurse practitioners. *Image: The Journal of Nursing Scholarship, 25,* 281–284.

Keane, A., Richmond, T., & Kaiser, L. (1994). Critical care nurse practitioners: Evolution of the advanced practice nursing role. *American Journal of Critical Care, 3*(3), 232–237.

Keller, P. A., Hosokawa, M. C., Bruce, T. A., Huntington, C. G., & Lassiter, P. G. (1985). Rural practice: How do we prepare providers? *The Journal of Rural Health, 1*(1), 13–27.

Lanier, J. O. (1993). Restructuring military health care: The winds of change blow stronger. *Hospital and Health Services Administration, 38*(1), 121–132.

Legters, L. J., & Llewellyn, C. H. (1992). Military medicine. In J. M. Last & R. B. Wallace (Eds.), *Maxcy-Rosenau-Last public health and preventive medicine* (pp. 1141–1157). Norwalk, CT: Appleton & Lange.

Lukasik, S. D. (1993). *Nurse practitioners in the United States Navy: A historical perspective.* Unpublished master's thesis, University of Washington, Seattle.

McFadden, E. A., & Miller, M. A. (1994). Clinical nurse specialist practice: Facilitators and barriers. *Clinical Nurse Specialist, 8*(1), 27–33.

Mitchell, A., Hunter, D., Blackhurst, D., Strand, D. and Lee, B. (1994). Hospice care: The cheaper alternative. *JAMA, 271*(20), 1576–1577.

Naylor, M., Brooten, D., Jones, R., Lavizzo-Mourey, L., Mezey, M., & Pauley, M. (1994). Comprehensive discharge planning for the hospitalized elderly: A randomized clinical trial. *Annals of Internal Medicine, 120*(12), 999–1006.

Nice, D. S., & Hamilton, S. M. (1990). Determinants of the delegation of health care aboard ships with women assigned. *Military Medicine, 155,* 546–548.

Noyer, B. (1989, Winter). Medical services: You can count on Carol Dorsey, Jeannene Cramer—they're among the new breed of Foreign Service nurse practitioners. *State Magazine,* 10–12.

Rakel, R. E. (Ed.). (1994). *Conn's current therapy.* Philadelphia, PA: W. B. Saunders.

Richmond, T. S., & Keane, A. (1992). The nurse practitioner in tertiary care. *Journal of Nursing Administration, 22,* 11–12.

Selby, M., & Gonzales, J. M. (1978). The pediatric nurse practitioner in the Army health care system: A description of three roles. *Pediatric Nursing,* July/August, 20–25.

Schafer, D. D., Vanlandingham, D. A., Millington, P. A., Fry, J. G., Herterich, D. K., & Stephens, V. G. (1990). A nurses' wellness clinic. *Navy Medicine,* 12–13.

Snyder, J. V., Sirio, C. A., Angus, D. C., Hravnak, M. T., Kobert, S. N., Sinz, E. J., & Rudy, E. B. (1994). Trial of nurse practitioners in intensive care. *New Horizons, 2,* 296–304.

Story, P. (1994). *Primer of palliative care.* Gainesville, FL: Academy of Hospice Physicians.

Trible, L. (1993). National Health Service Corps needs more than 8000 health professionals. *Public Health Reports, 108*(2), 264–265.

U.S. Department of Commerce, U.S. Public Health Service. (1992). *Opportunities in the National Oceanic and Atmospheric Administration.* (Available from National Oceanic and Atmospheric Administration, Rockville, MD 20852)

U.S. Department of Health and Human Services. (1988). *Public Health Service Commissioned Corps.* (Available from U.S. Public Health Service Recruitment Branch, 320 First Street, NW, Room 1034, Washington, DC 20534)

U.S. Department of Health and Human Services, Agency for Health Care Policy and Research (1995). *Management of Cancer Pain, Clinical Practice Guidelines #9* (Pub. No. 94-0592). Washington, D. C: U. S. Government Printing Office.

U.S. Department of Justice. (1994). *Do your career justice. Health services.* (Available from the Federal Bureau of Prisons, U.S. Publich Health Service Recruitment Branch, 320 First Street, NW, Room 1034, Washington, DC 20534)

U.S. Public Health Service. (1994). *Career opportunities: United States Public Health Service nurse resource manual.* (Available from U.S. Public Health Service, Division of Commissioned Personnel, Room 4-35, Rockville, MD 20857).

U.S. State Department. (1993). *Career opportunity: Foreign service nurse practitioner.* (Available from U.S. State Department, Box 9317, Rosin Station, Arlington, VA 22219)

Vaught, W. L. (1994, March). In defense of America: Women who serve. *USA Today, 122,* 86–92.

Women's health, other benefits subject of Vets bills. (1993). *Congressional Quarterly Weekly Report, 51*(46), 320.

20

Advanced Practice Nursing: Moving Into the 21st Century in Practice, Education, and Research

Joanne V. Hickey

Predicting the future of advanced practice nursing is perhaps a presumptuous exercise. On the other hand, we would be remiss not to look ahead with concern and hope in a text heralding a new frontier for nursing. Unless we assume the risk of interpreting the present and anticipating the effects of healthcare trends and professional practice, we deprive ourselves of the possibility of influencing and shaping our own destiny as advanced practice nurses (APNs). More important, we relinquish our professional responsibility and accountability for active involvement in restructuring and redesigning quality healthcare for all Americans. Because trends only point a direction for a probable course given current circumstances, they are amenable to the influence of new forces or circumstances; thus, the course can, and most likely will, be altered in many ways. Therefore, the future is never certain; new possibilities always exist. As we strive to achieve new goals and excellence in practice, change is inevitable. Pursuit of excellence, especially in these times of tight budgets, requires courage, fortitude, imagination, creativity, commitment, visionary thinking, tireless energy, and leadership to create something better. Advanced practice nurses must exercise their growing power to deliberately choose and create their collective futures.

The preceding chapters and exemplars described current trends, issues, and barriers influencing advanced practice nursing, enticing us with visions of the future and opening to us the realms of possibility and probability! Currently, the most powerful factor influencing healthcare and advanced practice nursing is economics and the demand for cost-effective care. In our consideration of the future, this current preoccupation must not overwhelm the importance of other major political, social, cultural, and environmental factors that are concurrent active forces in the tapestry. Legal limitations imposed on scope of practice for APNs, for example, and third-party reimbursement are barriers to practice that are also tied to political is-

Hickey JV: ADVANCED PRACTICE NURSING: Changing Roles and Clinical Applications © 1996 Lippincott–Raven Publishers

sues. Removal of legal and financial barriers to advanced practice nursing is essential to actualizing the full potential of APNs. Accomplishing this goal requires a multifaceted approach that includes political action. The preceding chapters and exemplars have set the stage for this discussion of advanced practice nursing in the 21st century, which focuses on practice, education, and research.

ON THE THRESHOLD OF THE 21ST CENTURY:
A BROAD PERSPECTIVE

Before addressing specific aspects of APN practice, education, and research, consider four general trends in society, healthcare, and nursing that will affect advanced practice nursing. These trends reflect the unparalleled complexities and uncertainties accompanying profound change in many aspects of contemporary U.S. culture. Systems theory tells us that change in one part of any system influences reactions in other subsystems. The effect may be subtle or profound, but the ripple effect is felt in some way. Likewise, changes in the overall society affect healthcare and, through it, advanced practice nursing.

The first discernible major trend in society, globalization, is likely to have a profound effect well into the future. Rapid travel, communication highways, and information networks have shrunk global distances and communication barriers. We are fast becoming citizens of the world with more commonalities than differences. This broad perspective of a global citizenship changes how we, as health professionals, think about healthcare and illness within the context of cultural blending. For example, new understandings have fostered an appreciation for the value and compatibility of Eastern and Western healthcare practices, although we simultaneously recognize the limitations of each system. Western medicine has always focused on cures and treatments. From other medical traditions, we are gradually incorporating more global approaches to good health that emphasize health promotion and disease prevention. Such a proactive, health-conscious perspective is fundamental to creating models of care that focus on staying healthy rather than models that are activated after disease and illness are apparent.

The second enduring societal trend, the knowledge explosion, is profoundly influencing healthcare and professional practice. There is so much more to know, especially in science and technology. This naturally leads to increasing specialization in more narrowly focused areas. For healthcare to make the best use of ever more specialized knowledge for the benefit of the largest number of people, the system must be organized to efficiently and effectively identify and direct individuals along the continuum of care. The challenge to provide holistic, sensitive care within a humanistic and ethical–moral context will continue to become more complicated. It is a struggle for balance between quality of life and science, which often appear as dichotomous extremes. At what point in healthcare and treatment do we say that enough is enough, and when is going beyond a certain point a violation of the human spirit? These general questions will surface repeatedly in the form of specific ethical decisions as new breakthroughs are implemented. They will continue to spark debate and discussion in many circles, but are likely to remain contentious and divisive, however they are incrementally resolved.

The third important general trend pertains specifically to nursing and is, in essence, a countertrend to that occurring in the general society. Professional nursing, it seems, will continue to be a female-dominated profession. As such, it may become one of the few, perhaps the only, major profession identified as such. Chinn (1991) describes a vision of nursing as grounded in two distinct philosophical perspectives: nursing philosophy and feminist philosophy. The fundamental tenet of nursing philosophy is "health as wholeness"; that of feminism is "the personal is political" (p. 251). Basic to the philosophy of nursing is the idea that, as nurses, women are socialized to promote harmony and eschew controversy in the interest of placing another person's welfare first. According to feminist philosophy, on the other hand, women and nurses, as feminists in a patriarchal system, are encouraged to be personally assertive on behalf of their own self-interests. Chinn, who acknowledged the limitations imposed by these seemingly contradictory philosophies, has suggested that the nursing profession remove the limitations imposed by patriarchal ideology to create a new paradigm that provides a stronger base for autonomous advanced practice nursing for the predominantly female practitioners.

Chinn's suggestion points to the need for a seminal change in how nurses are socialized and in how they plan their careers. Most women, even highly educated women, enter their professions without well-reasoned career trajectories. By comparison, men typically have well-planned and clearly defined career goals and trajectories. A major reason for this difference is that women generally do not have mentors who assist them in developing a career plan or who are willing to "open doors" to assist junior members of a profession in ascending to the next level of a career path. This must change for women to achieve the highest levels in their careers. Mentoring is critical for APNs as they move into new levels of practice and responsibilities. As more APNs assume visible leadership roles in healthcare networks, they will be able to establish new trends in career development for nurses. As such, they have a responsibility to assist, direct, and act as mentors to new practitioners as they ascend their career paths.

The fourth trend with great implications for the future of advanced practice nursing is a long-standing one that has worked to limit APNs' scope of practice and income potential. Barriers to scope of practice revolve around turf and competence issues that will slowly be resolved as APNs demonstrate their ability to provide high-quality advanced care in multiple settings. Because advanced practice requires longer preparation and more insightful knowledge and skills than other levels of practice, it deserves to be compensated accordingly. Third-party reimbursement for independent APN services will follow when, and only when, major providers view APNs as a cost-effective alternative. It is imperative for APNs to actively participate in activities designed to remove barriers to practice. Without the latitude to practice and receive third-party reimbursement, the growth of advanced practice nursing will be stymied.

FUTURE OF ADVANCED PRACTICE NURSING

The practice–education–research triad provides an organizational framework for the following discussion that explores the current forces likely to affect the further development of advanced practice nursing. Predictions are made on the courses along which practice, education, and research for advanced practice nursing are likely to proceed; the discussion is also based on a compilation of APNs' observations, experiences, and thoughts about key issues, trends, and projections. No particular order of priority is implied, nor is there an attempt to be inclusive. In addition, although certain predictions are listed in one category (e.g., practice), there will often be implications and ramifications of that prediction for the other categories (i.e., education and research) as well. Readers are invited to add, delete, and modify the list according to their perspective and ability to read tea leaves or interpret Bayesian theory.

Practice

Practice in a Cost-Containment Environment Is Here to Stay

"We have no more money . . . now we must think." This oft-quoted remark by a British politician whose budget had been severely cut reminds us that unlimited resources over long periods generally lead an enterprise to be riddled with waste, fraud, and abuse. When the backlash comes, and it has arrived in healthcare as in many other areas of society, the pain is not always fairly distributed. However, the rethinking of traditional ways of doing things that inevitably results is usually a healthy and productive process. Cost-containment, which has become an integral and permanent part of practice for all healthcare professionals, has forced us to think differently. We are constantly challenged to think creatively and forced to question whether each component of a care plan is cost-effective. What information will be gained by ordering a test or procedure? How will that information affect the treatment plan? Is there a more economical way to meet the patient's needs? Attention to cost containment has become a leading measure in the standards of practice by which practitioners are judged. Economic considerations are forcing APNs to think creatively and to factor cost into every decision made about patients and patient care.

Managed Care Environments Are Here to Stay; Care Will Be Provided Through Mega-Health Networks That Will Result From Mergers of Health Providers

The "bigger is better" theme that is taking over the private healthcare business runs counter to the current populist sentiment playing out in government and private industry. The momentum of consensus elsewhere in society is to reduce size, turn back decision making to the lowest level, and encourage independent small enterprises. Witness the rejection in 1994 of legislation perceived as establishing federal government control of private healthcare. Despite this anomaly, it seems clear that almost all healthcare in the near future will be provided through large managed care environments. Mega-health networks are developing: major hospitals are buying out primary care practices, home care services, and multiple other components of the continuum of care to manage subscribers in cost-effective ways. Although there will initially be many health network organizations, most will succumb to mergers or buyouts by a few meganetworks. The private healthcare business has temporarily put aside monopolistic fears and populist sentiment in the interest of stemming the enormous increases in healthcare costs. As a result, the future undoubtedly will reveal relatively few giants who will emerge as the major providers of U.S. healthcare.

Mission of Healthcare Is Being Redefined

Healthcare, as the term is applied to the U.S. system, has been a misnomer. Given the actual mission and orientation of services provided, the more appropriate term is *illness care.* There is strong evidence (e.g., primary-care gatekeepers and collaborative practice models) that a true healthcare system is beginning to emerge that will emphasize optimal wellness for all individuals and provide real incentives to focus on health promotion and disease prevention. Why is healthcare being redesigned to place its mission more in sync with its name? With the average life span continuing to increase and with the demographic bubble reaching the age of increased chronicity, there is a greater incentive and demand for care models that will manage chronic illness better and keep people as independent as possible and free of complications for as long as possible. Consequently, rehabilitation and support services will need to be increased and education and counseling of patients and their families will become routine and more elaborate. Advanced practice nurses will continue to play a key role in health promotion and disease prevention because they have knowledge and skills that uniquely qualify them to assist patients to manage their chronic illness and enjoy an optimum quality of life.

Client Demands Are Being Met for Increased Patient Satisfaction

As signified by the gradual replacement of "patient" with "client," healthcare providers are realizing that customer satisfaction is becoming a major determinant of success in the new competitive healthcare world. It has become fashionable to listen to the patient to hear what is important to him or her. Based on this feedback, care is being restructured and redesigned to provide for such novel ideas as flexible scheduling of appointments, simplified language in patient education, and emphasis on hotel comforts. As this trends takes hold, APNs will continue to articulate the needs of patients and their families and assume a greater patient advocacy role. The input of APNs will be sought and integrated into the reengineering of healthcare to meet patient needs and demands more effectively .

Environments for Bedside Care Are Changing

Home is where the bedside healthcare of the future will be centered as hospital-based care inevitably shifts to community-based care. The number of beds left in hospitals will continue to shrink until hospitals become little more than giant intensive care units and surgical suites supported by radiology and laboratories. Indeed, many would argue that, by most standards, they already are. Hospital care will continue to use ever more complex and elaborately interfaced technology that requires increasingly specialized and sophisticated training for those providing care. Concurrently, the realities of the technological production line will suggest that proven equipment and procedures be transferred to the home environment, supported by community-based facilities to provide ancillary services. It will be the APN's job to find ways to safely accomplish this transition as high technology in the home environment becomes commonplace. Only the most sophisticated and experimental technology will be located in the hospital environment. Home healthcare will be the major growth area in healthcare well into the future, and APNs will be at the forefront of providing home care by developing new models of practice and adapting their well-developed, high-tech hospital skills to the home environment.

Care Is Shifting From Hospital-Based to Community-Based Care

The shift to community-based care as the context for most care is a signal phenomenon of our times, which is already occurring at a dramatic pace. In the past, hospitals, as the central institutions of care, received the bulk of resources and were an impediment to the development of community-based services. The change to community-based care as the predominant mode has been underway for some time and will continue to develop for the foreseeable future. The pieces of the care complex that were missing in the community are steadily being developed. New entities of care delivery are appearing, such as day hospitals. Nursing homes are being redefined as places where people go for short stays to recuperate and then return home. As discussed in the exemplars, APNs have developed and implemented many community-based health services. Programs for the chronically ill and geriatric populations are emerging as important centers of care and health promotion, and school health is an expanding area of practice. Perhaps there is no more obvious area where increased community-based health services are needed than in rural communities. Many more rural nurse practitioners will be needed to meet the diverse needs of patients in rural settings.

Hospital Nursing Will Continue To Become More Selective and Specialized

Given that hospital care is becoming more dependent on high technology and oriented toward shorter stays, those nurses who continue to be employed in hospitals will require more ongoing education in technology and its application to patient care. The downsizing of hospitals means a shrinking workforce in the hospital, which includes the need for fewer nurses. Those nurses who remain will take over functions that require advanced clinical reasoning skills as well as specific skills in the use of high-tech equipment and protocols. They will require not only an increased understanding of the pathophysiology of their areas of specialization, but also more background in the basic biologic and physical sciences, instrumentation, and computer technology. A new breed of APNs, called *acute-care nurse practitioners* and *critical care nurse practitioners,* will have an increased presence in hospital settings, helping to fill the void created by a projected decrease in specialty residency programs as more physicians are trained in primary care. With hospital care changing and the nature of the required nursing skills shifting, there will be a periodic need for retooling and reeducation of the nursing work force (see the section Education).

Transitional Care Will Become a Major Growth Area

In today's healthcare world, hospitalized patients either receive an intensive care unit–level of care or they are out of the hospital environment. Recovery now takes place in special short-stay units or in the home where patients are sent "quicker and sicker." *Transitional care* refers to care that bridges the gap between acute- and convalescent-care environments. It is designed to meet the needs of the patient and family during the rapid movement from one phase to another along the continuum of care, whether in the same setting or between healthcare environments. Transitional care is currently an undeveloped area. With their special knowledge and skills, APNs are well positioned to create the bridges needed to guide patients and their families through these difficult transitions while enhancing the recovery process and achieving better patient outcomes.

Development and Use of Practice Guidelines Will Increase

Both professional accountability to consumers and eligibility for third-party reimbursement are tied to attaining measurable outcomes within a given time frame. This reality is driving practice for all health professionals. National practice guidelines and practice standards will become the norm. The practice recommendations from patient outcomes research team programs, national practice standards such as *Clinician's Handbook of Preventive Services: Putting Prevention Into Practice* (American Nurses Association, 1994), and care maps (discussed in Chapter 1) have been and will continue to be implemented by APNs to provide quality care to patients.

There Will Be New Emphasis on Primary Care, Which Will Be Redefined

Chapter 5 discussed the important renaissance and redefinition of primary care in contemporary healthcare. Primary care health professionals, called *gatekeepers* in current parlance, will control and often monitor the patient's interaction with specialty care. Although there will still be need for both, the ratio of generalists to specialists will increase. Many APNs will be providers of primary care, most often in collaborative practices, with some choosing independent solo practice. Other APNs who will provide care for special populations (e.g., patients with heart failure or strokes) will continue to include aspects of health promotion and disease prevention within their scope of practice.

Collaborative, Interdisciplinary Practice Models Will Come Into Vogue in All Settings

Collaborative and interdisciplinary models are now recognized as the cornerstone for providing efficient, cost-effective, high-quality care and for ensuring continuity of care. By bringing together the expertise of many different healthcare professionals who work together collaboratively, outcomes are optimized for the patient through the continuum of care. Advanced practice nurses will continue to work in collaborative models in hospitals and community-based facilities and will take on new responsibilities as the boundaries of practice are renegotiated with physicians. Nurses will assume roles and responsibilities traditionally held by the physician as physicians take on new roles and responsibilities demanded by advancements in technology and medical practice. This is not a new phenomenon, but will proceed much more rapidly than in the past. Consider, for example, the progress that has been made since the sphygmomanometer was introduced into practice in 1901 (Fulton, 1946, p. 250), when taking the blood pressure was the sole responsibility of the physician. Imagine how roles and responsibilities will be renegotiated and redesigned in the 21st century.

Communications, Computers, and Information Networks Will Erase Boundaries Created by Distance and Inaccessibility to Physical Facilities

Excellent interpersonal and verbal communications skills have always been essential for APNs as well as for other health providers. In the 21st century, however, computer literacy will also be an absolute requirement. Electronic technology has enormously expanded our access to information and people, through such advances as voice mail, electronic mail, Internet, fax, and beepers. Direct applications of electronic technology to practice will become pervasive. For example, the very portable notebook computers will allow healthcare providers to enter histories, physicals, and progress notes in a standard format directly into a central database from the patient's bedside. Computer technology also provides rapid access to the latest scientific articles and clinical texts through on-line literature searches. Currently, medical reference texts can be accessed easily by way of the computer to check specific topics. Computers, video cameras, and remote electronic sensors provide a means for specialists to examine patients hundreds of miles away. Communication highways and computer networks connect urban and rural settings, generalists and specialists, national and international centers, and individuals and the medical libraries or special networks of the world. The bad news is that knowledge is exploding at an almost indigestible rate. The good news is that it is instantly available—to the computer literate person—at a work station or notebook computer. Computer technology becomes more user friendly all the time, and APNs will continue to integrate computer technology into practice. Major challenges will be to preserve patient privacy and to limit nonessential access to personal information.

Programs for Special Needs and Vulnerable Populations Will Increase

Niche marketing, a successful trend that has recently been growing in the overall economy, certainly has its equivalent in the healthcare industry. Competition for market share and new sources of revenue will drive providers to experiment with innovative specialized programs designed to attract clients suffering from focused healthcare problems or seeking to prevent specific problems. The rapid pace of the development of new knowledge will be reflected in the rate at which new information is transferred from research to practice. Today's news story about a revolutionary health breakthrough or newly discovered health problem will be followed almost immediately by a clinic to address the problem. This need not be a predominantly negative trend, because only well-founded programs are likely to gain longevity. Successful efforts will identify valid special needs in truly vulnerable populations and design meaningful and reasonable care plans that are specially tailored to address real needs. Advanced practice nurses will develop and implement many of these programs. Examples of such programs that have already proven to be successful are breast clinics and menopause clinics as subdivisions of women's health programs, geriatric day care centers as part of geriatric care, and sick child care sections in day care programs.

Greater Emphasis Will Be Placed on the Ethical Component of Care

Technology has taken medical care so far that "a natural death," within the context of healthcare, has become a complicated and difficult event, as have decisions about the allocation of transplant organs and the viability of genetically flawed fetuses. These and other equally value-laden ethical conundrums can only become more complex as technology scales new heights. With more medical and technological breakthroughs on the horizon, there will be a greater emphasis on integrating ethical decision making into care plans based on quality of life outcomes. Advanced practice nurses have always understood the ethical component of care and have been advocates for patients and families' wishes. In the future, APNs will need to continue to apply frameworks for ethical decision making to new technology and medical therapies and assist other health professionals in including this dimension of care.

Education

As is apparent from the preceding chapters, APNs face the 21st century on a threshold of opportunity and change seldom experienced in a profession. Doors are opening, taboos are crumbling, and administrators are saying, " Okay, you asked for it. Let's see what you can do." Advanced practice nurses must be educationally prepared to meet this challenge. New knowledge and clinical skills will be required to assume the evolving advanced practice roles in primary care, tertiary care, and all areas between these anchors on the continuum of care. Curricula will need to be revised and updated, and the educational process of preparing APNs will need to be revamped. Curricula and APN education will need to provide better methods of developing the critical thinking skills that will be so important in performing at new levels of responsibility and accountability. The following are predictions about formal academic programs and continuing education programs for APNs.

Major Academic Curricular Changes for Graduate Nursing Education Will Be Necessary

Four areas of APN education must be strengthened to meet the coming challenges. These areas are the biologic sciences, computer literacy, clinical reasoning, and health policy and financial management.

Traditionally, nursing education has emphasized curricula directed toward holistic care for patients, with major attention given to coping with illnesses of the psyche as well as those of the body. As such, nurses have been well grounded in the behavioral sciences, allowing less room for biologic science content. A further detour in this direction was taken when nursing curricula began to be influenced by the national trend in medical education toward a decreased emphasis on a broad knowledge base in the biologic sciences. Thus, nursing graduates entered graduate programs with a less-developed understanding of the biologic sciences at a time when a strong science base was essential in order to keep up with the knowledge explosion in the medical sciences.

If APNs are to assume responsibility for aspects of diagnoses and for treatment planning—formerly the province of physicians—their knowledge of the biologic sciences and medicine must be strengthened. Advanced practice nurses must have a better grounding in anatomy, physiology, pathophysiology, immunology, genetics, and pharmacology than had been previously expected in less clinically demanding roles. This provides not only a better understanding of disease processes and treatment, but also a common ground for communicating effectively with physicians and other health professionals. This strengthening of the biological sciences component of curricula must not be accompanied by a deemphasis on a broad knowledge base in the behavioral sciences. Holistic care, which is still the differentiating hallmark of nursing, is the patient's best hope for an optimum outcome and can only be provided by the blending that results from an integration of both the biological and behavioral aspects of care.

To practice in an information society, nurses must be computer literate and comfortable with computer applications to clinical practice and documentation of patient data. They must also be able to use computer technology for rapid access to the most current information on patient management as well as communication with other health professionals and centers. In addition to understanding clinical applications of computer technology to patient care, nurses will need to understand basic concepts involved in the interpretation of data produced by clinical instrumentation. Terms such as *hertz* and basic physics concepts involved in the analysis of waveform data are two examples of important information not generally emphasized in courses for APNs. Advanced practice nurses are going to be expected to answer questions such as, Are the physiological data observed on the monitor screen real values or calculated values? What is the difference between the two? What is the significance of the difference? Advanced practice nurses must be taught the concepts and terminology they need to know to be able to understand and properly interpret the data they will be expected to apply in making clinical decisions.

Another curricular area in need of strengthening involves the critical thinking skills necessary for clinical reasoning. This area must become the fundamental core of APN graduate education. The ability to process clinical data quickly and accurately is imperative for making excellent decisions related to patient care. This learning focus provides APNs with a model similar to that used by physicians and other health professionals. Clinical reasoning then becomes the common denominator in collaborative practice and decision making related to patient care. The old adage "Give a man a fish and he will have one meal, but teach a man to fish and he can eat for life" applies to the teaching of critical thinking. It will be a basic survival skill for professional life in the 21st century. The nursing profession cannot expect that the thoughts and ideas given APNs will prepare them for lifelong practice because treatment protocols change and new technology necessitates new knowledge. However, teaching APNs how to think, identify what they need to know, and make decisions is vital if they are to maintain themselves as effective practitioners.

Regardless of which direct patient care focus is chosen, to practice effectively, APNs must be well versed in health policy and financial management. Health policy and cost containment are the context of healthcare delivery for the future, and healthcare professionals who ignore the details of this context will do so at their own peril. Advanced practice nurses will be expected to integrate this knowledge in planning and implementing programs and administering care. Ethical decision making in the context of evolving healthcare policy is an area in which APNs must be prepared to participate in preserving patient quality of life and dignity.

Educational Pathways for Advanced Practice Nurses in Clinical Practice Will Become More Distinct

Graduate education for nurses parallels special career paths for nurses. The career path of the nurse manager has evolved from that of the head nurse, who was often an experienced expert practitioner. The nurse manager role requires advanced skills oriented toward fiscal, budgetary, personnel, and program management. The APN in a clinical tract has a need for different skills to meet his or her responsibilities, although some interdependent skills complement those of the nurse manager. As career paths become further delineated, educational needs will become more apparent. Fewer basic core courses will be needed as more specialized courses are developed. Educators must design courses in which nurse managers and direct patient care providers can learn and interact together in a way that supports their socialization as nurses who work together for common goals.

Only One Category and One Basic Curriculum Will Exist for Advanced Practice Nurses

Despite some resistance and controversy, the clinical nurse specialist and nurse practitioner roles will be blended into a single role called the *advanced practice nurse*. Credentialing bodies will be slow to accept this change in nursing practice. However, cost containment and the demand for expanded skills in nurses who are assuming advanced practice roles will facilitate this trend. In the meantime, many APNs will continue to be certified as both clinical nurse specialists and nurse practitioners in an area of specialized practice. With the skills of both the clinical nurse specialist and nurse practitioner embodied in one APN, patient care will be more holistic to the benefit of society.

New Specialized Advanced Practice Nurse Graduate Programs Will Be Offered

As new roles develop for APNs, new academic programs will be developed to prepare APNs to meet these needs. Currently, acute-care nurse practitioner and critical care nurse practitioner programs are being developed at major centers to meet shortages of house officers and attending physicians to staff intensive care and intermediate units. In addition, APNs in tertiary care are prepared and willing to assume greater responsibility and accountability for patient management. These trends will continue, and other focused APN programs will be developed. Programs to prepare APNs with a focus on home health management and rural care will be the next big areas of demand for preparation.

Combined Education of Advanced Practice Nurses, Physician's Assistants, and Medical Students Will Become Commonplace

Selected courses open to APNs, physician's assistants, and medical students will become more common. Teaching and clinical supervision will increase interdisciplinary involvement of educators and clinicians from these fields. This combined education has already been implemented successfully in some institutions and is proving to be a cost-effective approach to teaching the many basic courses needed by all health providers. Additional benefits derive from the introduction of different health providers to each others' roles and from the resulting socialization that will facilitate future collaborative practice.

More Doctorally Prepared Nurses Will Provide Direct Patient Care as Advanced Practice Nurses

More APNs who have been prepared as clinical nurse specialists and nurse practitioners will obtain doctorates and assume the role of the academic clinician discussed in Chapter 1. Research programs emerging from their clinical practice will result in important findings applicable to direct patient care.

Distance Learning Will Assist Advance Practice Nurses in Lifelong Learning

Knowledge today has a short half-life that will continue to grow shorter in the future. Advanced practice nurses will need to be lifelong learners through continuing education programs. New cost-effective methods of teaching and learning using interactive technology will become accessible to APNs in their homes and workplaces through personal computers, interactive teleconferences, and other not yet contemplated forms. Continuing education will no longer be a "once-in-a-while" requirement but a constant part of professional practice. Educators, as well as practitioners, need to prepare for this onslaught by completely redesigning and restructuring continuing education to meet the needs of these lifelong learners.

Research

What new innovative things should nurses be doing? Are current practices cost effective and are they making a difference in terms of patient and family outcomes? These types of questions, vital to justifying the future of nursing, cannot be answered without well-designed and conducted nursing research. Thus, the future of APNs is linked to the development and testing of current practice and new knowledge through research. The body of knowledge called *nursing science* and the growth and development of professional nursing depend on clinical research undertaken by nurses. There is a need to demonstrate the efficacy of nursing management through well-designed research programs. There are also many one-time nursing studies that need to be replicated because of small sample size, design flaws, or limited generalizability. Research that is inaccessible or that is never widely applied to practice is useless. Therefore, nurses must learn to be savvy consumers of research through education in research use that emphasizes the skills necessary for interpreting and applying research findings.

The establishment of the National Institute for Nursing Research as an independent institute within the National Institutes of Health was a milestone affirming the viability and importance of nursing research to the nation. Funding for research through the National Institutes of Health is competitive, however, and the requests for funding far outstrip available funds. Therefore, nurses need to pursue other sources of support and funding to conduct research. Many organizations provide seed money for pilot work, and some provide major support for promising studies in special areas of practice or for special health problems. The following are key trends and predictions for the 21st century for nursing research.

More Researchers Will Apply for a Relatively Small Pool of Funds, Which Is Not Expected To Increase Significantly

Unless nurses have promising pilot studies in priority areas of research, they will not be competitive for funding of independent studies through the National Institutes of Health. However, more nurses will be able to conduct pilot studies through small grants from a variety of sources. It will be important for nurses to carefully explore possible sources through their professional organizations and private foundations. Use of computer networks to assist researchers will be another avenue for locating potential funds.

Research Priority Will Be Outcome Measurement Studies That Demonstrate Cost-Effective Care

There is, and will continue to be, a critical need to conduct research that not only focuses on measurable and improved outcomes for patients but also demonstrates cost effectiveness. Research will need to be conducted to demonstrate the efficacy of the many nursing procedures that have not been investigated. Comparison studies will also be needed to demonstrate which of several effective interventions for a particular condition is the most cost-effective. Because APNs who provide direct patient care will know which important research questions need to be studied and because they will be positioned to obtain the necessary data, they will assume major roles in clinical application studies.

Emphasis Will Be on Collaborative, Multidisciplinary, and Multicenter Research Studies

Well-designed collaborative, multidisciplinary, multicenter studies will have a greater chance of funding. Through collaboration across disciplines, a variety of research questions can be answered for each discipline in the same well-designed study. Because so many studies have small sample sizes due to a limited study population, multisite studies will be conducted to increase sample size while completing the study in a shorter time frame. These studies have the added advantage of increased power and reliability of the findings for generalizability. Many APNs will participate in various roles in collaborative, multidisciplinary, multicenter research.

*More Advanced Practice Nurses Will Develop a Career Plan
for a Research Program in a Specific Area*

As APNs learn to plan their careers, they will choose an area of interest and will plan a program of research with each study building on a previous study. This will result in generation of new knowledge and will increase their competitiveness for research funding.

CONCLUSION

It is easier to predict what advanced practice nursing will be like in the year 2000 than what it will be like in the year 2020, 2050, or beyond. A nurse reading this book somewhere in the distant future may contemplate, in utter amazement, how primitive advanced practice nursing was at the end of the 20th century and how far it has come. It would be a sad scenario, however, if our nurse of the future were to read this book and wonder, Who were these so-called advanced practice nurses and when did they become extinct? The future of advanced practice nursing is in our hands; let us use our collective power to make that future exceed our most optimistic hopes and dreams.

References

American Nurses Association. (1994). *Clinician's handbook of preventive services: Put prevention into practice.* Washington, DC: Author

Chinn, P. L. (1991). Looking into the crystal ball: Positioning ourselves for the year 2000. *Nursing Outlook, 39*(6), 251–256.

Fulton, J. F. (1946). *Harvey Cushing: A biography.* Springfield, IL: Charles C Thomas.

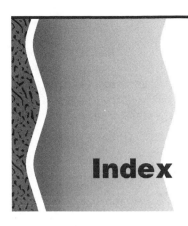

Index

Page numbers followed by *f* indicate figures;
those followed by *t* indicate tabular material.

W

Wellness
    demand for, 8–9
    workplace programs for, 274
Women's issues, in reformation of healthcare, 11–12
Workplace, primary care in. *See* Healthcare in the
               workplace: SAS Institute Health Care
               Center